THE OLDER ADULT

A process for wellness

It's What You Do– Not When You Do It

Ted Williams, at age 42, slammed a home run in his last official time at bat. Mickey Mantle, age 20, hit 23 home runs his first full year in the major leagues. Golda Meir was 71 when she became Prime Minister of Israel. William Pitt II was 24 when he became Prime Minister of Great Britain. George Bernard Shaw was 94 when one of his plays was first produced. Mozart was just seven when his first composition was published. Now, how about this? Benjamin Franklin was a newspaper columnist at 16, and a framer of The United States Constitution when he was 81. You're never too young or too old if you've got talent. Let's recognize that age has little to do with ability.

THE OLDER ADULT
A PROCESS FOR WELLNESS

ELIZABETH JANE FORBES, RN, C, NHA, EdD

ANA Certified Gerontological Nurse; Professor of Nursing,
Department of Baccalaureate Nursing, College of Allied Health Sciences,
Thomas Jefferson University, Philadelphia, Pennsylvania;
formerly Associate Dean for Continuing Education,
College of Nursing, Rutgers—The State University of New Jersey,
Newark, New Jersey

VIRGINIA MACKEN FITZSIMONS, RN, C, EdD

ANA Certified Gerontological Nurse; Assistant Professor,
College of Nursing, Rutgers—The State University of New Jersey,
Newark, New Jersey

with 77 illustrations

The C. V. Mosby Company

ST. LOUIS • TORONTO • LONDON   1981

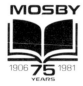

MOSBY

1906 **75** 1981
YEARS

A TRADITION OF PUBLISHING EXCELLENCE

Editor: Diane L. Bowen
Manuscript editor: Teri Merchant
Design: Diane Beasley
Production: Stella Adolfson

Printed in the United States of America

The C.V. Mosby Company
11830 Westline Industrial Drive, St. Louis, Missouri 63141

Library of Congress Cataloging in Publication Data

Forbes, Elizabeth, 1934-
    The older adult.

    Bibliography: p.
    Includes index.
    1. Geriatric nursing. 2. Aged—Care and hygiene.
3. Health. I. Fitzsimons, Virginia, 1943-   joint
author. II. Title. [DNLM: 1. Geriatric nursing.
2. Preventive medicine—Nursing texts. WY152 F692o]
RC954.F66   613'.0438'024613   80-39513
ISBN 0-8016-1631-X

GW/VH/VH 9 8 7 6 5 4 3 2 1   02/B/211

To

our loving parents

Elmer and **Agnes Forbes**

James and **Nora Macken**

Foreword

An increasing proportion of our population in the future will be longevous. This age structure will have a significant impact on the health care system and nursing, because older people use a disproportionate share of expensive drugs and medical services. The national concern to contain health care costs and to make health care services accessible to all has led to the formulation of a preventive strategy that will lessen dependence on sick care services and place more responsibility on individuals to develop healthy living styles and to obtain information and skills necessary for health promotion and health maintenance. For example, Joseph Califano, while Secretary of the Department of Health, Education, and Welfare, received a mandate from President Carter "to improve the health of Americans by reducing environmental and occupational hazards and encouraging health-enhancing personal behavior, as well as improving the effectiveness •of our medical care system." Califano stated that "A new and vigorous prevention strategy—which seeks to keep people healthy rather than cure them after they become sick—is critical if we are to gain firm control over health costs and to achieve continued improvement in the nation's health" (Public Health Rep. **93**:600-601, November-December 1978).

This push for a preventive strategy will apply to all age groups from the beginning to the end of life. It is never too late to help people increase health-conducive behaviors, minimize and compensate for health-prejudicial losses and the impairments of aging, and preserve and restore function in the context of coping with various diseases and disabilities. The nurse prepared for preventive nursing intervention based on the concept of wellness can help people age successfully by using a systematic process. This preparation will reduce negative stereotypes of aging and establish a more positive view of the value of health promotion, preservation, and maintenance.

A growing emphasis is being placed in the training of various levels of personnel to provide service to older adults. Specialization in the health professions is being encouraged. Highly educated and skilled nurses can make a significant impact on the quality of life and health through teaching, advising, and counseling older persons, and by applying current knowledge and research findings in a hands-on approach to practice.

The challenge to nurses working with older adults is to promote wellness in addition to their traditional role in providing care during illness. The focus of this book is on nursing's role in working with the older adult to maintain wellness and to attain the highest level of health and functioning possible at a particular time. The information provided addresses real problems encountered by older adults as well as the use of the nursing process, including step-by-step practical and humane approaches to help them cope with these problems, thereby enhancing the quality of life. Respect for persons and their rights is emphasized, as is the importance of nurses tending to their own developmental problems. Information is also provided to give direction and to help solve selected problems in governance, such as quality assurance and ethical issues. This book is designed to meet educational needs of all types of nursing personnel working with older adults. It will help nurses meet the challenge of providing high-quality care to older persons in their homes, in communities, and in institutions. By using this book, nurses can increase their professional competence and client satisfaction and enhance their own self-esteem.

Laurie M. Gunter, PhD, RN

Professor of Nursing and Human Development, The Pennsylvania State University, University Park, Pennsylvania

Preface

Two decades of exaltation of the youth culture shortchanged the older persons in our population during the 1960s and 1970s. Decreased emphasis on older adults lowered the status of agencies and persons involved in their care. Demographic changes have shifted the spotlight; persons over 65 comprise the fastest growing segment of our population. In the 1980s and beyond, greater numbers of older adults will give that group new visibility.

Nursing has long been associated with the care of older adults who were ill. Now, nurses are in the uniquely exciting position of being front-line advocates of vigorous health maintenance planning, health teaching, maximum independence in activities of daily living, and illness prevention. *The Older Adult: A Process for Wellness* offers current, practical information to make that advocacy as powerful as possible in the community, in the hospital, and in long-term-care facilities. The latest research data and theories on many aspects of the older adult's life gleaned from the literature of nursing and other disciplines, both in the United States and other countries, are discussed as a basis for sound nursing decision and illustrated in action by the use of vignettes. These vignettes were collected by nurses as they worked with older adults in their clinical practice.

The nursing process serves as the organizing framework of this book. The American Nurses' Association has used the nursing process as the base for its Standards for Gerontological Nursing Practice to outline quality assurance guidelines. Since quality care is the goal of all nurses, the steps in the nursing process are valuable tools in the delivery of care.

The four components of the nursing process—data collection, care planning, intervention, and evaluation—comprise the four units of this book. Each unit is subdivided into chapters that address specific aspects of that particular component of the process.

Unit I, Data Collection, discusses various theories on the aging process and models of care for the older adult. These chapters form part of the knowledge base section of the data collection unit. As the advantages and limitations of each of these nursing models are outlined, the nursing process comes across as the most appropriate model for effective contemporary nursing. The chapter on nursing health assessment leads into the chapter on the nursing diagnosis, concluding the first component in the nursing process, data collection.

Unit II, Care Planning, presents care planning based on nursing through objectives. By accentuating the positive and planning the care on an ethical base, the nurse can utilize the strengths of the older adult as well as her own strengths as a basis for quality, ethical care.

Unit III, Intervention, is a hands-on approach to care that builds on the nurse's knowledge of communication skills and fundamentals of care. Its unique approach is based on modifications in the fundamental techniques of nursing necessitated by the normal physiological changes in the older adult. Recommendations of other professional groups such as dentists, podiatrists, physical therapists, and occupational and recreational therapists, as well as personal grooming specialists, such as cosmeticians and hair stylists, have been included. Information from these sources specific to the older adult helps the nurse incorporate a broad knowledge base as she gives care.

Unit IV, Evaluation, is particularly important to meet today's regulations for quality assurance for Medicare and Medicaid. Evaluation tools that have been used widely and have proved useful have been included. In addition, the evaluation unit serves as a base for developing mechanisms for the peer review process.

Many textbooks on geriatrics are available to the nurse. This one is different, however, because it does not follow the medical model's emphasis on disease entities and handicaps. Instead, it uses the nursing model of health maintenance through the nursing process. Therefore, this book can serve as a valuable resource for the student in courses related to care of the older adult as well as to the nurse in clinical practice. The nurse interested in continuing education will find this book an important part of her independent study.

Issues involving consumer rights come across loud and clear in virtually every aspect of business encounters today. Persons buying goods and services expect quality for their money and will go elsewhere if the provider of the service does not meet their needs. People have the right to know what they are getting and to have input into the contract agreement. Whether they are purchasing a refrigerator, a car, or household repairs, it is anticipated that satisfaction is guaranteed or their money is refunded. This is the least that is expected from a reputable business person. Nurses are providers of health services. When nurses engage in providing nursing care, they in effect have a contractual agreement with the person receiving the care. A person needing legal services engages a lawyer and becomes the lawyer's client. A person needing accounting services engages an accountant and becomes the accountant's client. In both cases, they want input into the decisions made on their behalf; they want to know all the predictable consequences of the decisions made, and they fully understand that they can go elsewhere if they are not satisfied with the services given. Consider the definition of the words *client* and *patient*.

Client	*Patient*
Customer	Enduring without complaint
Consumer	Calmly tolerating delay
Patron	Passive
	To keep oneself in check
	Persevering

These characteristics describe the behaviors of a client compared with those of a patient. Persons receiving nursing care are purchasing services and participating in the planning of their own care. In addition, they have the right to quality assurance regarding that care, and so these persons are customers or clients. If we expect the persons to whom we give care to endure without complaint, to calmly tolerate delay, and to be passive, then they are patients. It is our philosophy that persons should be intimately involved in their care planning and have consumer rights regarding the quality of that care. Therefore, the world *client* will be used throughout this book to describe the person to whom we give nursing care.

The term *older adults* rather than *the elderly* or *the aged* has been used because they are adults and should be given all of the rights of adults. These rights follow:

To share their knowledge and experience
To be recognized as individuals
To make their own decisions
To have control of their own destiny
To strive for self-esteem and self-actualization
To be recognized for their strengths
To be independent
To be creative
To follow their own spiritual inclinations
To follow their own life-styles
To follow their own cultural ethnic beliefs
To be productive within their own physical and mental limitations
To have dignity

Suggested readings provide the reader with further sources of information. The appendices provide the reader with additional resources useful to the nurse caring for the older adult.

Special thanks and acknowledgment must be given to the following persons whose work and support were a great help to us during this project.

Nancy and Tom Reilly got the project off to a flying start by putting us in touch with Carleen Lucus for the typing of the first draft, and Nancy was always available to tie last-minute odds and ends together.

Without readers and their comments, no book is possible. We called upon our friends, professionals in the field, and colleagues: Maureen Tobias, Diane Fitzsimons, Paula Bloom, Reggie Hepner, Anne L. Saletta, Arliss Thompson-Willis, Elizabeth Severino, Sharon Oswald, Kay Dodds, and Jean Alfgren were most helpful.

To Nancy Evans, whose early guidance and encouragement were invaluable in helping us get this project off the ground, and to Teri Merchant, whose expertise and sense of humor helped us land safely, we offer our deepest and sincerest thanks.

We thank AID Health Care Centers, Inc., Mr. Earl Woomer, Senior Vice President, and Barbara Rexrode, Vice President of Operations, for sharing their quality assurance program with our readers.

Betty Goon was a conscientious research assistant for us. Glen Rowe was the artist for several of the illustrations.

The final drafts were entrusted to Patricia Sutherland and Elaine Tandy for typing.

Jackie Price, a most professional secretary, must have our special thanks also.

We appreciate Julio J. Amadio, MD for his clinical expertise and compassion for the older adult.

To Neil and Christine Fitzsimons, the world's best 5- and 2-year-old, our special love and thanks.

Without Conny Fitzsimons' patience, parenting skills, good ideas and helpful suggestions, sense of humor, and perfect timing in bringing us snacks and drinks during crucial moments, this book would not be possible. Our special love and thanks to him.

Elizabeth Jane Forbes
Virginia Macken Fitzsimons

Contents

I

DATA COLLECTION

1 Aging: the theories

NURSING PROCESS

What is the nursing process, and why should it be used? A process is a continuing development involving many changes, using a number of steps in order to reach a conclusion. It provides the user with a systematic approach to a situation and provides particular steps for the course of action taken. Flexibility is built into this approach because of the cyclical nature of the steps. The steps in the nursing process are: data collection, planning, intervention, and evaluation. These four steps are useful and inclusive. Some authors designate that the nursing process has four steps; some outline it as having three steps. The titles of each step may vary slightly; however, the scientific process involved is the same (Fig. 1-1).

The term *data collection,* rather than assessment, is used as the title for the first step because it is more descriptive.

The output of one step in the nursing process is equal to the input of another. This means, for example, that in order to have good planning, the data collection must be rich with information. If the information is scanty, the planning will limit the nurse's choices for intervention. If nursing intervention is limited, evaluation will expose that intervention as less than optimum nursing care. The feedback system in the nursing process frees the nurse to swing back to an earlier step to fill in the gaps in her information and to redesign her care plan and intervention. Emphasis on data collection encourages the nurse to expand her knowledge of the person she is caring for as an individual. Also, it gives the nurse the basic theory needed for the care, whether it be in health maintenance of a particular organ system or supportive intervention during illness.

Data collection goes beyond the data found in the chart of the client or in the physician's orders exclusively. The nurse is encouraged to reach out to many sources for information. Intellectual growth is achieved by expanding one's knowledge base, and this growth is demonstrated in the precision of the nursing diagnoses. Because a nursing diagnosis is a summary of the data collection findings, it *demands* that the nurse have autonomy and accountability in planning.

The nursing process has direct advantages for the clinical nurse. With the nursing process, the nurse can state the purpose of her activities, demonstrate that she has an organized approach, and channel her creative ideas into benefits for the client. It gives her an easy, systematic way of thinking and solving health problems and functioning so that she is not caught up in random activity. Her actions have a purpose; they are goal directed. Job satisfaction for the nurse increases as her clients and supervisors acknowledge her organization and thoroughness.

The time spent in nursing care is shortened by using the nursing process. There is little waste of nursing personnel, effort, and equipment. The client gets care directly and effectively from the nurse who is able to identify and solve his health problems.

With the nursing process, the intellectual functions dominate over the technical "get the job done, get the tasks completed" approach. The caregiving phase of nursing gets the support of good planning and the prestige of documented, validated evaluation. Nursing has always wanted to do this, and now quality assurance mandates that care be delivered and evaluated in a systematic way. The nurse now gets recognition and job satisfaction for the successful outcome of nursing intervention. The advantages cited are for the individual nurse, but the overall profession of nursing benefits. As every nurse becomes personally involved in using the nursing process, the nursing diagnoses made form a basic language for nursing. This

3

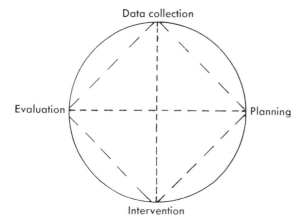

Fig. 1-1. The nursing process is cyclical and flexible. At any time the nurse can move from step to step to collect more data, evaluate the care, and adjust the nursing plans and interventions as appropriate.

Table 1-1. Comparison of scientific method of thinking and nursing process

Scientific method	Nursing process
Identify area to be investigated	Identify area to be investigated
Data collection	Data collection
	Knowledge base
	Nursing history
	Nursing assessment
	Nursing diagnosis
Generate hypothesis	Planning
Testing hypothesis	Intervention
Evaluate outcome	Evaluation

language facilitates the communication of nursing problems so that nurse researchers have unified themes for investigation. The information gained from nursing research enables nursing to keep abreast of other disciplines as technological advances permit mushrooming of information in every sphere of knowledge. Nursing research provides the individual nurse with tested information to improve day-to-day care. Having our own body of tested knowledge reinforces our right to autonomy and accountability in our nursing practice. In addition, it documents the need for nursing manpower and job descriptions.

Data collection

Science has made great advances in the past several hundred years because of its organized and rigorous use of the scientific method. Instead of using guesswork and intuition, the scientist begins by stating the area to be investigated. He gathers all known information about the topic, lists possible solutions to the problems, tests the solutions to find the best one, and then uses that solution to solve the problem. After the problem appears to be solved, the scientist evaluates the results of the work done to determine if it was successful enough to meet his expectations. If it is not successful, he goes back and looks at his problem statement to see if it is clearly stated. He collects

more information so that he can list more possible solutions, then tests those solutions again. This process is repeated over and over again until the right answer is found. Sometimes it is a long and difficult procedure. By recording each step as he goes along, the scientist is able to go to a colleague and share the problem and solution with him. This is another source of expanding his information on the problem. His colleague can give him ideas for possible solutions or point out mistakes he may have been making but has not noticed.

Using this style of solving problems, Louis Pasteur discovered the process of pasteurization, Edward Jenner developed the method of vaccination to prevent smallpox, and the Wright Brothers invented the airplane. Because the problem being investigated was clearly stated and the solution written down in specific steps, other persons were able to pasteurize milk, manufacture smallpox vaccine, and build airplanes. The scientists shared their new information for the benefit of everyone.

Business persons, seeing that the scientific method is such a successful way of thinking, use the technique to solve management and business problems and call it *decision making*. Both scientists and businesspersons agree that the most important step is the information-gathering, or data collection, step. The more information they have regarding all aspects of the situation under study, the more possible solutions are available. The chances for a successful outcome for the problem or decision are increased.

Nursing uses the scientific method to solve nursing problems and make nursing decisions and calls this method the *nursing process* (Table 1-1). Data collection is the first step in the nursing process. Several sources of the nurse's information are her knowledge base, the nursing history, and the nursing assessment. The nursing diagnosis completes the data collection step of the nursing process.

The knowledge base is the information that the nurse has learned from nursing and the biological, psychological, and social sciences. The nurse adds to her knowledge base through clinical experience, reading textbooks and journals, and attending continuing education programs. Consulting with other nurses and persons from other areas of practice also enriches her knowledge base.

The nursing history is taken to obtain an individualized picture of the client. The nurse asks the client to tell her in detail about his past and present health problems and life-style, and what types of things are causing difficulty at the present time. Parts of the nursing history are taken by direct interview with the client, his family, and/or significant others. Information can also be obtained from the records of various agencies the client uses.

The nursing diagnosis identifies those physical and psychological signs and symptoms of the client that can be prevented or relieved by nursing intervention. It is the last part of the data collection step in the nursing process.

Information about the process of aging is an important part of the nurse's knowledge base. The nurse uses theories on aging from the biological, psychological, and social sciences to understand the client's response to the aging process. She shares this information with the client as a part of health teaching and health counseling, as she and the client plan for care.

BIOLOGICAL THEORIES OF AGING

A theory is a way of looking at something and speculating. Scientists from various disciplines have looked at aging and examined the phenomena that interest them. The sifting and sorting out of relationships among the phenomena lead to a statement of principles. These principles are usually verified to some degree.

Scientific inquiry has led to the development of theories of aging from the disciplines of biology, sociology, and psychology. Each discipline has proposed its explanation for the changes that occur with the aging process. Some theories have been verified, whereas others have been subjected to little testing. Not all theories have been accepted; however, they generate questions for further investigation and controversy among the scientists.

The theories on aging describe the reasons why people age. To broaden the nurses' knowledge base, the theories of aging are examined in terms of their nursing application. These theories on aging will help the nurse understand the client's behavior and aging process. The nurse can then generate her own questions and research answers for the nursing problems of the older adult.

The specific cause of aging is not known. Death is inevitable in all living things. The goal of scientific research is to understand the aging process so that the quality of life of the older adult can be improved to an optimum level.

Research is a method of careful investigation. Some scholars say that the most important step in research is to ask the right questions, because the right question will send the researcher down the right path as information is being gathered and solutions are being evaluated. In a way, every person is a researcher at some time. A mother trying to coax a child to eat can use research methods to solve the problem. She can read Dr. Spock, talk to a nurse at the clinic, speak with neighbors, and review articles on children's eating habits in current women's magazines. Each of these sources will offer her possible alternative solutions. The goal is to get the child to eat. After trying the suggestions, she evaluates the child's food intake to determine if the goal was accomplished. This is an elementary example, but similar to the scientific method used by the biologist or social scientist. A question or problem is raised, and then the researcher tries out many different possible solutions.

The primary methods of investigating the aging process are laboratory studies, longitudinal studies, and autopsy. Laboratory investigation can involve the study of the life cycles and aging of laboratory animals. Characteristics of aging animals are compared with those of younger animals. Although results cannot always be generalized to humans, they often do apply. Laboratory study can also be the basic study of the cells with the electron microscope. Much information has been discovered regarding the aging of individual cells grown in tissue cultures in the laboratory. Longitudinal studies are investigations of groups of people over periods of many years—some as many as 25 years. They are difficult to control and expensive because of the long time span involved.

One approach that overcomes the time span obstacle is in the use of the human placenta as a model in the study of aging. Placental growth patterns are the same as other organs; however, it is an aging organ in a young body. After the initial cell division, it has a period of rapid growth followed by a slowing of cell mass growth. The physiological changes in the placenta are similar to changes found in aging organs. As the placenta is being studied, it might be used as a model to study the aging process. The effects of malnutrition in the placenta and its effects on biochemical actions within the cell, such as cell division, RNA metabolism, and blood perfusion, might be the same as those seen in aging.

Autopsies also are a source of information on aging. Autopsy reports give researchers information regarding the condition of various organs at different ages. Aging is the accumulation of many changes over time. Researchers get much information when they can connect the condition of an organ with the age and general health or illness of a person. For example, an autopsy demonstrates that many persons in their early twenties have obvious changes in their arteries due to arteriosclerotic plaques. Their life-styles and habits are reviewed and compared with the life-styles and habits of persons whose arteries show no such plaque formation. Assumptions can be made and questions raised regarding age of death, condition of arteries, and former life-styles; these assumptions and questions are then taken to the laboratory, and tests are completed on laboratory animals. The animals (mice or monkeys, for example) are divided into two groups. The control group will have the life-style of a person who does not have arteriosclerosis. The experimental group will have the life-style of a person who has arteriosclerosis, including stress, high-fat diet, and family history of hypertension and smoking. If autopsy reveals

that the experimental group has the arterial change, then the researcher will conclude that there is a correlation between this life-style and arteriosclerosis. The nurse then takes this research data and uses it as information for health teaching and health counseling.

The study of the aging process is relatively new. Technological breakthroughs in the last decade now permit the investigation of biochemical structures as they change with age. Although the focus has traditionally been on the study of diseases of aging (called geriatrics), a newer approach, gerontology, studies all the processes of the body as it ages. This includes health adaptations and changes that occur and can be seen in a positive light.

Considerable investigation has been done on the molecular level to find the fundamental mechanisms of aging. The research cited in this chapter is research that is repeatedly seen in the literature on aging. There are many theories of aging because no single cause has been found to be *the* cause of aging; the number of theories reflects the complexity of the subject. The investigations seek an understanding of the aging process both in the internal and external environment. The research cited in this chapter reports first on internal and then on external factors. The goal of present-day research is to add years to the life of the older adult as well as to add life to those additional years.

Knowledge of the theories of aging helps the nurse to reduce negative environmental factors and support positive aspects. Nurses used similar planning with infectious diseases. Mortality rates dropped dramatically when public health nurses and other health professionals checked water supplies and taught hand washing and sanitary principles. Altering the external environment maintained and improved public health.

Laboratory researchers depend on nurses to apply the theory learned and test research data as a part of their clinical practice. For example, researchers stated that high blood pressure was related to strokes. Nurses were involved in massive campaigns to screen for hypertension. Many persons found to have hypertension were treated. Nurses helped these clients reduce external factors when dietary intake predisposed them to hypertension. A therapeutic regimen of dietary changes, health teaching, and medication therapy altered the course of a disease process. Nurse researchers have added to the literature on hypertension prevention by studying the relationship between obesity, ethnicity, and hypertension.

Homeostasis is the fundamental drive of all organisms for life-supporting balance within the organism. When balance is maintained, life is prolonged significantly.

Researchers have determined that aging is part of development in general and is species-specific. Humans have the longest life span of all mammals. Cells grown in tissue cultures in the laboratory indicate that all cells are programmed to die eventually. The environment has some influences on the life span. The National Institute of Aging, founded by the federal government in 1974, has funded much basic cell biochemical research in universities throughout the country. The Rand Corporation predicts chemical control of aging by the year 2025. Biochemical stimulation of new organs and limbs is foreseeable also. Microsurgery now repairs small vessels and restores limbs and nerve functions. Research in the field of mechanical engineering led to the development of the cardiac pacemaker. Organ transplants of skin and kidneys are common. Data from the immune system research make these possible.

As often happens with scientific advances, philosophical and moral issues arise. Are these advances consistent with our respect for human life? How much interference with the process of aging is right? Does this research diminish or support our respect for aging persons? These and other questions are work for the philosopher and moralist studying biomedical ethics.

The role of theory in science is to look for similar patterns of actions that can explain events. As attention is focused on particular questions, in-depth study is possible. There are 20 to 30 theories on aging; continued research will eventually narrow these to a few most probable causes. In actuality, these theories are hypotheses, that is, below thesis or theory level. The objective is to prove facts experimentally. A hypothesis becomes a theory when the results of the same phenomenon can be repeatedly demonstrated and statistically verified.

Because of progress in the fields of biology and chemistry, techniques are available to test the theories experimentally. In years past, theories were available but could not be tested because equipment had not been developed. Today, most theoretical ideas are tested in the laboratory using delicate and ultraprecise instruments and measuring apparatus.

The National Institute of Aging's major focus is on biochemistry, cytology, and physiology; it does not support research in psychology and social aspects of aging. Its goals are to promote health and reduce the incidence of illness in the older adult. Illness is costly both in dollars and in human suffering. One who studies the older adult learns about the younger years also. All persons should do everything possible in the early years of life to prepare for old age. For example, studies on nutrition and the older adult demonstrate that faulty nutrition at any age can cause problems.

Genetic theories of aging

The theories on aging describe the reasons why we age. The general genetic theory holds that the life span is programmed within the genes. This means that an individual will inherit his family's tendencies for short or long life. Persons fortunate enough to choose long-lived parents and grandparents will live approximately 6 years longer than those persons whose parents die before age 50.

The function of DNA in the cells is to produce enzymes and protein in a particular chain. If this chain is altered, the cell is not programmed for cell function and reproduction, and it dies. Some researchers believe that life span is programmed before birth into the genes in DNA molecules.

The error theory of aging maintains that death of the cell occurs because of changes in the sequences of information transfer. Cell structure and function are programmed in the cell in the DNA molecule. Decoding is done by RNA molecules in specific portions of the DNA chain. If the new protein or enzyme is not exactly the same as the one before, it cannot do precisely the same function within the cell. This leads to the deterioration of the cell, aging, and death. Initially, the error rate is low, but with time and the reduced cell reproduction in the adult, errors become more frequent and more harmful to the cell. Since the exact process of information transfer in the DNA and

Table 1-2. Stress units for life events[*]

Event	Mean value
Family constellation	
Death of spouse	100
Divorce	73
Separation	65
Death of a close family member	63
Marriage	50
Marital reconciliation	45
Change in family member's health	44
Pregnancy	40
Gain new member to family	39
Sexual difficulties	39
Arguments with spouse	35
Children leaving home	29
Trouble with in-laws	29
Change in living conditions	25
Move or change in residence	20
Change in schools, recreation, and church activities	20
Change in social activities	19
Change in sleeping habits	16
Change in number of family get-togethers	15
Change in eating habits	15
Vacation	13
Holidays	12
Individual changes	
Jail term	63
Personal injury or illness	53
Death of a close friend	37
Outstanding personal achievement	28
Revision of personal habits	24
Minor violation of the law	11
Employment and/or social	
Fired at work	47
Retirement	45
Business readjustment	39
Change in job	36
Change in work responsibility (promotion or demotion)	29
Spouse begins or stops work	26
Begin or end school	26
Trouble with boss	23
Financial	
Change in financial status	38
Mortage or loan over $10,000	31

[*]From Burges, A. W., and Lazare, A.: Community mental health: target populations, Englewood Cliffs, N.J., 1976, Prentice-Hall, Inc.

Table 1-2. Stress units for life events—cont'd

Event	Mean value
Financial—cont'd	
Foreclosure	30
Mortgage or loan under $10,000	17

Suggested score interpretation

150-199	Mild stress	37% of the population will become ill
200-299	Medium stress	51% of the population will become ill
300 and over	High stress	79% of the population will become physically ill

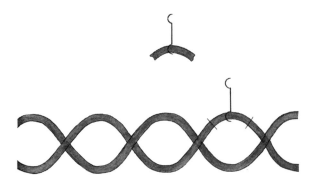

Fig. 1-2. The DNA helix is the core of cell reproduction. When a cross-linkage molecule attaches itself to one side of the DNA structure, it can be excised and no damage is done.

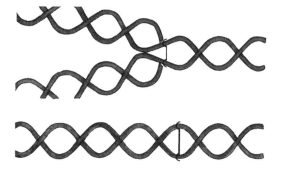

Fig. 1-3. When the cross-linkage molecule attaches itself to both sides of the DNA structure, the cell is doomed. The DNA can neither divide nor return to normal.

RNA molecules is unknown, the nature of the error cannot be specifically described. Studies are now investigating RNA differences in young and old tissues.

Wear and tear theory

The wear and tear theory views the body as an energy field or a machine. As cells of the body respond to stress and wear out, they must be replaced if the work of the body is to continue. The used cells are replaced through the process of cell reproduction. New blood cells are continually being made in the marrow of the long bones and sternum. Skin cells are shed and replaced by new cells.

Muscle and nerve cells, which do not reproduce, have internal mechanisms for repair and replacement of molecules within the cell. Stresses accumulate over time, and the ability of the body to maintain its reproduction and repair functions decreases. An individual's available energy for coping or adapting determines to a great extent the impact of the stress on the body. Chronic exposure to stress leads to such diseases as hypertension, arteriosclerosis, and myocardial infarction. Studies show no changes in the ability of the adrenal cortex to produce adrenalin in response to stress, but the receptor organs do not respond to the stimulation; they seem to be "worn out" from repeated exhaustion of stimulation. It is possible that the external environment can be modified to reduce stress and so decrease the adaptation demands on the older adult's body. Any change in the life of a person will be stressful. These changes can be happy or sad events. The older adult can respond to the stress, but needs more time than a younger person to make the adaptation to the stress situation (Table 1-2).

Lipofuscin accumulation theory

An end product of cell metabolism is called lipofuscin. It is insoluble, and its increasing amounts are associated with the aging process. They accumulate in neurons and myocardium and often take up one third of the cell volume. Current investigations are exploring what damage these lipofuscins or age pigments do in the cell. It is thought that they might interfere with cell wall diffusing ability. This alters the cell's ability to handle electrolytes.

Researchers have demonstrated that vitamin E and selenium break the chain of lipofuscin production. They inhibit the destruction of the fatty membrane, and the cell is protected. Vitamin E, an antioxidant, is a nutrient. Studies with animals have shown that it can be added to the diet to produce a reduction in lipofuscin accumulation. Further investigation is needed to determine minimum daily requirements for humans.

Cross-linkage theory

Cross-linkage has been named a primary suspect as a cause of aging. Consider a double helix strand of DNA. Between two strands is a cross-linkage molecule with a chemically active access on each end. The DNA strand should divide in the normal cell reproductive cycle. Fig. 1-2 illustrates a strand of a cross-linkage molecule in a state that causes

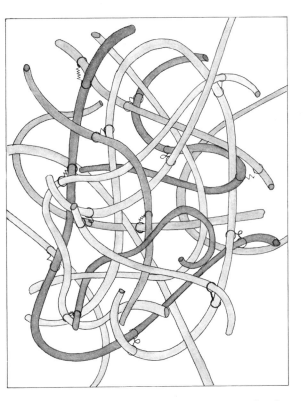

Fig. 1-4. Age-related inelasticity of tissue is considered to be a result of accumulated cross-linkage processes.

no damage. However, the cross-linkage molecule prevents the division. Repair of the strand is impossible, and the cell dies. Cross-linkages are stable molecules and accumulate over time. Fig. 1-3 illustrates the cross-linkage molecules attached to DNA. They affect proteins in elastin and collagen. The cell deaths resulting from these produce the decrease in elasticity of blood vessels and skin commonly seen in the older adult. As illustrated in Fig. 1-4, thickened cross-linked cells form, and up until recently, seemed impenetrable. Enzymes from the organism *Bacillus cereus* have been shown to be able to penetrate these thickened cross-linked cells and soften them. So far, this has been done in laboratories on agar plates and on a small study with mice. The mice that were given the enzymes were less gray and more active than the mice who did not receive the *Bacillus cereus* enzyme injections. More studies on greater numbers of mice are now under way.

Cell death theory

The cell death theory holds that cell division is a finite process. The total number of cell reproductions is programmed into the cell. This can be demonstrated in the laboratory. Tissue cultures of human cells show that the end of cell reproduction can be predicted. A human tissue cell will divide about 50 times in culture media in the

laboratory. The embryo tissue from a turtle species whose life span is 175 years lives twice as long in cultures as human embryonic cells do. Extracellular environmental factors such as the condition of surrounding tissue, blood, neuron, and hormonal supply greatly influence the viability of the cell.

Immunological theory

The immunological theory holds that aging is an autoimmune process. As cells change with age, the body's immune system fails to recognize its own cells. Autoimmune responses damage cells and lead to cell death. Changes in the thalamus lead to dependence on less specific types of immune cells. In addition, the overall susceptibility to infections and to cancer increases with age.

The immunological system defends the body from external microorganisms as they enter the body, and also defends against mutant cells that form inside the body. Recognition might occur, but the aging body might not be able to produce mature antibodies or phagocytic cells. Errors might develop in the antibodies so that they react to normal as well as to abnormal cells. Testing is being done with older animals being given the stem cells' antibody cells of younger animals. The immune ability of the older animal increases. Success in this area of research will improve the qual-

Table 1-3. Expectation of life at birth, 1920 to 1973*

Year	US population			White population			Black population and others		
	Total	Males	Females	Total	Males	Females	Total	Males	Females
1920	54.1	53.6	54.6	54.9	54.4	55.6	45.3	45.5	45.2
1930	59.7	58.1	61.6	61.4	59.7	63.5	48.1	47.3	49.2
1940	62.9	60.8	65.2	64.2	62.1	66.6	53.1	51.5	54.9
1950	68.2	65.6	71.1	69.1	66.5	72.2	60.8	59.1	62.9
1955	69.6	66.7	72.8	70.5	67.4	73.7	63.7	61.4	66.1
1960	69.7	66.6	73.1	70.6	67.4	74.1	63.6	61.1	66.3
1965	70.2	66.8	73.7	71.0	67.6	74.7	64.1	61.1	67.4
1970	70.9	67.1	74.8	71.7	68.0	75.6	65.3	61.3	69.4
1971	71.1	67.4	75.0	72.0	68.3	75.8	65.6	61.6	69.7
1972	71.1	67.4	75.1	72.0	68.3	75.9	65.6	61.5	66.9
1973	71.3	67.6	75.3	72.2	68.4	76.1	65.9	61.9	70.1

*Source: US National Center for Health Statistics, Vital statistics of the United States (annual). In US Bureau of the Census, Statistical abstract of the United States. 1975, p. 59, No. 82.
NOTE: Before 1960, Alaska and Hawaii are excluded.

ity of life of the older adult. Debilitating diseases such as rheumatoid arthritis, maturity-onset diabetes, thyroiditis, some anemias, and multiple sclerosis are thought to be autoimmune diseases.

Some believe that the cross-linkage theory and the autoimmune theory are closely related. It is possible that the decrease in the immune response in the older adult is the result of random uncontrolled cross-linkages. Cross-linkages may (1) form a network that hinders intracellular transport and so inhibits the functions of the immune system, (2) hamper the function of essential molecules, and (3) cause destruction of the DNA, which controls immunological functions.

Genetic patterns and longevity

Statistical data shed some light upon genetic inheritance for longer life spans. If a person's parents live into their 80s, there is a greater likelihood that he will have a longer-than-average life span also.

Gender makes a difference in longevity predictions. In the United States, a woman has approximately 6 more years of life than a man. This holds true for all countries. Built-in genetic material advantages seem to favor the female in all species from birth. Race also is a significant factor in predicting longevity. Although women have the longer life spans in both groups, whites have up to 7 years more expected life at 60 years than blacks. Black men are at considerably more risk than any other group (Table 1-3). External environmental factors, densely populated living conditions, lack of health screening and health maintenance facilities, and all the stresses of poverty affect the homeostasis of the organism. More knowledge regarding how to maintain that stability internally and externally will maximize the life span and the quality of life. The longevity-assurance hypothesis is the humanistic approach.

Conclusion

These theories of aging sum up the biological research currently in progress. Repeatedly the effects of the environment are stated because environmental conditions affect the cells by speeding up or slowing down the aging process. Nursing addresses the internal and external environments of man. By manipulating or not manipulating the environment, nursing slows down or speeds up the aging process.

PSYCHOLOGICAL THEORIES OF AGING

Psychological theories of aging have been based on developmental theories. Some theories have been clinically tested, while others are being refined. The following selected theories present an overview of the most prominent writings that have significance for nurses caring for the older adult.

Freud's psychoanalytic theory

The psychoanalytic theory of Sigmund Freud (1962) is more concerned with humans' thoughts and feelings than their behavior. The establishment of identity and gratification of instinctual drives at an early age frames subsequent behavior and personality throughout life. Three structures—the id, ego, and superego—describe the personality. The id is governed by the pleasure principle, as compared with the ego, which controls inner drives to achieve realistic aims. Two major influences set limits on gratification of drives: reality and social rules as mediated by the superego.

The ego psychology of Hartmann, which views outer social conditions, permits the extension of the theory to study adulthood and aging. However, Freud himself recommended that psychoanalytic theory not be used on older adults. Other studies include the individual psychology of Alfred Adler and the sociological extensions by Horney, Fromm, and Sullivan. Dibner (1971) identifies psychological aging as a preference for simplicity, which includes an attitude of conservation, self-protection, redundancy, and security. The most frequently used adaptive mechanisms by the older adult are unmodified anxiety, depression-withdrawal, projection, somatization, and denial (Table 1-4). These mechanisms are responsible for the specific clinical syndromes seen in later years.

Sullivan's interpersonal theory

Sullivan (1953) theorizes about phenomena not addressed by Freud and posits the following developmental stages of personality: infancy, childhood, juvenile era, preadolescence, late adolescence, and adulthood. Both Sullivan and Erikson (see pp. 13-14) agree that a satisfactory resolution

Table 1-4. Most frequently used adaptive mechanisms

Adaptive mechanism	Definition	Example
Unmodified anxiety	A magnified feeling of apprehension, uncertainty, fear, terror, and panic	The older adult is afraid of his house being robbed, and being mugged. He may add all kinds of locks to his doors and windows, buy a dog and still be afraid to sleep at night, hear all kinds of strange noises, and have palpitations as soon as it gets dark.
Depression/withdrawal	A state of mind in which the client experiences sadness, pathos, and withdraws physically and verbally from society and social activities	An older adult's wife dies, and he loses interest in his personal hygiene and has intermittent crying spells. He feels helpless, guilty, and can't get out of bed in the morning; in fact, he sleeps a lot some days and has insomnia other days. He has general physical complaints of fatigue, headache, anorexia, GI disturbances, and constipation. He slumps in a chair, lacks voice and facial expression, and refuses to leave the house and accept invitations from his friends and family.
Projection	Attribution of one's own ideas and shortcomings to others	The older adult feels that he has to live on a low pension because of his family. Years ago he turned down an executive position in Arabia because his wife refused to move there with the children.
Somatization	A mental state of mind that is converted into bodily symptoms	An older adult voices many discomforts regarding his body systems. He attributes his discomfort to arthritis. The pain is particularly distressing when he attempts to pay the monthly bills and balance his checkbook.
Denial	Refusal to acknowledge painful anxiety-producing occurrences and feelings	Arrangements have been made for an older adult woman to move in with her daughter. The older adult goes out and buys all new draperies for her own house.

is needed at each stage for optimal development and prevention of abnormalities. Sullivan is noted for the development of the interpersonal theory of psychiatry. Maturity is the establishment of satisfactory interpersonal relationships within the personal environment of the individual. He also places great emphasis on the interpersonal relationships between the caretaker and the client. The importance of therapeutic and nontherapeutic aspects of an interpersonal relationship is addressed in staff conferences and in-service staff development programs. This is an early development of milieu therapy and an innovative approach for hospitalized clients. Sullivan posits anxiety as the disruptive obstacle to the establishment of an interpersonal relationship and the development of problems in living. His theory is founded on the assumption that human behavior is positively directed toward goals of collaboration and mutual satisfaction and security unless interfered with by anxiety.

Sullivan's concepts of anxiety and interpersonal relationships are particularly important for the nurse caring for the older adult. Interpersonal security, especially in view of the client's changing roles, such as retirement and widowhood, the establishment of new relationships, and the relief of anxiety need to be recognized by the nurse in implementing the components of the nursing process. The theory has application for resolving interpersonal problems between older adult parents and middle-aged children. The establishment of rapport and interpersonal relationships and decrease in anxiety are addressed in Chapter 9.

Maslow's hierarchy of needs theory

Abraham Maslow (1962) proposes a theory that identifies psychological and physiological needs. His theory posits a hierarchal order for universal basic human needs. People are motivated to meet these needs in order to maintain physiological and psychological homeostasis. The physiological needs, such as food, water, oxygen, rest and sleep, elimination, and absence of pain have to be sufficiently satisfied in order for the next level of needs, safety and security, to emerge. The need for love and belonging will receive attention and motivate the individual's behavior when the need for safety and security is satisfied. The individual must experience an acceptable degree of satisfaction of love and belonging and self-esteem before he can address satisfying self-actualization, the highest need of Maslow's hierarchy (Fig. 1-5).

Maslow's theory is of particular interest to nurses caring for the older adult. Application of the five levels of needs is explored in depth in Chapters 10 and 11. Nurses are in a unique position to help the older adult adapt appropriate responses for satisfying his basic needs and maintaining homeostasis. Hulicka (1972) has studied the basic needs of institutionalized older adults and identified obstacles to meeting those needs. Physical and environmental limitations combined with depersonalization, task orientation, dependency, authoritarianism, staff convenience, and staff insensitivity are factors in institutional life that militate against the fulfillment of basic human needs.

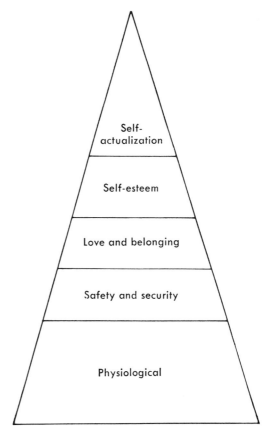

Fig. 1-5. Maslow's hierarchy of needs.

Erikson's theory of developmental stages

Erik H. Erikson (1963), a developmental theorist, suggests a developmental approach to aging that starts with birth and continues through death. He outlines eight tasks placed in stages of development that the individual must confront during his journey along the road of life (Fig. 1-6). An age sequence and two alternatives are designated for each developmental task. The tasks of stages 7 and 8 are the ones that will be confronted in caring for the older adult. However, resolutions for earlier developmental tasks have a significant influence on resolutions at stages 7 and 8.

The time frame designated for the Generativity vs. Stagnation stage is years 25 through 65. The seventh stage covers many events that happen within a 40-year period. This is the period in life when most people set courses to accomplish career goals, lifetime dreams, and ambitions. Productivity and creativity in work play major roles in this stage.

It is theorized that *generativity* is satisfied through establishing an interest in or guiding the next generation. Having offspring to leave behind in the next generation is not necessary for satisfying this developmental task. Other contributions through work and feelings of self-satisfaction and fulfillment are equally important for accomplishing this stage. An unsuccessful journey through this phase of life Erikson calls *stagnation*. It refers to a sense of unsuccessful accomplishment, sluggishness, boredom, and inactivity.

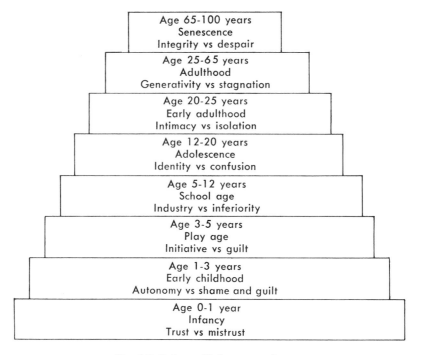

Fig. 1-6. Erikson: Eight stages of man.

The eighth and final stage of Erikson's theory is called Integrity vs. Despair. The time span for this stage is from 65 years through 100 years. It encompasses senescence, which is the term applied to normal aging. Erikson posits that as life is growing to a close, the individual looks for a semblance of meaning to his life. He evaluates his accomplishments and failures and gets a sense of *integrity* from his life: what was to be, was to be.

The older adult who evaluates his life as having no meaning, a waste of time, or a total loss, gives up hope. This older adult is ending his journey in life with a sense of *despair*.

As the older adult uses reminiscence and life review (Butler 1963), the nurse will receive cues about how he resolved Erikson's eight developmental tasks. These data will give the nurse a historic perspective that can help her understand the client's present coping mechanisms. Nursing plans, intervention, and client goals will vary, depending on the client's resolution of the Generativity vs. Stagnation and Integrity vs. Despair stages of adulthood developmental tasks.

Peck's developmental theory

Peck (1955) expanded Erikson's theory because he felt that the last two stages address adulthood in a global manner. He proposes four stages for middle age and three stages for old age (Fig. 1-7).

The stages Peck identifies for middle age expand the Generativity vs. Stagnation stage of Erikson. The four stages examine the developmental tasks that occur within a middle-age time frame. For example, in Valuing Wisdom vs. Valuing Physical Powers, people use knowledge (wisdom) gained through experience instead of physical powers that are lost through aging. Men and women view each other as individuals and companions with a close interpersonal bond, and sex becomes less significant as the children leave the home in the Socializing vs. Sexualizing in Human Relationships stage. When parents die, middle-aged adults shift emotional ties to new friends and their children's family; this stage is called Cathectic Flexibility vs. Cathectic Impoverishment. Mental Flexibility vs. Mental Rigidity sees humans' minds as open to new experiences and innovative ways to solve

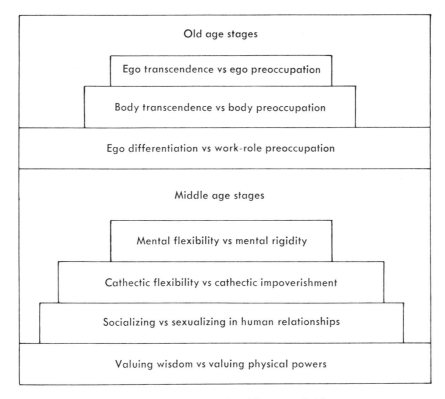

Fig. 1-7. Peck: Stages of middle age and old age.

problems or as closed and rigid to problem solving.

The three stages identified for old age expand Erikson's Integrity vs. Despair stage. Ego Differentiation vs. Work-Role Preoccupation examines the replacement of work and parenting roles that are lost because of retirement and children's leaving home with meaningful activities and new roles that lead to a sense of satisfaction. Body Transcendence vs. Body Preoccupation explains that satisfying relationships and creative activity enable older adults to transcend illnesses and preoccupation with their bodies. The last stage for old age examines Ego Transcendence vs. Ego Preoccupation. Life satisfaction is achieved through one's contributions to society, children, and friendships; this satisfaction transcends ego and extends beyond death. This overcomes a preoccupation with the ego and withdrawal.

Erikson's and Peck's theories are applied to nursing practice in Unit III, Intervention.

SOCIOLOGICAL THEORIES OF AGING

Sociological studies have been interested in the older adult's interaction with society, cultural influences, attitudes, relationships, family structures, and socioeconomic factors that influence longevity. Sociologists have combined the developmental theories and the sociostructural theories to develop psychosocial concepts of aging. The influence of the aging process on social roles was one of the earliest areas to be studied by sociologists. Several of the sociological studies and their conclusions are presented to whet the appetite of the nurse for further investigation and future nursing research in gerontology.

Disengagement theory

The theory on disengagement was developed by Cumming and Henry in 1961 after a 5-year study. It is one of the earliest theories on aging and the most controversial. Controversy has focused on the sample being neither large enough nor a diversified representative of all socioeconomic levels in society. Interest in the theory is such that it has been revisited on numerous occasions, and is under scientific investigation even today. The premise of the theory is that, with aging, people disengage from society. This is viewed as a mutual phenomenon on the part of society and the individual. It is suggested that disengagement starts in middle life when the individual realizes that his own death is inevitable. The individual and society continue to mutually disengage as his roles change with aging. For example, with retirement, the worker disengages from the business world. Disengagement is supposed to free the individual from the many mundane emotional ties and activities and offer greater equilibrium as a result of independence and solitude. He has a new-found freedom, since he is released from pursuing opportunities for socialization.

Engagement is the opposite of disengagement and is viewed as continued interaction of the older adult within society. The engaged person is seen as bound, committed to society, and the disengaged person free, without restricting ties to society. Considering all things equal—health, energy, and resources—this new-found freedom, the theorist posits, gives the disengaged person the capability to enjoy old age. The individual who can use this freedom to his best advantage is the one who will delight in old age. The orientation for this theory is expressed well by a man who worked all his life as a mechanic. The day he retired he said, "I have no intention of working ever again. My hands have been dirty my whole life, and now my hands will be clean." He literally retired to a life of leisure, and leisure for this man is a form of activity.

The disengaged older adult now looks over his priorities and reorders them to fit his increased freedom. The disengaged person may still maintain some very select activities. A characteristic of disengagement is its tendency to take a self-perpetuating course. For example, one telephones friends less frequently; then the friends stop calling.

Cumming and Henry view disengagement as a satisfactory life-style for the older adult. Their evidence finds the disengaged adult 65 and older with a higher morale than those who do not disengage. In no way does the theory imply that the older adult disengages from the value system of his society. Data continue to be collected even today, and more sophisticated research designs and sampling are being used to validate patterns of interaction and adaptation for the older adult. However, given the right ingredients, the older adult will seek the most satisfying degree of disengagement and activity that is within his realm of personality development, self-concept, and life satisfaction.

Cumming states that disengagement permits the older adult to die without causing major social changes. She compares this with the young adult who dies and leaves many uncompleted social and business commitments because of his engagement. As he advances in age, the very old adult may find himself with severed friendships and no family ties because of death. At this point in life, his situation can be compared with that of an orphaned child. There are no familiar ties; no one is available to look after his social or physical needs. He becomes a ward of society.

The disengagement theory was altered in 1965 by Henry, who places it in a progressive developmental framework rather than in the tasks of old age. Cumming sees the older adult as being permitted the freedom and self-expression similar to that of an adolescent. The old-old* are allowed the dependency and distinctness of a small child, who is the beneficiary of needed help and support.

Freedom, expressiveness, dependency, individuation, adolescent, and child behaviors have significant implications for nursing practice. Nurses are in a unique position to collect data to verify the behaviors and characteristics postulated in the theory. Nurses can test out the postulates during their nursing intervention.

For instance, the nurse may look for similar behavior and socioeconomic backgrounds or differences among disengaged clients. Disengagement is the rationale for those clients who do not wish to participate in bingo and other social activities. It is a matter of respecting the individual values and rights of the client. The nurse may suggest other options and let the client make his own de-

---

*The old-old are adults 75 years and older who are particularly feeble and vulnerable to disease because of their frail condition.

cisions. However, the nurse must be alert and able to differentiate signs and symptoms of a state of depression and withdrawal from disengagement. Nursing research can contribute much to expand, modify, and verify existing scientific inquiry. For example, in 1975, Cumming suggested that neurophysiological findings be investigated as causes of disengagement. In 1978, two nurses, Edsall and Miller, investigated the relationship between loss of auditory and visual acuity and social disengagement. Their research did not measure the quality or stresses of interpersonal relationships. Two conclusions from their research study follow.

1. Disengagement may be present in conjunction with neurophysiological deficits that make social interactions less satisfying although not completely eliminating them.
2. There is no significant relationship between loss of visual and auditory acuity and social disengagement.

The investigators made recommendations for duplicating the research with modifications for examining other neurophysiological factors. Interested nurse researchers can use these recommendations as a basis for future investigations.

Activity theory vs. disengagement theory

Every nurse has had some kind of firsthand experience with the disengagement and activity theory. Almost any nurse can name an older adult who is a member of the church senior citizen's group. The individual is very active in church affairs and probably belongs to one or two other groups. She goes to all the functions and enjoys days trips, weekend trips, and vacation trips. She is called a very active person because she is engaged in activities.

The activity theory (Havighurst, 1963) supports the belief that the older adult should remain active and engage in society's activities. New roles, new friendships, new hobbies, and new interests should replace discontinued ones. A basic supposition of the theory is that activity promotes well-being and life satisfaction. The activity theory is one of the most acceptable theories of aging. Our culture also seems to sanction and support activities for older adults. Three factors—high status, good health,

and employment—are present in 75 percent of older adults who rate their morale as high.

The older adult's interest in remaining active and the relationship between barriers that prevent activity, such as poor health and lack of financial, psychological, and social resources, need to be addressed. The cause and effects still need to be studied.

Continuity theory

The continuity theory, also known as the developmental theory of aging (Neugarten, 1964), may be sandwiched in between disengagement and activity. Neugarten studied the personality of older adults and found that, as people age, their personality makeup does not change and their behavior becomes more predictable. For instance, a housewife who always worried about insignificant things is likely to find more things to worry about as an older adult. An assertive young woman may become an active member of the Gray Panthers in older adulthood.

The theory also endorses the notion that, with aging, the older adult develops his own system of relationships that he can turn to for emotional and psychological support when needed.

Neugarten individually and with others further studied the influence of age on the structure and change in personality. She found that the personality processes that change are a decrease in ego energy, ego style, and sex-role perception. Men and women seem to switch roles. The woman takes on the leadership, aggressive role while the man assumes the nurturing, tolerant role. The man passes on to his wife the household decision-making authority, while he is perfectly happy being waited on by his wife. Spouses play the more significant role of companion.

The older adult no longer is controlled by peer pressure, fads, and keeping in step with the Joneses. Instead, he is concerned with his inner self, introspection, and his own individuality. Neugarten (1968) labels this change in the personality *interiority*. Interiority had its beginning in the 1950s and picked up momentum through the years. Kimmel (1974) suggests that it may be a precurser to the reminiscence and life-review process identified by Butler (1963).

Kimmel states that developmental research

needs to study the interaction and influence of variables, such as biological changes, sociological and cultural influences, attitudes, and personality processes on age, rather than age per se. Nurses caring for older adult individuals and couples should assess the extent of these variables and plan nursing intervention to meet the individual client's adaptation to aging.

Having assimilated this knowledge into our practice, the nurse can anticipate the needs identified with developmental and personality process theories. She can use her knowledge base to help the older adult identify realistic goals to meet his health needs. Nurses are then better able to plan and execute suggested nursing intervention strategies for individual clients.

The passages theory

In 1974, Gail Sheehy wrote a best-selling book, *Passages: Predictable Crises of Adult Life,* that addresses adult developmental stages and identifies various patterns of adult life. Sheehy's in-depth research and interviews of men, women, and couples describe practical situations of real people applying the social and psychological developmental theories. Although she is an author and not a scientist or theorist, she did for the adult what Spock did for the child. Finding a void of information on how the individual progresses from adolescent to adulthood and middle age, she set out to unravel the mystery of growing up from ages 18 to 55. She took each decade of adulthood and studied what occurred in the life of the woman and the man. Using the same design, she studied married couples at each decade of adulthood. Her research reveals that men and women's developmental stages at each decade are not synchronized. Each passes through a decade to the beat of a different drummer, reaching his or her peak of individuality at a different time. Crises that occur at each period of life were fully explored. The author feels that once these crisis can be predicted, a pattern for adulthood can be developed that will enable the individual to better manage his life.

The research sample used was the educated middle class. The author believes that this group is motivated, healthy, the translators of social values, and the generators of new life-styles and attitudes. It is the group in society with the most choices for initiating change and life improvement.

Even though the book is not the culmination of a controlled scientific study, it has relevance for the older adult. Passages through each chronological life cycle, including its resolutions, are significant for the older adult. Many of the crises during the generativity stage are presented in case histories not as problems but as a continuation of changes that occur within the life cycle. Sheehy was instrumental in getting the average person to read about adulthood and identify with or reject the personality changes common to his decade of life.

NURSING STUDIES ON PSYCHOSOCIAL THEORIES OF AGING

As early as 1952, nursing investigators had completed research in psychosocial gerontology. Mack (1952) reports in *Nursing Research* the results of a study entitled Personal Adjustment of Chronically Ill Old People under Home Care.

Since the 1950s, research has centered around psychosocial nursing studies and clinical studies. The areas of health needs reported in *Nursing Research* have been incontinence, attitudes of nursing personnel, and psychosocial nursing interventions focusing on meeting the needs of the older adult. However, there is a gap in the research regarding the development of measurement tools that focus on aging and describe older adult developmental behaviors. Nursing has this rich, fertile area to study the behaviors of older adults within the various environments in which nurses encounter these clients. Gunter and Miller (1977) see a need for a framework for future studies and divide them into two groups: general nursing care research and specialized nursing care research.

General nursing care research includes investigating fundamental nursing skills and their application to the older adult. Health promotion, maintenance, rehabilitation, health teaching, and the evaluation of nursing intervention are included in this group. Specialized nursing care research includes the evaluation and comparison of three types of environments:

1. Institutional care
2. Home care
3. Community services

The requirements of various cultures, subcultures, and socioeconomic groups need to be identified within the three care settings. In addition, the roles of nursing education, continuing education, and staff development need to be explored for the improvement of quality care to the older adult. A spectrum of interdisciplinary theories, nursing theories, and gerontological theories may be used to design the studies.

SUMMARY

Some of the early theories of psychiatry and psychology have been found to be appropriate for the field of gerontology. Many have been expanded or modified in order to fit the older adult model. The disengagement and activity theories reported in the 1960s are still being used as examples for successful aging. Nursing became involved in gerontological research over 30 years ago. Today, nurse researchers are testing the significance of stress and changes in the neurosensory system on the disengagement and activity theories.

The older adult has the same needs as those in Maslow's hierarchy. The degree of assistance required to satisfy these needs depends on the individual and his support system.

Research is being done individually by psychologists and sociologists and jointly with psychiatrists in a multidisciplinary effort to develop a theory of adult development and aging. An area of interest in the past 20 years is that of personality and aging. It is anticipated that, with the increase in life span and the older adult population, new knowledge and cultural awareness will bring to light new realities that will demand new approaches to the study of aging, personality, and society.

We are at the tip of the iceberg in psychosocial research in gerontology. There is an army of nurses representing a vast resource who have not been tapped to collect data and participate in research. Nurses are in a unique position to study the older adult and contribute to the development of new concepts and knowledge in the field of gerontology.

REFERENCES

Adler, A.: The practice and theory of individual psychology, translated by P. Radin, New York, 1971, Humanities Press.

Ardrey, R.: The social contract, New York, 1970, Atheneum Publishers.

Beall, G. T., and Mulak, S.: Perspectives on the availability and utilization of foreign-source informational materials in gerontology, Gerontologist 17:537, December 1977.

Birren, J. E., and Schaie, K. W.: Handbook of the psychology of aging, New York, 1977, Van Nostrand Reinhold Co.

Blau, Z.: Old age in a changing society, New York, 1973, New Viewpoints.

Britton, J. H., and Britton, J. O.: Personality changes in aging, New York, 1972, Springer Publishing Co., Inc.

Browning, M. H.: Nursing and the aging patient, New York, 1974, The American Journal of Nursing Co.

Butler, R. N.: The life review: an interpretation of reminiscence in the aged, Psychiatry 26(1):65, 1963.

Cumming, E.: Engagement with an old theory, Int. J. Aging 6(3):187, 1975.

Cumming, E., and Henry, H.: Growing old: the process of disengagement, New York, 1961, Basic Books, Inc.

Davison, A. N.: Biochemical aspects of the aging brain, Age Ageing Suppl:4, 1978.

de Beauvoir, S.: The coming of age, New York, 1972, G. P. Putnam's Sons.

Dibner, A. S.: Psychological aging as preference for simplicity. Unpublished paper presented at 24th annual meeting of the Gerontological Society, Houston, Texas, October 1971.

Edsall, J. O., and Miller, L. A.: Relationship between loss of auditory and visual acuity and social disengagement in an aged population, Nurs. Res. 27:296, September-October 1978.

Erikson, E. H.: Childhood and society, ed. 2, New York, 1963, W. W. Norton & Co., Inc.

Ferris, S., Crook, T., Sathananthan, G., and others: Reaction time as a diagnostic measure in senility, J. Am. Geriatr. Soc. 24:529, December 1976.

Freeman, M. J.: Don't lose your senses, Nurs. Times 73:137, January 1977.

Freud, S.: The ego and the id, edited by J. Strachey, translated by J. Riviere, New York, 1962, W. W. Norton and Co.

Fromm, E.: The crisis of psychoanalysis, New York, 1970, Holt, Rinehart and Winston, Inc.

Gelperin, A.: Our elderly. Who are they? J. Am. Geriatr. Soc. 26:318, July 1978.

Greene, J. A.: Science, nursing and nursing science: a conceptual analysis, ANS Adv. Nurse Sci. 1979, October 2(1):57.

Gröer, M. E., and Skekleton, M. E.: Basic pathophysiology: a conceptual approach, St. Louis, 1979, The C. V. Mosby Co.

Gunter, L. M., and Miller, J.: Toward a nursing gerontology, Nurs. Res. 26:208, 1977.

Guyton, A.: Textbook of medical physiology, ed. 6, Philadelphia, 1979, W. B. Saunders Co.

Harper, A. E.: Recommended dietary allowances for the elderly, Geriatrics 33:73, 79, May 1978.

Harbert, A. S., and others: Growing old in rural America, Aging 291-292:36, January-February 1979.

Harman, D.: Free radical theory of aging: effect of free radical reaction inhibitors on the mortality rate of male lab mice, J. Gerontol. 23:476, 1968.

Harris, A. J., and Feinberg, J. F.: Television and aging: is what you see what you get? Gerontologist 17(5 Pt 1):464, October 1977.

Hartmann, H.: Essays in ego psychology, New York, 1964, International Universities Press.

Havighurst, R.: Successful aging. In R. H. Williams, C. Tibbitts, and W. Donahue, editors: Process of aging, vol. I, pp. 299-320, New York, 1963, Atherton.

Henry, W. E.: Engagement and disengagement: toward a theory

of adult development. In Kastenbaum, R., editor: Contributions to the psychology of aging, New York, 1965, Springer Publishing Co., Inc., pp. 19-35.

Henthron, B.: Disengagement and reinforcement in the elderly, Res. Nurs. Health **2:**1, March 1979.

Hoff, L.: People in crisis, Reading, Mass., 1978, Addison-Wesley Publishing Co., Inc.

Horney, D.: Self-analysis, New York, 1942, W. W. Norton and Co., Inc.

Hulicka, I. M.: Understanding our client, geriatric, patients, J. Am. Geriatr. Soc. **20:**438, 1972.

Kastenbaum, D. S.: New thoughts on old age, New York, 1964, Springer Publishing Co., Inc.

Kent, S.: Antiaging therapy in the USSR, Geriatrics **34:**99, May 1979.

Kimmel, D.: Adulthood and aging, New York, 1974, John Wiley & Sons, Inc.

Krohn, P. L., editor: Topics in the biology of aging, New York, 1966, John Wiley & Sons, Inc.

LaMonica, E.: The nursing process: a humanistic approach, Reading, Mass., 1979, Addison-Wesley Publishing Co., Inc.

Linn, M. W., and Hunter, K.: Perception of age in the elderly, J. Gerontol **34:**46, January 1979.

Mack, M. J.: Personal adjustment of chronically ill old people under home care, Nurs. Res. **1:**9, June 1952.

Marriner, A.: The nursing process: a scientific approach to nursing care, ed. 2, St. Louis, 1979, The C. V. Mosby Co.

Maslow, A.: Toward a psychology of being, Princeton, N.J., 1962, Van Nostrand Reinhold Co.

McKenzie, S.: Aging and old age, Glenview, Ill., 1980, Scott, Foresman and Co.

McNulty, B.: The elderly: a challenge to nursing—longevity and loss, Nurs. Times **73:**1967, 15 December 1977.

Metress, J., and Kart, C.: A system for observing the potential nutritional risks of elderly people living at home, J. Geriatr. Psychiatry **11**(1):67, 1978.

Moon, M.: The measurement of economic welfare: its application to the aged poor, New York, 1977, Academic Press, Inc.

Mountcastle, V. B., editor: Medical physiology, ed. 14, St. Louis, 1980, The C. V. Mosby Co.

Naus, P.: The elderly as prophets, Hosp. Prog. **59:**66, May 1978.

Neugarten, B. L., and others: Personality in middle and late life, New York, 1964, Atherton Press.

Neugarten, B. L.: Adult personality: toward a psychology of the life cycle. In Vinacke, E., editor: Readings in general psychology, New York, 1968, American Book Co.

Neugarten, B. L.: Middle age and aging, Chicago, 1968, University of Chicago Press.

Neugarten, B. L., and Hall, E.: Acting one's age: new rules for old, Psychol. Today **13:**66, April 1980.

Peck, R. C.: Psychological developments in the second half of life. In Anderson, J. E., editor, Psychological aspects of aging, Proceedings of a conference on planning research, Bethesda, Md., April 24-27, 1955. Washington, D.C.: American Psychological Association, 1956. In Neugarten, B. L., editor: Middle age and aging, Chicago, 1968, University of Chicago Press.

Rawson, J. G., and others: Nutrition of rural elderly in southwestern Pennsylvania, Gerontologist **18:**24, February 1978.

Reinhardt, A. M., and Quinn, M. D., editors: Current practice in gerontological nursing, St. Louis, 1979, The C. V. Mosby Co.

Rockstein, M.: Theoretical aspects of aging, New York, 1974, Academic Press, Inc.

Sands, J. D., and Parker, J.: A cross-sectional study of the perceived stressfulness of several life events, Int. J. Aging Hum. Dev. **10**(4):335-341, 1979-1980.

Seefeldt, C., Jantz, R. K., Galper, A., and Jerack, K.: Using pictures to explore children's attitudes toward the elderly, Gerontologist **17:**506, December 1977.

Selye, H.: The physiology and pathology of exposure to stress, Montreal, Canada, 1950, Acta, Inc., Medical Publishers.

Selye, M., and Heuser, G.: Stress, 1955-56 5th Annual Report, New York, 1956, M.D. Publications, Inc.

Sheehy, G.: Passages: predictable crises of adult life, New York, 1976, E. P. Dutton & Co., Inc.

Sullivan, H.: The interpersonal theory of psychiatry, New York, 1953, W. W. Norton & Co., Inc.

Timiras, P. S.: Developmental physiology and aging, New York, 1972, Macmillan Publishing Co., Inc.

Yura, H., and Walsh, M. B.: The nursing process, assessing, planning, implementing, evaluating, ed. 3, New York, 1978, Appleton-Century-Croft.

2 Effects of aging on body systems

The process of aging affects each organ system of the body. Because the body is an integrated whole, change in one organ system affects other organs and systems. Understanding the physiological mechanisms that alter the function of individual organs, and the interrelationships of those mechanisms, helps the nurse plan realistically.

Depending upon the state of vigor of the older adult, he may consider himself young-old or old-old. This makes a truism of the expression, "You are as young as you feel." A person feeling alert and active can be young-old at 90.

This section presents the anatomy and physiology of each organ system. Because of space limitations, only those areas of each system that are most frequently seen as limitations for the older adult are discussed. More extensive information can be obtained from the references at the end of the chapter.

Overall, older adults maintain a steady balance of all organ systems. Even in the presence of considerable functional decline, the body strives for homeostasis. This balance is precarious at best, and damage to one system will affect other systems. Stresses and environmental changes outside the body can induce the loss of homeostasis. The nurse has the opportunity to minimize internal and external stresses in the environment and enable the individual to keep organ systems functioning normally. Hans Selye believes that disease causes aging, rather than age causing disease. His research demonstrates that drugs, hormones, and dietary alterations can affect the progress of a disease. His position is that the environment should be manipulated to support optimum health.

Many incidental problems of the aged, if not addressed, can make the last years of life miserable. Very common things such as dyspepsia or sinus infections can make the day-to-day existence of an older adult most uncomfortable. Anything that im-mobilizes the older adult is a priority that should be attended to by the nurse. Any problems with the feet, knees, and hips, and anything such as dizziness that would stop the person from moving about can have a profound effect on all the organ systems. These uncared for problems are the sources of the infirmity of old age. If a common problem such as pernicious anemia is treated, the older adult recovers very well, just as quickly as a younger person would. The recovery makes a dramatic effect on the life-style of that person. Although some implications for nursing intervention are introduced with the discussions of the characteristic changes occurring with aging, an in-depth presentation of nursing intervention is found in Chapter 10.

NERVOUS SYSTEM

The nervous system comprises the central nervous system, the peripheral nervous system, and the autonomic nervous system. The central nervous system includes the brain and spinal cord. The peripheral nervous system includes 12 pairs of cranial nerves and 31 pairs of spinal nerves. The autonomic nervous system is divided into sympathetic and parasympathetic divisions, which integrate the internal and external environments, and has been described as the "fight or flight" response system.

Cells of the nervous system are laid down in the first weeks of embryonic life. Cell division continues into the second year, then stops. There are 10 to 12 billion neurons in the human brain. The cellular structure of the nervous systems is highly complex, with highly differentiated groups of cells; that is, each group has specific actions. The cerebral cortex integrates the complex tasks of learning, language, memory, and memory skills. There are motor areas for body movement and sensory areas for perceptual tasks. Association areas connect sensory and motor areas and transmit impulses from one neuron to another within the spinal cord and brain. The nervous system components are particularly interdependent.

Microscopically, the nervous system consists of nerve cells or neurons, supporting cells, or glia, and extracellular space. The basic unit of the nervous system consists of the neuron and glia. The neuron comprises dendrites, the cell body, and the axon. Dendrites transmit impulses to the cell body. Neurons become glial in the older adult. Glial or neuroglial cells are passive, nonnervous cells that form a dense network among the nerve cells. The network serves as the mechanical support system for the nervous system tissue and acts as part of the system that transports nutrition to the neurons.

The dendrites carry impulses the the cell body. The axon carries impulses away from the cell body. The autonomic nerve fibers lead to sweat glands, blood vessels, erector muscles of the hair, or to each of the organs. The myelin sheath covers the cranial nerves with white matter in the brain and spinal cord, and helps transmit nervous impulses.

The autonomic nervous system governs the activities of the heart, lungs, digestive tract, glands, blood vessels, urinary bladder, uterus, and some endocrine organs. It is not actually automatic or independent of the central nervous system, but it is a part of the overall orchestration of body function.

After neuron cell division ends at 2 years of age, protein is synthesized and excreted in enormous amounts by each individual cell. Errors occur as the protein production continues, and errors have a cumulative effect over time. Pathological conditions in aging neurons include:

Accumulation of lipofuscin pigment

Decrease in cytoplasmic RNA

Changes in neuron shape

Neuron death

Interrelated in nervous systems changes are changes in the blood vessels and cerebrospinal fluid systems. The systems supply the nervous tissue with oxygen and nutrients and remove waste products. If oxygen or nutrition supplies are compromised, cell change in the neuron is inevitable. Since neurons do not reproduce, the damage is permanent.

Lipofuscin is a fat-based, brown waste material that collects in nervous tissue and selected other tissues such as cardiac muscle, skeletal muscle, smooth muscle, liver, spleen, epididymis, seminal vesicles, pancreas, and adrenals. It is possible that the inner cell becomes congested with these residues, which restrict the activity of the cell. The cell may lose its ability to maintain itself. There is some evidence that the more active the cell, the less lipofuscin is deposited. In a study on guinea pigs, lower lipofuscin deposits were shown on active cranial nerves and more deposits on less active cranial nerves. External factors affect the accumulation of lipofuscin pigment. Drugs, oxygen depletion, lower vitamin E intake, and cirrhosis each predispose the neuron to lipofuscin deposits.

The electroencephalograph (EEG) of the older adult is within the normal limits of other age groups with the exception of being about one cycle slower. This gives evidence of a somewhat slower pace of electrical impulses in the brain. There is a decrease in frequency of the dominant alpha rhythm, and an increase in the slower theta and delta waves. It must be noted, however, that the individual differences in EEG patterns are far greater in the adult population than in other age groups. A healthy status is the key factor. Illness, especially in the central nervous system, causes marked changes in the EEG reading. Often, cardiovascular disease causing hypoxia will cause EEG changes. An individual in a healthy state has EEG readings that correlate closely with good levels of learning ability, memory status, and perceptual and sensory motor functions. Shifts to lower functions are demonstrated on EEG readings and are related to severe intellectual debilitation.

Some research has shown that reaction time of the older adult is somewhat slower than that of the younger adult. This is a response of a slower velocity in the transmission of impulses along the nervous conducting system. Movement time decreases the time that is needed to physically respond to a situation. More time is needed to perform complex sensory motor skills or tasks. It is possible that older adults may require more time to do tasks because they have a higher level of caution and a low risk-taking preference. This might also be a coping mechanism for their declining perceptual senses, since it is most often seen in new or strange environments rather than at home. For example, if you go into an older woman's home and she offers you a cup of tea, she can be quite efficient in getting the kettle boiling and assembling the teacups and the tea, completing the task very comfortably. She may even be able to speak and move about at the same time. The same woman in a new situation such as a hospital or nursing home seems ill at ease, uncoordinated, and very slow in her movements. What the nurse can do is set an environmental tone to meet the slower pace of the individual. Don't overload the person with stimuli. This helps her avoid having to tap her limited reserve capacities and to risk stress vulnerability. Permit the person to progress slowly and to feel comfortable with her tasks. She will most often finish what has to be done, and will be comfortable doing it at a slower pace. The loss of ability for fine motor coordination and the rapid initiation of movement can be compensated for with a slower pace of activities.

The central nervous system can be viewed as a transmitter that sends and receives signals from the brain to the body parts. Because of the number of cells that decrease with age, the transmission strength decreases. The signals are slightly blurred. The threshold for arousal of an organ system may be higher, but this has yet to be actually demonstrated in research. What has been seen and can be observed in the older population is that overstimulation leads to anxiety and tension.

Muscular weakness is not caused by central nervous system or peripheral nervous system deterioration. Most of the weakness can be attributed to disuse atrophy. In addition, it is often pharmacological side effects and decrease in hormone secretion that cause the muscular weakness. The actual rate of speed of the nervous impulses decreases only 10 percent. This decrease in the rate of speed could possibly be due to vascular changes leading to ischemia, the general lowering of basal metabolic rate, and the temperature changes in the nerve fibers, which are created by changes in the surrounding tissue.

With age, there is increase in recovery time within the autonomic nervous system. It takes an organ longer to return to base level activity after

stimulation. Such sensitivity of tissue substances can be seen when drugs are taken that alter the heart rate, the blood sugar levels, and other endocrine activities. Aging tissue is very sensitive and requires far lower drug levels.

The aging of the central nervous system dramatically affects the general aging process of the individual. The central nervous system is intimately related to the cardiovascular system because of its dependency on oxygen. A state of hypoxia can contribute enough disequilibrium in the central nervous system to endanger general body homeostasis.

Intelligence is not affected with increasing age. Adults who are well show normal distribution of IQ ranges. Verbal abilities change very little as a person grows older; only the performance aspects seem to be diminished. These aspects relate to psychomotor skills, those tasks we perform with our hands. It is not that the person decreases in skill, but that the skill requires a longer period of time to perform. Verbal skills can actually increase with age. Solving new problems can be difficult if past experience is not involved in the solution. This is often seen in laboratory examinations or when a person has to fill out a medicare form. This is not a difficulty felt exclusively by the older adult. Younger persons often have this problem in new situations too. Ability to solve new problems based on past experience is a valuable asset to the older adult in a work situation. They have a decided advantage over a younger person because of their years of experience.

Long-term memory remains intact, so that older memories are often recalled and reviewed. The physiological process of storage and retrieval mechanisms of memories is not well known. It appears that these machanisms are more efficient for long-term than for short-term memory. Because the short-term memory is not very efficient in the older adult, learning can be difficult. Short-term memory is imperative for new learning to occur. When the individual's self-pacing is taken into account, learning can occur fairly effectively. The central factors to success in learning are motivation, level of interest in the topic, and general past experience that can be related to the new learning. The central nervous system has to address the mental status also. Depression is a very common problem with the older adult; suicide rates of men over 75 are among the highest of any age group.

CARDIOVASCULAR SYSTEM

The cardiovascular system provides the metabolic requirements of all tissues of the body over a wide range of activities. At rest, the needs for oxygen and nutrients are at a physiological minimum. Increased activity of any cell, tissue, or organ results in a greater need for these products and in the formation of additional carbon dioxide and other metabolic waste products. The cardiovascu-lar system responds to the need by sending a small increase in blood flow to the local area of activity or a widespread increase in blood flow.

The myocardium or cardiac muscle is different from skeletal muscle, in that all of the fibers act together upon neuron impulse. It consists of bands or layers of muscle that make up the atria and ventricles. These cardiac muscle layers are relatively thin in the atria but can be up to three times as thick in the left ventricle. Their structure is suited to function. The right ventricle has a comparatively thin wall muscle to expel blood to the

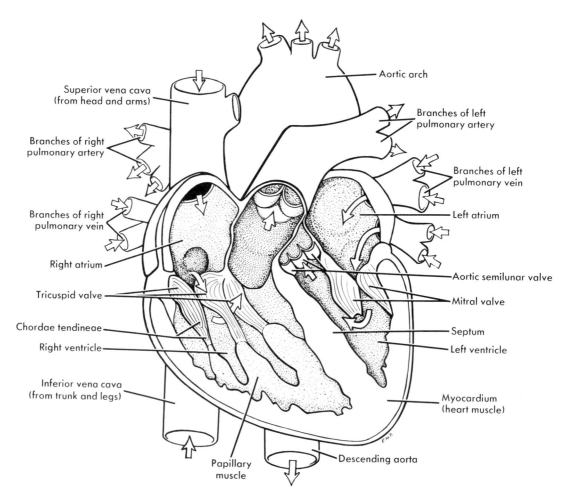

Fig. 2-1. Frontal section of heart showing the four chambers, valves, openings, and major vessels. Arrows indicate direction of blood flow.

pulmonary system at low pressure. The far thicker left ventricle chamber forces blood into the aorta against considerable resistance (Fig. 2-1).

The atria and ventricles are connected by a band of specialized muscle, the atrioventricular bundle of His. Electrical impulses arising from the sino-atrial (SA) node, the pacemaker of the heart, travel in atrial walls and cause the atria to contract. The atrioventricular (AV) node in the lower inner wall of the atria picks up the impulse and transmits the impulse through the bundle of His to contract the ventricles.

The ability of the myocardium and its nerve tissue to serve as an adequate pump depends on the blood supply to it from the coronary arteries. Cardiac tissue receives blood first; the left coronary artery is the first branch off the aorta. A block in a major coronary artery serving any part of the nerve conduction system threatens the ability of the myocardium to contract, and the pumping action can cease. The aging myocardium has the advantage of an alternate blood flow system called collateral circulation. Over the years, arteriosclerotic plaques narrow the arterial wall. To compensate for diminished blood supply, anastomoses between arteries open, permitting diversion of the blood around the obstruction. Even in the presence of a full arterial obstruction, the individual may remain symptom free. The so-called silent heart attack is relatively pain free, because ischemia (tissue death) is prevented by an adequate supply of blood through the collateral circulation.

The cardiac output is the amount of blood ejected from each ventricle in 1 minute. The average amount is 5 liters/minute (5000 ml/minute).

By 80 years of age, this amount may be reduced by one half. Stroke volume is the amount of blood ejected from each ventricle with every beat. The total amount of blood the heart can pump to the cells of the body is a relationship between the heart rate and stroke volume.

Cardiac output equals heart rate times stroke volume ($CO = HR \times SV$). Adequate stroke volume depends on (1) the ability of the myocardium fibers to stretch during ventricular filling, (2) the ability of the myocardium to contract, and (3) the amount of tension during systole if the ventricle is to open the semilunar valve and eject blood.

Just as a rubber band snaps back with force when stretched, so does the myocardium contract with vigor when stretched with blood as it fills the ventricle. The amount of blood available to fill the ventricle depends on the venous return of blood to the heart. The better the venous return, the more complete is the filling and stretch of the ventricles and the more efficient the contraction.

Contractility refers to the chemical activities within the myocardial cell that cause the muscle to contract or shorten. Some drugs, such as epinephrine, increase contractility, as does stimulation by the sympathetic nervous system.

The ventricular tension or overload depends on the size of the ventricle and the arterial pressure. Normal tension is 120 mm Hg. When the arterial pressure is elevated in hypertension, the ventricle meets increased resistance as it contracts and attempts to eject blood. The ventricle dilates to meet the increased tension demands. After a time, the ventricle becomes permanently overdistended and is less efficient. Because its contractility is reduced,

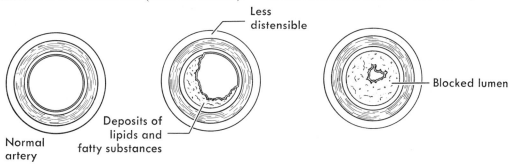

Fig. 2-2. Atherosclerotic vessel changes. (From Groer, M., and Shekleton, M.: Basic pathophysiology: a conceptual approach, St. Louis, 1979, The C. V. Mosby Co.)

the stroke volume and thus the cardiac output are reduced. Circulation to body tissue is decreased.

Generalized systemic hypertension is considered a physiological process of aging caused by narrowing of the arteries and arterioles (Fig. 2-2). A combination of factors causes this constriction. Reduced elasticity of vessel walls is caused by arteriosclerotic lesions and hyperfunction of adrenal hormones, which cause vasoconstriction. Such factors as race (blacks are more at risk with increasing age), family history, living environment, and level of activity all contribute to the risk of hypertension in the older adult. Smoking places an additional burden on the aging cardiovascular system because nicotine is a vasoconstrictor.

The lowest or basal blood pressure occurs upon awakening in the morning. The pressure rises with stress or activity. A blood pressure taken on a client in a sitting or standing position rather than lying down will show an increase in the diastolic levels. Exercise and states causing oxygen depletion (hypoxia) cause a rise in the systolic pressure. Women generally have higher blood pressures than do men; however, men exhibit more adverse signs and symptoms of the hypertension.

With aging, the myocardium shows an accumulation of lipofuscin and deterioration of the cells because of atrophy. Fat globules and connective tissue replace the myocardial fibers, and the valves develop areas of calcification. It is possible that these changes occur because of lack of exercise and myocardial activity. Like all muscles, the myocardium is subject to disuse atrophy. This progressive decline in myocardial vigor is seen in the lower cardiac reserve of the older adult.

Cardiac reserve is the heart's ability to respond to increased oxygen needs by increasing pump efficiency. The heart rate and strength increase, and after the immediate need has passed, the rate returns to normal. In the younger person the cardiac reserve is such that, on demand, the heart can increase output fivefold. The older heart has a significantly lower cardiac reserve. The output cannot be increased as much on demand, and when the heart rate has increased, it takes much longer to return to a predemand state. An older adult cannot run around a track as fast as a younger person because of physiology: the increased oxygen needs of the muscles cannot be met as

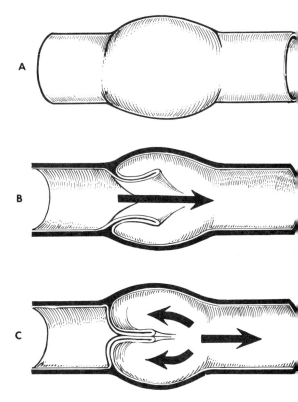

Fig. 2-3. Action of venous valves. **A,** External view of vein showing dilation at site of valve. **B,** Interior of vein with semilunar flaps in open position, permitting flow of blood through valve. **C,** Valve flaps approximating each other, occluding cavity, and preventing backflow of blood.

efficiently by the heart of a 70-year-old as by the heart of a 17-year-old.

Arteries have walls consisting of three layers: (1) the tunica intima, a smooth inner lining for the vessel, (2) the tunica media, the middle muscle layer, and (3) the tunica adventitia, or external coat. With aging, the intima becomes thickened and less smooth as arteriosclerotic streaks are accumulated. Muscle fibers in the media are replaced with collagen or connective tissue and calcium material. These changes in the layers of the arteries result in a decreased ability to expand or stretch. The young artery has the potential of increasing its length by 60 percent; in older arteries the stretch is 30 percent. The combination of decrease in the interior diameter of the artery and

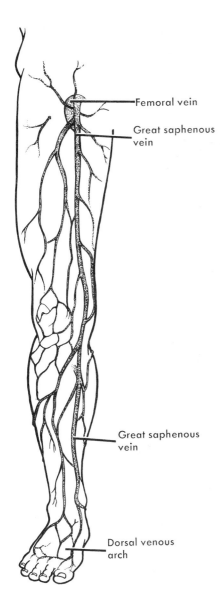

Femoral vein

Great saphenous vein

Great saphenous vein

Dorsal venous arch

Fig. 2-4. Anterior view of main superficial veins of lower extremity.

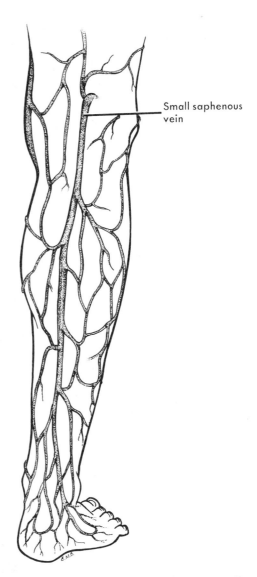

Small saphenous vein

Fig. 2-5. Posterior view of main superficial veins of lower extremity.

diminished stretch ability results in the normal finding of higher blood pressures in the older adult.

The veins are the blood collection system; they resemble arteries in structure, having an intima, media, and adventitia. They differ from arteries in that the walls are thinner and less elastic because the media has little muscle. To compensate,

the intima falls into semicircular folds whose edges lie across the direction of the blood flow. These valves permit little interference with blood flowing toward the heart, but prevent a reversal of the direction of the flow (Fig. 2-3).

The lower extremities have three sets of veins: (1) superficial (Figs. 2-4 and 2-5), (2) connecting,

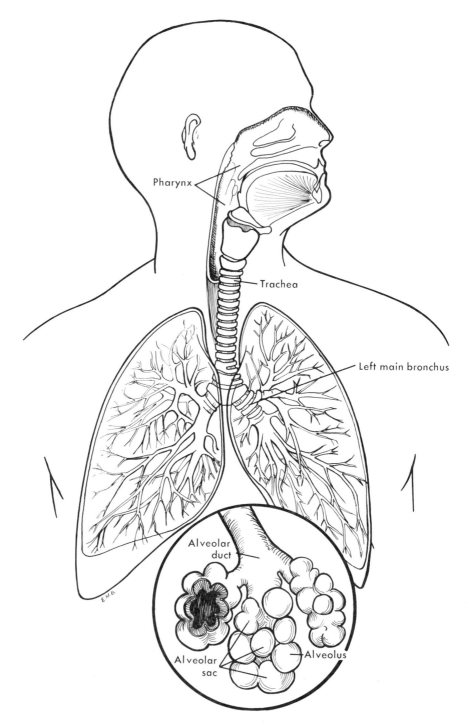

Pharynx

Trachea

Left main bronchus

Alveolar
duct

Alveolar
sac

Alveolus

Fig. 2-6. Pharynx, trachea, and lungs. Inset shows grapelike alveolar sacs where inspired air and blood exchange oxygen and carbon dioxide through thin walls of alveoli. Capillaries (not shown) surround alveoli.

and (3) deep. Muscle contraction in the legs provides an upward propelling force for venous return. Moderate exercise (walking for instance) effects a 30 percent increase in blood volume returned to the inferior vena cava. Familial predisposition to varicosities and the toll of inactivity and constricting clothing and leg positions (crossing legs at the knees) rupture the valves. Varicose veins are a common occurrence in the older adult, and venous stasis leads to diminished mobility of the individual.

RESPIRATORY SYSTEM

Respiration is a number of processes that serve to supply all the cells of the body with oxygen and remove carbon dioxide from the cells. The mechanisms of respiration are capable of a wide-range variation in their response, resulting in a respiratory exchange that closely correlates body activities.

Although respiration is essentially an involuntary process, voluntary control can be initiated in a number of ways. The breath is regulated when whistling and singing. Involuntary respirations automatically respond to a significant rise in blood carbon dioxide level, as when the breath is held.

The structure of the respiratory system relates specifically to its function. Air passes through the nose, pharynx, larynx, trachea, bronchi, and bronchioles. The ciliated mucous membranes filter the air of dust and debris and add humidity. The cough reflex serves to remove the thick exudate of the irritated mucous membrane caused by infection, smoking, air pollution, or any other noxious substances. Through this mechanical cleansing and moisturizing, the air reaches the bronchi relatively dust free and 100 percent humidified.

The bronchi divide into smaller and smaller segments called bronchioles. Alveolar sacs are the terminal end of the bronchioles. It is within these sacs that the exchange of oxygen and gaseous waste materials occurs (Fig. 2-6). The wall of each alveoli is a single layer of cells. This ultrathin pattern permits easy passage of the gas molecules across the wall to the capillary beds on the other side. Any structural or fluid alteration in the alveoli affects the exchange process by increasing the distance between the gas and capillary beds on either side of the alveolar wall. Unless the gas/wall/capillary connection is made, no oxygen–carbon dioxide exchange occurs. The exchange of gases at the alveolar level is called external respiration. The amount of air inhaled with each breath depends on the ability of the rib cage and diaphragm to expand in a bellowlike action.

Internal respiration occurs at the cellular level in each organ system throughout the body. Like the alveolar wall, the capillary wall is one cell thick and permits oxygen and carbon dioxide exchange.

With aging, structural changes in the respiratory system diminish the efficiency of the external respiratory process. Because of aging, the alveolar sacs enlarge as the walls weaken and stretch. When the alveolar walls rupture, they fuse with neighboring walls, and new larger alveolar sacs are formed. The new sacs appear to have the character of emphysematous sacs and have an increased residual volume. It is believed that increased collagen cross-linking occurs, reducing lung flexibility and vital capacity, resulting in the emphysemalike changes. Dilatation occurs in bronchioles and alveolar ducts leading to the alveolar sacs.

The capillary beds serving the alveolar sacs exhibit changes with aging also, and gas exchange is altered. Lung vital capacity is reduced as a result of diminished chest movement from skeletal changes of osteoporosis and kyphosis.

Since internal respiration requires patent arteries for blood and gas transport, the presence of arteriosclerotic plaques hampers the delivery of oxygen to the organs for exchange.

GASTROINTESTINAL SYSTEM

Absorption of foodstuff into the bloodstream is the overall purpose of the gastrointestinal system (Fig. 2-7). Food is prepared for absorption through chemical and mechanical actions, which are controlled by the central nervous system and the autonomic nervous system. Elimination of food residue by defecation is a conscious action under voluntary control.

The teeth bite and grind food. Salivary glands empty their secretions into the food, giving moisture and beginning the breakdown of starch. The tongue aids in the mechanical action of mixing the food and is the receptor for taste. Papillae, or taste buds, are innervated by the seventh and ninth cranial nerves. The esophagus, about 10 inches long, transports food from the pharynx to the stomach. At each end of the esophagus is a muscle band. The muscle band or sphincter at the lower end of the esophagus serves as a barrier to prevent the backup of stomach contents into the esophagus. It is usually closed, but opens as food passes into the stomach and during belching and vomiting. The mucus secreted by the walls of the esophagus speeds the passage of food to the stomach and protects the wall lining from injury. Peristaltic waves move the food along at about 2 to 4 cm/second.

The stomach is a dilated segment of the tract

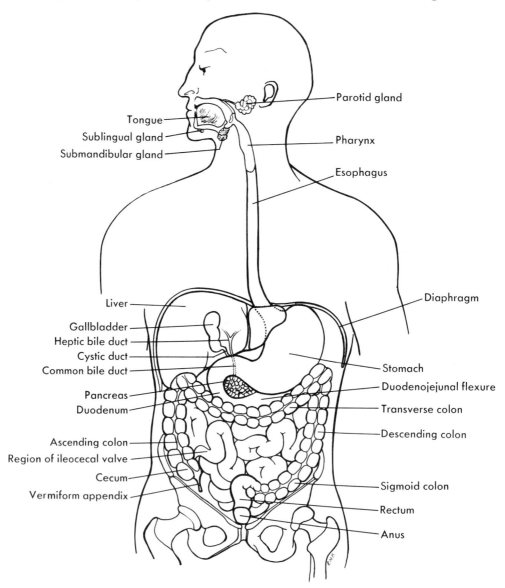

Fig. 2-7. Organs of digestive system.

and serves as a retaining mixing reservoir in which some chemical digestion occurs. Digestive enzymes are secreted from the inner mucosal layer of the stomach wall.

The small intestine, divided into duodenum, jejunum, and ileum, digests and absorbs nutrients and water. Bile and pancreatic ducts open into the duodenum and begin the digestive process in earnest. Peristalsis continues to move the food bolus along as absorption continues through the walls of the ileus and jejunum.

The large intestine extends from the cecum to the anus and is the area of the final processing of the bolus. Water and electrolytes are reabsorbed. The remaining fecal mass is 75 percent water and 25 percent food residue, bacteria, cells, and unabsorbed minerals.

Vitamin K and some B vitamins are synthesized by the bacteria in the large intestines. The peristaltic action is slow. Two or three times a day the fecal mass is moved along in the ascending and transverse colon to the descending and sigmoid colons. Once every 24 to 72 hours the peristaltic action of the intestine propels the fecal mass into the rectum, distending the rectal wall. The rectal muscles relax, and the defecation urge is felt by the individual. Voluntary contraction of the abdominal muscles and glottis closure, a bearing-down movement (the Valsalva maneuver), facilitates evacuation of the bowel. Defecation can be stopped by voluntarily contracting the levator ani and external sphincter muscles. Rectal evacuation can occur from twice a day to once in 72 hours and still remain within the normal range. If the defecation urge is ignored, the bowel continues to absorb water, and the stool becomes dry and firm. Difficulty is then encountered with the next urge for a bowel movement.

With normal aging there are some characteristic alterations in gastrointestinal anatomy and physiology. Table 2-1 outlines the digestive process in the older adult. The grinding surface of the molars wear down, reducing the mechanical effectiveness of chewing. Reduced salivary gland secretion, volume, and acidity result in diminished ptyalin action on starch digestion. Less salivation diminishes the moisture otherwise added to the food in the mouth. Also, a thickening of the mucin component of saliva, an inadequate fluid intake, and

mouth breathing can result in a distressfully dry mouth, a common discomfort in the older adult. It is possible that the decrease in salivary gland activity is a result of decreased stimulation. Social changes in the life-style of the older adult force changes in eating environment and menu. Disuse atrophy applies to gland secretion also. Root absorption and transparency of the teeth produce an appearance of receding gum line. Once a tooth is lost because of decay or trauma, adjacent teeth are affected. These nearby teeth become more mobile in the bony foundations within the gums, move out of alignment, and are subject to additional stresses during chewing. Professional dental care can save the remaining teeth through proper support, bridgework, and crowns. In addition, dental consultation promotes gum care. Large proportions of older adults are found to have gum disorders such as leukoplasia and sublingual mucosal varicosities.

There is a characteristic decline in the number of taste buds on the tongue of an older individual. From a total of 248 circumvallate papillae in a young child, these laterally distributed taste receptors number 88 in the average 75-year-old adult. The resulting decline in the taste appeal of food fosters poor appetite, and the commonly occurring malnutrition. Muscle atrophy in the mouth, cheeks, and tongue makes eating and speaking a slower process. Although all the changes in the mouth are common and present few significant clinical signs, they alter the quality of life of the older adult, because enjoying food and mealtime conversation meet the needs of an individual on physical, psychological, and social levels.

The wall of the esophagus thins out and becomes more sensitive because of reduced production of the protective mucin. Peristaltic activity slows, and the older adult might have a sensation of fullness or heartburn after meals. Acidic gastric juices can flow up through a relaxed stomach muscle band into the esophagus, causing a burning sensation in the throat or in the retrosternal area. This occurs in almost 65 percent of older adults and even more frequently in obese women.

Cell changes in the lining of the stomach lead to atrophic gastritis in up to 50 percent of all people by age 70. There is a progressive decrease in

Table 2-1. The digestive process in the older adult

Structure	Digestive fluid	Enzyme(s)	Substance acted upon	Product formed	Where absorbed	Use in body
Mouth	Salivary ptyalin	Amylase	Cooked starch	Dextrins, maltose	Broken down further, then absorbed in jejunum	Meeting energy needs of cells, stored as reserved energy, protein-sparing regulates fat metabolism
Stomach	HCl		Pepsinogen	Pepsin		Digestion of proteins
			Ferric iron	Ferrous iron		Major component of hemoglobin for oxygen transport; required in many enzyme activities
			Bactericidal			Destruction of invading bacteria entering GI tract
		Pepsinogen		Pepsin		Splitting protein chains into small parts
		Pepsin	Proteins	Proteoses, peptones, polypeptides	Jejunum	Digestion of proteins; splitting peptide linkages
			Vitamin B_1 (thiamin)		Upper third of duodenum	GI tract tone, good appetite, mood, cardiac tone
			Vitamin B_2 (riboflavin)		Upper half of small intestine	Mucous membrane integrity in mouth, tongue, lips, eyelids; Krebs cycle
			Niacin		Small intestine	Needed for fat digestion and absorption, tissue respiration, integrity of nervous tissue
			Vitamin B_6		Small intestine	Active in protein metabolism, antibody formations, hemoglobin molecule formation
			Vitamin B_{12}		Very complex A. Begins in stomach with gastric acids and enzymes B. Binds with intrinsic factors in stomach fundus and cardiac	Participation in DNA synthesis; essential in RBC production and in nervous tissue

	Mucin	Stomach and duodenal walls			Lubrication and protection of wall linings
	Lipase	Fats	Fatty acids	Small intestine	...cosa in unbound form; older persons absorb about 5% of available B$_{12}$; younger persons absorb 10%. Essential for absorption of fat-soluble vitamins; source of stored energy; lecithin and other phospholipids are essential components of nervous tissue
Liver	Intrinsic factor	B$_{12}$			Essential for absorption of Vitamin B$_{12}$
	Bile	Acids			Neutralizing acids in duodenum
		Fats	Emulsified fats		Fats prepared for lipase action
		Vitamin A components		Small intestine	Maintenance of integrity of tissue that lines all body cavities and skin; maintenance of dim light vision; facilitation of fat-soluble vitamin and fat absorption
		Vitamin D		Jejunum and ileum	Necessary for calcium and phosphorus absorption and use
		Vitamin E		Small intestine	Maintenance of cell walls; reduction of oxidation of polyunsaturated fatty acids; essential channel for cholesterol excretion

Continued.

Table 2-1. The digestive process in the older adult—cont'd

Structure	Digestive fluid	Enzyme(s)	Substance acted upon	Product formed	Where absorbed	Use in body
Pancreas	Pancreatic juices	Amylase	Starch	Dextrins, maltose		Readily available energy
		Chymotrypsin, trypsin	Proteins	Proteoses, peptones, polypeptides		Protein is the basic building and repair material of the body; chief solid material of muscles, organs, and endocrine glands; major component of bones, teeth, nails and hair; regulation of body functions of osmotic pressure and water balance; basic to all enzyme and hormones; source of potential energy
		Lipase	Fats	Monoglycerides, fatty acids, glycerol	Jejunum	Supplying energy stored as adipose tissue; insulator of body heat; protection of vital organs, for example, fat pads that surround kidneys; lubricant in GI tract
Small intestine	Succus entericus (intestinal juices)	Enterokinase	Trypsinogen	Trypsin		Basic protein molecules available to cells
		Aminopeptidase	Amino acids	Amino acids		
		Dipeptidase	Dipeptides	Nucleotides		
		Nuclenase	Nucleic acid	Nucleosides, phosphoric acid		
		Nucleotidase	Nucleotides	Purine, pentose		
		Nucleosidase	Nucleosides	Diglycerides,		
		Leicthinase	Lecithin			

		tose		Carbohydrate molecules available to cells
Maltose	Maltose	Glucose and glucose	Small intestine	
Lactose	Lactose	Glucose and galactose	Small intestine	
		Vitamin C	Small intestine	Formation of collagen, the basis of intercellular substance in skin, bone, cartilage, and blood vessels
Large intestine	Bacteria	Vitamin K	Ascending and transverse colon	Essential in prothrombin formation; active in oxidative processes in body

hydrochloric acid (HCl) and enzyme production. Since vitamin B_{12} absorption depends on the intrinsic factor in HCl, pernicious anemia is a common finding. Dietary iron in the ferrous form is more absorbable than in the ferric form. A decreased acid environment in the stomach inhibits the reduction of iron from the ferric to the ferrous form and increases the risk of anemia. Liver cells continue to reproduce, the liver function remains stable, and its enzyme production is the same. There are some pancreatic cell changes; however, enzyme production is adequate, and the absorption of those foods affected by pancreatic enzymes remains good. Bile viscosity and cholesterol level increase; however, the total bile volume decreases. Many older adults form biliary tract stones but demonstrate no overt clinical signs.

Generalized lipofuscin pigmentation and widespread areas of calcium deposits occur throughout the large and small intestines. Reduced arterial supply to the intestine, through its splanchnic bed, is presumed to be a factor in many intestinal problems.

Polyps in the colon are also frequently seen, as are diverticuli. General muscle weakness in the intestinal wall leads to a higher incidence of these bulging sacs.

The volume of stool in the bowel movement reflects the amount of food ingested. An older adult who eats a small amount of food will have small bowel movements. Activity, fluids, dietary fiber, and sleep all foster bowel motility. Quick response to the defecation reflex promotes comfortable and complete bowel movements. Since laxatives and enemas dampen the reflex, they encourage bowel atony and constipation.

The gastrointestinal tract is often the focal point of the stress of psychological pressures. Resulting psychosomatic discomfort distresses the older adult, as it does other age groups.

URINARY SYSTEM

The kidneys perform the vital function of excreting metabolic waste products from the blood stream. They are also a primary organ in the fluid and acid base balance of the blood and thus the entire body. In addition to the excretory functions, the kidneys produce the blood pressure–regulating product called renin, are a factor in stimulating

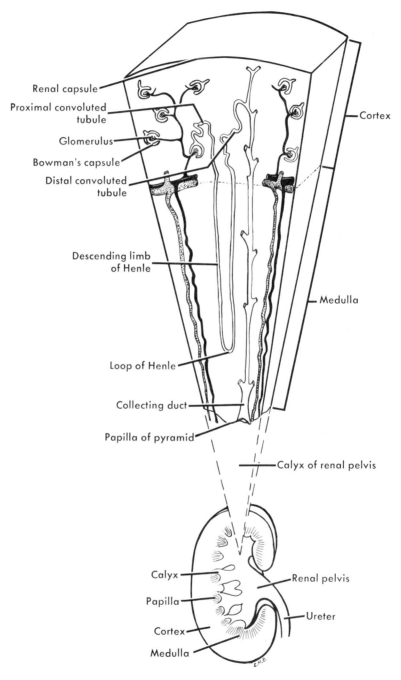

Labels on figure:
Renal capsule
Proximal convoluted tubule
Glomerulus
Bowman's capsule
Distal convoluted tubule
Descending limb of Henle
Loop of Henle
Collecting duct
Papilla of pyramid
Cortex
Medulla
Calyx of renal pelvis
Calyx
Papilla
Cortex
Medulla
Renal pelvis
Ureter

Fig. 2-8. Magnified wedge shows that renal corpuscles (Bowman's capsules with invaginated glomeruli) and both proximal and distal convoluted tubules are located in cortex of kidney. Medulla contains loops of Henle and collecting tubules.

red blood cell production by the bone marrow, and metabolize vitamin D. The urinary system organs are the kidneys (Fig. 2-8), the ureters, the urinary bladder, and the urethra.

The nephron is the functional unit of the kidney. Nephrons number about 1 million in each kidney. A nephron includes the Bowman capsule, capillary beds called the proximal and distal convoluted tubules, and collection ducts. Urine is formed as blood is filtered in the Bowman capsule. About 1,200 ml is filtered per minute. Most of the fluids and solids filtered in the Bowman capsule are reabsorbed in the convoluted tubules. The final output of the kidneys is 1500 ml urine/day.

The urine from each nephron collects in the renal pelvis. The ureters serve as transport ducts from the renal pelvis to the urinary bladder. Urine is stored in the bladder then excreted through the urethra.

Some normal physiological changes in the urinary system occur with aging. Overall, there is a general loss of nephrons. Because kidney cells divide but do not form new multicellular units, by the age of 75 only 65 percent of the nephrons remain. Age age 90, 53 percent are left. Because of this loss of nephron mass, the kidneys do not concentrate urine as well. In addition, there are some degenerative changes in the remaining nephrons. Even with all this decline in nephron numbers and these changes in the remaining nephrons, the kidneys are still able to maintain the acid balance under normal circumstances. When the general circulation decreases, the renal filtration rate decreases also at about a 6 percent decrease per decade. Reabsorption of fluid and solids is also impaired. Renal arterioles become constricted with the general arteriosclerosis that is occurring throughout the body. Blood is diverted to other parts of the body and does not filter through the glomerular filtration system.

Even in the presence of these physiological and anatomical changes, the kidneys of an older adult can still respond to emergencies almost as well as those of a young person. During periods of stress, the vasoconstriction mechanisms in the renal arteries disappear, and the kidneys respond to the systemic need. However, at rest, there is considerable vasoconstriction. In general, the kidneys have more difficulty restabilizing after a stressful

situation or changes in the body homeostasis. Even minor changes can disrupt the renal function. The general size and weight of the kidneys decrease with the aging process.

There is an accumulation of fatty deposit between the nephron cells. Although the effects of these fatty changes are not known, they are visible as gobs of fat in the intracellular connective tissue of the kidneys.

Although the cells decrease in number, the remaining cells appear to be able to maintain intracellular enzyme and protein levels.

Nocturia is a frequent event with the older adult. The normally functioning kidneys of a younger person decrease filtration rates at night. Their bladders do not become distended with urine. However, with the less efficient filtration of the nephrons of the older adult, this nightly decrease in activity does not occur. The urine output of the older adult continues day and night, and so the bladder becomes filled, and the person has the desire to void during the night.

Bacteria in the urine is not the norm for the younger person. However, with the older adult, high levels of bacteria are frequently seen in the urine, in the bladder, and even in the renal pelvis without clinical signs and symptoms being noted. It is believed that these high concentrations of bacteria are detrimental to the nephrons of the older adult. The bacteria hasten the onset of nephron deterioration and weaken the function of the kidneys.

The kidneys' function as the maintainer of the acid balance in the body remains satisfactory well into the advanced years. The normal serum pH serum bicarbonate levels remain unchanged in the older adult. The BUN (blood urea nitrogen) shows an increase of about 5 mg/100 ml, so the rates for an older adult run from 10 to 25 mg/100 ml.

GENITAL SYSTEM

Sexuality is a strand intricately woven into the fabric of life. If the nurse is to acknowledge the wholeness of an individual, then his sexuality cannot be ignored. An understanding of human sexual function enables the nurse to be helpful to the older adult as questions regarding sexuality arise. Some alterations in sexual function are an inevitable part of the physiology of the older adult.

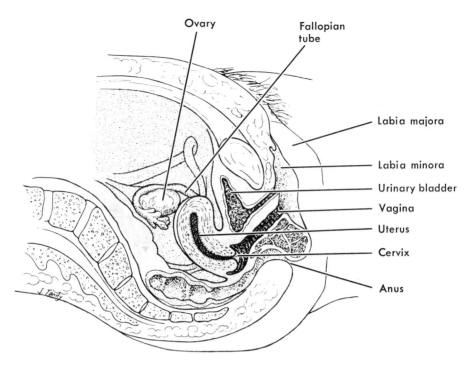

Fig. 2-9. Midsagittal view of female pelvic organs with subject on back. (From Jensen, M. D., Benson, R. C., and Bobak, I. M.: Maternity care: the nurse and the family, St. Louis, 1977, The C. V. Mosby Co.)

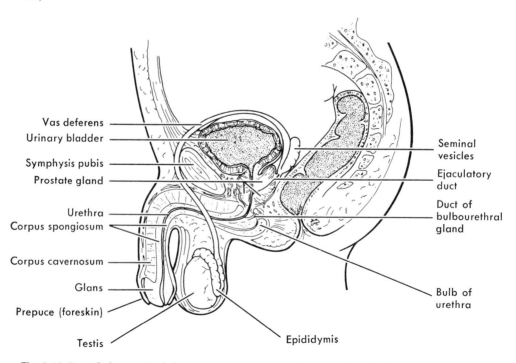

Fig. 2-10. Fascial planes of male lower genitourinary tract. Relationship of bladder, prostate, seminal vesicles, penis, urethra, and scrotal contents. (Modified from Smith, D. R.: General urology, ed. 9, Los Altos, Calif., 1978, Lange Medical Publications.)

The nurse who has the knowledge base to provide anticipatory guidance and comfortably answer questions regarding sexuality can add considerably to the quality of life of her clients.

Not all persons regard their sexuality in a positive light, and the topic may cause them to be uncomfortable. Discussions of sexuality are individually designed to use the beliefs and life-style of the clients as guidelines. Often, the coping mechanisms of denial, repression, or rationalization are the basis for apparent lack of interest in sexuality, especially in the face of the stresses of illness. On the other hand, active participation in sex is not an absolute prerequisite for a full and healthy life. It is the choice of the individual.

Female genital structures

The structures of the female genital system are the ovaries, fallopian tubes, uterus, vagina, labia minora and majora, and the clitoris (Fig. 2-9).

The ovaries have two functions: production and release of the ova, and production of hormones, especially estrogen and progesterone. The outer layer of the ovaries contains estrogen-producing follicles holding ova in various stages of maturation. Estrogen, the female sex hormone, gives the female feminizing characteristics such as curved hips, enlarged breasts, and the female distribution of pubic hair. It also increases vagina size and vaginal wall tissue thickness. Progesterone prepares the uterus for pregnancy.

The fallopian tubes are closely connected to the ovaries and serve as the connection ducts for the ova in transport to the uterus.

The uterus is a muscular sac that provides the site and conditions for implantation for the fertilized ovum. The walls of the uterus are particularly sensitive to ovarian hormones.

The vagina is a slightly curved muscular canal about 7 to 8 cm (3½ to 4 inches) long. The muscular wall of the vagina falls into folds called rugae. These rugae permit vaginal tissue to stretch during the birth process, and they give the vagina resiliency during sexual intercourse.

The central nervous system and the anterior pituitary gland regulate the production of hormones in the ovaries. The pituitary gland secretes a follicle-stimulating hormone (FSH) and a luteinizing hormone (LH). FSH and LH are responsible for the follicle activity. The central nervous system orchestrates the ebb and flow of the glandular and hormonal interactions.

Central nervous system regulation of ovarian hormones

Central nervous system
(specifically, cerebral cortex and hypothalamus)
stimulates and regulates secretions of
↓
Anterior pituitary gland,
which secretes

FSH	LH
Follicle growth	Follicle maturation
Estrogen production	Estrogen and progesterone production

Male genital structures

The male genital structures consist of the scrotum, the testes, a system of excretory ducts with their auxiliary glands, and the penis (Fig. 2-10).

The testes are two ovoid bodies that lie in the scrotum. They produce spermatozoa in addition to the male androgen hormones. The anterior pituitary gland regulates the activities of the testes in much the same way that it regulates the actions of the ovaries. The FSH and LH produced in the pituitary gland of the male increase the size of the testes and stimulate androgen hormones, such as testosterone.

After the spermatozoa are produced, they are stored and then transported through a series of ducts, including the epydidymis, ductus deferens, ejaculatory ducts, and urethra.

The auxiliary structures of the male genital tract are the seminal vesicles, the prostate gland, the bulbourethral glands, and the cavernous bodies of the penis. The seminal vesicles produce a thick, alkaline, globulin-containing secretion that is added to the spermatozoa during ejaculation. The prostate gland is located beneath the bladder and surrounds the first portion of the urethra. The ducts of the gland open into the urethra, secreting a thin liquid that stimulates the movement of the spermatozoa. The two bulbourethral glands lie on either side of the urethra and secrete a slimy, viscid material that lubricates the urethra. The

Table 2-3. Female and male sexual response phases

Phase	Female response	Male response
Excitement		
Physical or psychological stimulation	Vaginal lubrication	Penile erection
	Vaginal canal widens	Skin of scrotum smooths out
Long or short in duration	Cervix and uterus are elevated	Testes are elevated
Marked increase in sexual tension	Labia majora flatten and elevate	
	Clitoris increases in size	
Any distraction can decrease the build-up of sexual tension	Nipples become erect; may be increase in breast size	Sometimes nipple erection
Plateau		
Increases in sexual tension level off	Much vasocongestion in outer third of vagina	Minor increase in diameter of penis
	Opening appears narrow	Deepening of penis color
High degree of sexual arousal has been reached	Clitoris retracts against pubic symphysis	Testes increase in size
Duration varies widely	Measlelike rash (in 50%-75% of women) called *sex flush*—starts on chest and may also occur on buttocks, back, face, and extremities	
Orgasm		
May be triggered by a neural reflex	Rhythmic contractions of uterus, outer third of vagina, and rectal sphincter	Accessory sex organs begin contractions
Is a total body response		Seminal fluids pool in prostatic urethra; sensation of ejaculatory inevitability
EEG shows changes in wave rates and activities, especially hemispheric laterality		Rhythmic contractions of the prostate, the perineal muscles, and the shaft of the penis combine during ejaculation
Heart rate, blood pressure, and respiratory rates increase		
Multiple orgasms are possible for the female		
Males have one orgasm, then begin resolution phase		
Resolution		
Physical changes of excitement and plateau phases return to preexcitement state	No refractory period; can continue into next orgasm at once	Refractory period, a waiting time before which another ejaculation is possible; lasts for a few minutes or for hours; great variability within and between males
	Tissue engorgement is relieved	
	Uterus lays back into pelvis	
	Vagina shortens and narrows	Erection diminishes; normal blood flow returns
	Clitoris returns to position	Testes decrease in size

cavernous bodies of the penis are the erectile tissue, which is spongelike with large open spaces. In the relaxed state, the cavernous spaces are collapsed and contain little blood. During an erection, these spaces become filled with blood, which causes the penis to become enlarged and rigid. The filling of the spaces is controlled by a network of nerves stimulated in the central nervous system.

Sexual response cycle

Masters and Johnson have contributed much important information to the literature regarding the physiology of the sexual response. The sexual

Table 2-4. Sexual response phases in the older adult

Phases	Female	Male
Excitement	Vasocongestion in breasts reduced or absent More limited distribution of sex flush Vagina less expansive Vaginal lubrication in lesser amounts and needs longer period to stimulate (these changes are accentuated by periods of sexual inactivity in postmenopausal years)	Longer time period needed Needs more direct stimulation of genitals Modest decrease in firmness of erection
Plateau		
Orgasm	Remains the same Some decline in generalized myotonia	Intensity of ejaculatory experience diminished because of reduced volume of ejaculate and changes in prostate gland and nerve supply Ejaculation not necessary at each sexual opportunity Feeling of stimulation and satisfaction remains
Resolution	Multiorgasmic ability continues	Lengthens with increasing age

response is described in four phases: the excitement phase, plateau phase, orgasm, and resolution phase (Table 2-3). Each of these phases may overlap somewhat. In general, they are characteristic of the findings of the Masters and Johnson Clinic in St. Louis.

Sexual response in older adults. Regular sexual intercourse maintains the optimal physical health and response of the genital organs. Each of the four phases of sexual response is fully attainable (Table 2-4).

When a sexual partner is available, women express a desire for greater frequency of sexual activity than men. This increased interest is attributed to the decrease in pregnancy risk in the postmenopausal years.

In general, patterns of frequency of intercourse in older adults correlate with the frequency of their twenties to forties. More important than the frequency is the psychodynamic aspect of sexual activity. The psychological beliefs and expectations give the feelings of pleasure and satisfaction to the older adult. Regular sexual arousal and intercourse ensure a lifetime of sexuality even when physiological changes occur. Sexual activity keeps the genital organs in optimum condition, avoiding the "if you don't use it, you lose it" syndrome.

When sexual partners are not available, mastur-

bation is found to be a channel for release of sexual tension through the sixth and seventh decades.

Older adults should be encouraged to explore aspects of their sexuality. Discussions can identify and help resolve problems. The reality of adult physiology is that the sexual organs are no less capable of functioning than any other organ. The functioning is somewhat slower in pace than before, but the meaningful pleasure of intimate interaction remains. A man would not expect to beat his grandson in swimming 10 laps in a pool, so he should not be concerned when the time to have an erection is a bit longer. He can still swim, and he can still have an erection. Arousal time increases, but orgasmic capability is not diminished.

A frank discussion of sexual physiology with adults in their fifties and sixties is useful. This type of information can prepare them to develop realistic expectations of sex in the older adult years. Sexual interest and capability are alive and well into the ninth decade in many persons.

Female genital physiological changes

The overall weight of the ovaries begins to decline after age 30. There is generalized ovarian atrophy and an increase in the growth of fibrous tissue and cysts. Unlike other mammals, the human female does not experience a loss of orgasmic abilities when ova production stops. In fact, her multiorgasmic capabilities remain as long as she is regularly aroused and is sexually active.

The estrogen level is stable until age 40 and then begins to decline. Progesterone production dramatically drops after age 30 because of the decreasing number of mature progesterone-producing follicles. The anterior pituitary increases rather than decreases the production of the gonadotropins. There is a decreased ovarian sensitivity to pituitary LH and FSH stimulation. The urinary excretion of these gonadotropins is seen in postmenopausal women until age 80, when it drops sharply.

The uterus decreases in weight by 50 percent and contains many fibrous networks. The vagina becomes smaller, and the walls become thinner. If the woman is not active sexually, the vagina can atrophy to half its former length and width. It takes on the appearance of paper-thin tissue. Rugal folds disappear. Vaginal secretions become less acid.

The external genitalia lose subcutaneous fat layers, and the labia and clitoris are somewhat smaller. Clitoris function as the seat of sexual orgasm is not affected. Pubic and axillary hair becomes thinner.

Glandular and fatty tissue in the breasts responds to lowered blood estrogen levels by becoming flaccid and drooping. The breasts can still remain lactating organs. Wet nurses continue to produce milk even after menopause.

There is no change in the female libido (sexual energy) or orgasmic ability after menopause, as long as the general health of the woman is good. The hot flashes experienced by some women are caused by vasomotor instability in the presence of changing hormone patterns. It is not known whether the psychological symptoms ranging from irritability to depression are based on physical causes or induced by social forces.

Male genital physiological changes

Although there is no significant weight change in the testes, there are cellular changes. The fat content of the cells increases, and cell numbers decrease. There is a progressive decline in the number of sperm ejaculated, up to 50 percent at age 90. Both the size and shape of the sperm change, reducing fertilization ability.

There is no sudden hormone change as in wom-

en. It is a more gradual reduction. Androgen production begins declining at age 30 and continues until the nineties. Testosterone level decreases somewhat after age 60. Some men with a serum testosterone level below 325 mg/100 ml show characteristics of the male climacteric or male menopause. They may feel listless and frequently fatigued and have appetite loss, weight loss, and decreased concentration and libido.

The prostate gland becomes slightly irregular, thickens, and becomes fibrous. The cause of benign prostatic hypertrophy, considered a normal physiological change, is not known.

Availability and interest in sex

Cultural stereotypes deny the older adult sexual feelings or sexual relationships. Social or health situations may alter the availability of a sexual partner, but sexual needs remain.

Sexual activity for women drops dramatically after widowhood. Lack of an available partner and the social attitudes regarding sex for an older woman limit her opportunities. Many women opt to sublimate sexual drives and deny any sexual interest. Male sexual activity after widowerhood continues at a steady rate as long as he is in good health and his socioeconomic level is maintained. Social custom permits men to maintain relationships with younger women. A 70-year-old man who dates a 45-year-old woman is tolerated, whereas a 70-year-old woman who dates a younger man raises eyebrows.

In the marriage partnership, it is usually the man who discontinues sexual activity. The cause is often ill health and the physical limitations imposed by it.

Often, however, the myths denying the sexual capabilities of the elderly become self-fulfilling prophesies. These myths hold that the older person is sexually inert and uninterested. Seeking out sexual partners is made most difficult as social and business ties are diminished in number.

In reality, there is an extremely wide range of individual differences in a group of older adults. Interest in sexual activity depends on past enjoyment and the frequency of sexual intercourse. If the person was active sexually in younger years, then most likely sexual intercourse will still be of interest. Those persons who have enjoyed active and fulfilling sexual lives often face their over-60 years with fear and discouragement. They believe the myth of the sexless older years.

Nurturing needs of the older adult

Sexual expression need not be only in the form of sexual intercourse. Other forms of expression of affection and tenderness must be available to the older adult. Nurturing is a special need of this age group for the feelings of well-being it brings. The need for love and affection increases rather than diminishes with increasing age. Psychological losses are being felt in social roles at work and as a parent. All forms of sexual expression can help the older adult cope with the losses and maintain a feeling of self-worth.

MUSCULOSKELETAL SYSTEM

Bones are the supporting framework of the body. They serve as the attachment points for the muscles, protect delicate organ structures, supply calcium to the blood, and are a part of blood-forming mechanisms. New bone cells form, and old cells are absorbed. Bone-forming cells are called osteoblasts; bone-destroying cells are called osteoclasts. Ongoing reconstruction of bone in adult life is dramatically less than in the early years. Calcium becomes available to the blood as the reconstruction proceeds. This physiological turnover maintains the plasma calcium level at a steady level. Calcium salts are laid down upon cylindric, cartilagelike bases called haversian canals. These canals supply the cells with blood vessels and nutrients. The pressure exerted on the long bones from standing and movement maintains the calcium at normal levels in the haversian system.

The joints of the hips, extremities, vertebral column, and jaw are elaborate structures that provide the free movement of the skeletal system. Two or more bones are encircled by a capsule of fibrous tissue. This capsule is lined with synovial membrane and filled with synovial fluid, giving lubrication and nourishment to the joint. This fluid has the colorless, viscid appearance of an egg white. Ligaments serve as bonds or cords to reinforce and strengthen the joint.

Muscles and skeleton as a unit

The periosteum, joint capsule, synovial fluid, cartilage, tendons, and muscles all work together as a unit to maintain the functions of the joints of the musculoskeletal system. This basic unit makes up the internal receptors and orchestrates movement, by means of the link with the perceptions of the eyes, ears, nose, mouth, and proprioceptors in the skin.

Body strength peaks in the twenties and then decreases. Muscle size and tone decrease. Older adults avoid heavy muscular activity; however, their muscle strength and capacity are ample for the routine tasks of daily living until the advanced years. Hand grip strength may decline, but hand function remains.

Stiff joints limit the older adult's full range of motion in the neck and limbs. These limitations in joint movement affect posture and gait. Stiff shoulder joints, for example, reduce an easy arm swing while walking. This in turn affects balance and skeletal flexibility.

Cartilage and joint capsules become calcified with age. Heberden's nodes are the bony spurs that form around joints. They occur on the distal joints of the fingers. Cell muscle fibers are replaced by adipose (fatty) and connective tissue.

Kyphosis is a posterior angulation of the spine, causing an asymmetry of chest leading to inadequate use of respiratory muscles. This decreases the size of the thoracic cavity and the amount of inspired air. Kyphosis is caused by cartilage changes in the intervertebral discs, which result in the decreased stature often seen in the older adult. A loss of ½ to 2 inches in height can be measured in older adults, giving them the appearance of having long limbs in relationships to their body.

Osteoarthritis is a degenerative joint disease caused by a breakdown of an essential element called chondrocytes in the joint cartilage. Weight-bearing joints of the hips, knees, and vertebral column are the joints most often affected, but joints in the fingers can be affected also. Osteoarthritis is more common in females than in males, and osteoarthritic changes can be seen in the x-ray films of 85 percent of persons over 75, even in the absence of pain and stiffness, the most frequent signs of osteoarthritis. Mild activity can loosen the stiffness in the joints. Plans should be made to keep a range of motion of all the joints of the body at the fullest. Bony overgrowths in the vertebral column can cause pain as nerve roots are irritated. Obesity is a factor in osteoarthritis, especially in the weight-bearing hip and knee joints. Weight reduction reduces the trauma to the joint cartilage. Range of motion activity, whether active or passive, is essential to maintain joint motion and muscle tone.

Activities can be alternated so that heavy tasks are interchanged with light tasks. Adequate periods of rest should be available between morning and afternoon activities. The day's activities should be paced appropriately, and materials for tasks such as stair climbing or the carrying of heavy loads should be organized to reduce unnecessary fatigue and stress. Proper body mechanics should be observed to reduce stress on muscles and joints, especially in the back.

Osteoporosis affects one third of all women over 60, and the age of onset is decreasing. Osteoporosis is essentially a decrease in bone mass. The declining bone matrix formation causes abnormally porous bone. The bone canals are enlarged, and abnormal spaces form. The bone becomes fragile, and there is an increase in the incidence of bone fracture. On a cellular level there is an increase of bone reabsorption in relation to the bone deposition. Weight-bearing parts of the bone are the last to be affected. The calcium is held in these parts of the bone with the stress of weight bearing. Calcium is essential for muscle contraction and nerve conduction. Calcium balance in the body is maintained by dietary calcium and the calcium stored in bones. (What is lost in the bone mass is calcium.)

Prevention and treatment of osteoporosis consist of encouraging an increase in bone mass. The stress of activity preserves bones and stimulates new bone growth. Calcium-rich foods should be included in the client's diet, since dietary needs for calcium and phosphorous and vitamin D are all known factors in bone growth. Studies are being conducted now regarding preferable calcium/phosphorous ratios in dietary consumption. In order for calcium to be absorbed, there must be a higher rate of calcium than phosphorous in the foods eaten. Junk foods and processed foods are usually calcium-poor and phosphrous-rich. Vitamin D regulates the absorption of calcium, so clients should be encouraged to have outdoor activities and not to be too heavily clothed so that they have exposure to the vitamin D of sunshine.

With osteoporosis it has been found that a high-protein, and especially meat-protein, diet reduces bone mass. Some studies relate the acid overload to bone mass loss. Denser bone is found in people on vegetarian diets.

Osteoporosis occurs most often in postmenopausal women. It is believed to be due to the decrease in estrogen production. Estrogen stimulates osteoblastic (bone growth) activity.

It is possible that osteoporosis can be prevented by fluoridation of the water. This is now being investigated by researchers. Increase in intake of calcium in childhood and early adulthood may also protect the female against osteoporosis in later life.

Some people equate mobility with health status. Americans are a mobile society, and in addition, mobility serves as a part of our nonverbal communication. The lack of mobility greatly increases the lack of a sense of security and protection against harm and the ability to flee in times of assault.

Decreased movement and speed are a result of the slow rate of decision making, not of decreased muscular limitations. People seem to move more slowly as they grow older because older adults are more cautious. Older persons can be put in a state of overload if too many complex stimuli are given to them at once. Stimuli must be interpreted one at a time. Older adults do very well on motor tasks if they are given preparation time.

INTEGUMENTARY SYSTEM

The integumentary system comprises the skin, hair, and nails. Skin serves the body in the function of protection, temperature regulation, excretion, absorption, and sense organ.

Skin protects deeper organs from injury and drying and forms a bacterial and mechanical barrier against microorganic invasion. Bacteria on the skin are sloughed off with the constant shedding of the keratinized layers. Normal flora on the skin are a decontaminating force. The mechanical barrier of multiple layers of skin presents a formidable barrier to outside organisms.

Skin presents a large radiating surface in the heat exchange process of temperature regulation. The percentage of heat exchange between the internal and external environments depends on the difference in body and environmental temperatures, blood flow in superficial vessels, evaporation of sweat, and air movement around the body.

The products of the sweat glands constitute the excretory function of the skin. Water, salts, and small amounts of urea are the principal products eliminated. Absorption through the skin is limited to a small number of products, such as methyl salicylate and mercury compounds.

The skin is the organ receptor for touch, pain, heat, and cold. Changes in the immediate external environment are monitored, and reflex responses are initiated and adapted to noxious sensations such as extreme heat or pain.

Accessory organs of the skin are the nails, hair, and sebaceous and sweat glands. The nails are modifications of the epidermis or outer layer of the skin. Hair arises from a pitting depression of the epidermis and receives nutrition from the vessels in the papilla or root.

Sebaceous glands secrete sebum or oil. Sebum keeps hair oiled and conditioned. On the skin surface, sebum forms a protective film, limiting water absorption and evaporation.

With aging, there is an overall decrease in skin turgor, and the skin has a dry, transparent, tissue-like appearance. Sweat gland secretions diminish. Brown pigmentation spots increase in number, size, and distribution.

The amount of hair loss depends on sex and family patterns. By age 65 generally the head hair distribution pattern changes are complete. Any further major hair loss is unusual. Hair texture is thin and may appear sparse. Almost universally hair color becomes gray, often beginning in the early thirties. Axillary and pubic hair decreases. Pigmentation changes in the face soften the complexion, and the skin color becomes lighter.

Sclerosis, hardening of the tissue, occurs throughout the body and is the process that causes the wrinkled appearance of the skin of the older adult. The dermis shrinks and becomes less elastic. Folds, or wrinkles, appear in the epidermis because it has a smaller underbase support.

Body fat declines, giving bony prominences a sharp, angular appearance under the skin. Nail growth on the fingers and toes slows.

As in any age group, the integument of the older adult reflects the overall hydration, blood-oxygen saturation, hygienic, and nutritional status of the individual.

SUMMARY

An overview of each system has been presented. With aging there are characteristic changes in the anatomy and physiology of the various body systems. There is a general slowing of cell division; however, system function remains.

The ability of the older adult's body to recover from stressful situations is prolonged. When in an environment that promotes body homeostasis, the older adult can adapt. Any alteration in the internal or external environment produces stress to which the older body reacts slowly.

Active use of each system of the body is one way to foster optimum health in the older adult. Disuse atrophy occurs in almost every organ of the body.

As in all persons, the various parts of the body of the older adult form an integrated whole. The function of each system is necessary for the function of the entire organism.

REFERENCES

Abramson, D. I.: Vascular disorders of the extremities, ed. 2, New York, 1974, Harper & Row, Publishers.

Andrew, W.: The anatomy of aging in man and animals, New York, 1971, Grune & Stratton, Inc.

Angel, R. W.: Understanding and diagnosing senile dementia, Geriatrics **32**:47, August 1977.

Blumenthal, M. T.: Some considerations regarding disease in old age (letter), J. Gerontol. **32**:642, November 1977.

Bozian, M. W., and Clark, H. M.: Counteracting sensory changes in the aging, Am. J. Nurs. **80**:473, March 1980.

Brower, H. T., and Tanner, A. L.: A study of older adults attending a program on human sexuality: a pilot study, Nurs. Res. **28**:36, January-February 1979.

Bunk, T. L.: Geriatric rigidity and its psychotherapeutic implications, J. Am. Geriatr. Soc. **26**:274, June 1978.

Comfort, A.: Non-threatening mental testing of the elderly, J. Am. Geriatr. Soc. **26**:261, June 1978.

Dall, J. L.: Management of confusional states, Age Aging Suppl.:77, 1978.

Davison, A. N.: Biochemical aspects of the aging brain, Age Ageing Suppl.:4, 1978.

Denham, M. J.: Assessment of mental function, Age Aging Suppl.:137, 1978.

Echocardiographic studies indicate that with age, left ventricular filling rate decreases substantially, from the NIH, J.A.M.A. **240**:2625, 8 December 1978.

Ernst, P., Badash, D., Beran, B., and others: Incidence of mental illness in the aged: unmasking the effects of a diagnosis of chronic brain syndrome, J. Am. Geriatr. Soc. **25**:371, August 1977.

Falk, G., and Falk, U. A.: Sexuality and the aged, Nurs. Outlook **28**:51, January 1980.

Ferris, S., Crook, T., Sathananthan, and others: Reaction time as a diagnostic measure in senility, J. Am. Geriatr. Soc. **24:**529, December 1976.

Gilleard, C. J., and Pattie, A. H.: The effect of location on the elderly mentally infirm: relationship to mortality and behavior deterioration, Age Ageing **7:**1, February 1978.

Greenblatt, D. J.: Reduced serum albumin concentration in the elderly: a report from the Boston Collaborative Drug Surveillance Program, J. Am. Geriatr. Soc. **27:**20, January 1979.

Gröer, M. E., and Shekleton, M. E.: Basic pathophysiology, a conceptual approach, St. Louis, 1979, The C. V. Mosby Co.

Guyton, A. C.: Textbook of medical physiology, Philadelphia, 1976, W. B. Saunders Co.

Hayslip, B., Jr.: Relationships between intelligence and concept identification in adulthood as a function of stage of learning, Int. J. Aging Hum. Dev. **10**(2):187, 1979-1980.

Heidrick, M. L., and Makinodan, T.: Nature of cellular deficiencies in age-related decline of the immune system, Gerontology **18**(5-6):305, 1972.

Hurst, J. W.: The heart, ed. 3, New York, 1974, McGraw-Hill Book Co.

Katz, M. M.: Behavioral change in the chronuity pattern of dementia in the institutional geriatric resident, J. Am. Geriatr. Soc. **24:**522, November 1976.

Kotler, M. N., and Segal, B. L.: The inflamed heart: pericarditis in the elderly, Geriatrics **35:**63, January 1980.

Linaker, B. D.: Aging and the small intestine, Lancet **2:**993, 4 November 1978.

Masters, W. H., and Johnson, V. E.: Human sexual response, Boston, 1966, Little, Brown and Co.

Masters, W. H., and Johnson, V. E.: Human sexual inadequacy, Boston, 1970, Little, Brown and Co.

Neurath, O.: Cardiovascular changes in/of old age, J. Am. Geriatr. Soc. **26:**286, June 1978.

Newman, G., Nichols, C. R.: Sexual activities and attitudes in the older person, J.A.M.A. **73:**33, 1960.

Palmore, E. B.: The effects of aging on activities and attitudes. Gerontologist **8:**259, 1968.

Pfeiffer, E.: Sexual behavior in old age, In Busse, E. W., and Pfeiffer, E., editors: Behavior and adaptation in late life, Boston, 1969, Little, Brown and Co.

Pfeiffer, E., and Davis, G. C.: Determinants of sexual behavior in middle and old age, J. Am. Geriatr. Soc. **20:**151, 1972.

Potvin, A. R., Syndulko, K., Tourtellotte, W. W., and others: Human neurologic function and the aging process. J. Am. Geriatr. Soc. **28:**1, January 1980.

Price, S. A., and Wilson, L. M.: Patho-physiology, New York, 1978, McGraw-Hill Book Co.

Ridley, J. C., Bachrach, C. A., and Dawson, D. A.: Recall and reliability of interview data from older women, J. Gerontol. **34:**99, January 1979.

Samis, H. V., and Salvatore, C.: Aging and the biological rhythms, New York, 1978, Plenum Publishing Corp.

Stare, F. J.: Three score and ten plus ten more, J. Am. Geriatr. Soc. **25:**529, December 1977.

Steel, K., and Feldman, R. G.: Diagnosing dementia and its treatable causes, Geriatrics **34:**79, March 1979.

Stevens, P.: Problems of Emily, Nurs. Times **74:**721, 27 April 1978.

Watkin, D. M.: Logical bases for action in nutrition, J. Am. Geriatr. Soc. **26:**193, May 1978.

Williamson, T.: Depression in the elderly. Age Ageing Suppl:35, 1978.

Wollner, L.: Postural hypotension in the elderly, Age Ageing Suppl.: 112, 1978.

3 Models of care

This chapter offers the nurse guidelines for viewing various styles of nursing practice models and life-style models for the older adult.

MODELS OF NURSING CARE

A model is a description or an analogy to help visualize numerous activities in a simplified, concrete way. For example, consider the architect who designs a house. He draws a blueprint and includes all the many components necessary for a building. The blueprint shows the walls and floors, the plumbing system, the electrical system, and other such important parts of the structure. Builders then can construct the house, down to the last detail. Any person wanting to assess the design of the house can either look at the actual building or the blueprint. Although a walk-through inspection of the structure would enable us to see the building itself, the blueprint does offer the same information in a concise, systematic way.

The primary use of models in nursing is to diagram nursing practice. A person wanting to know the style of a nurse's practice can go along with the nurse and view her as she gives care. Or, he can ask the nurse which model of care she uses for her nursing practice.

The nurse might outline her model of practice as focusing on one of the following examples.

EXAMPLE A
1. The individual and his disease, noting the limitations caused by the disease
2. Identifying deficits in functions
3. Understanding disease signs and symptoms
4. Carrying out prescribed treatments for care

EXAMPLE B
1. Environmental manipulation
2. Health maintenance
3. Health counseling
4. Observational skills
5. Fostering self-care

EXAMPLE C
1. Carrying out the doctor's orders
2. Passing the medications on time
3. Doing the treatments

The nurse who identifies with the focus on practice described in Example A would have the medical model as the framework of her care. Medical practice is legally defined as the diagnosis and treatment of human pathology. The four items listed in Example A are characteristics of the model for medical practice.

At the turn of the century when schools of nursing were tied in closely with physician-owned hospitals, the medical model became the content framework for the school of nursing. A doctor would lecture on the disease entity, the signs and symptoms of diseases, diagnostic tests, and treatment modalities. The nursing instructor would add a lecture about the nursing care for the disease. Later, nursing texts presented information in the same medical style. Many nurses find the medical model very familiar, because it is in the style of their own education.

Example B is the Nightingale model of nursing practice presented in 1860. She coined the phrase, "nursing the well." In her view, the primary role of the nurse is one of health conservation. She was the forerunner of today's public health advocate. Her main emphasis in instructions to nurses is the importance of adjusting the environment of the home and hospital. Given an environment free of stresses and health threats, the individual is in the best possible position for his own healing mechanisms to operate. In addition to recommending the removal of negative influences in the environment (poor sanitation, noise, stagnated air), she encouraged the adjustment of the environment to include positive aspects (variety of stimulation and good nutrition). The skill of scientific observation was the cornerstone of her practice. The data she collected through observational skills form the basis of the nurses' decisions. It is not a matter of just following orders. Her nurses worked from the premise of the Nightingale model, which is directed toward maintaining health. She speaks of health as the positive of which pathology is the negative. She posits that, through observation and experience, we learn more about the principle of health and nursing.

Model C is the bureaucratic model. Patient care is the primary focus. The model emphasizes a task-oriented approach and encourages adherence to specific agency routines. The bureaucratic style has decided advantages. Work in the agency is organized and delivered in a specified time frame. For example, lights are turned on at 6:30 AM, baths are completed by 11:00 AM, and medications are distributed at specific times. Limitations of the bureaucratic model are significant. Care is fragmented and largely depersonalized. Minimal flexibility is available for individualized care. Consider one patient, a person who works the night shift at the local factory. His time frame differs from the hospital's daily routine. This might not be a problem while he is acutely ill. As discharge time approaches, however, the nurse must try to gear him for his self-care at home (medications, colostomy care, or insulin injection). She has a most difficult time adapting the hospital routine to his life-style. Yet, if the transition from hospital to home is to be successful, this adaptation must be made before discharge.

If this night shift worker normally has a glucose peak at 4:00 AM, then his meal and insulin schedule will be different from the average day worker. Nightingale recognized this in 1860. She said a nurse must know the social background of the person in order to give adequate care. The bureaucratic model is efficient, but at the expense of individualization. One way to determine if an agency uses this model is to review the evaluation form used by the supervisors to evaluate the nurses. If such items as promptness, number of days absent, tidy uniform, organization of time and material predominate, then the bureaucratic model is in operation. The nurses are rewarded for carrying out the system's defined routine. Little time or rewards are available for other than the routine care.

The nurse striving for innovative care is in a difficult position. If she feels she has little time for individualized care, she is correct in her perception. The routines of a bureaucratic model take up an 8-hour shift. The bureaucratic style is cost efficient; fewer nurses are needed to complete the care tasks. The bureaucratic model is the predominant style used in health care agencies. It has contributed to the general improvement of care in hospitals over this century. However, the bureaucratic model does have significant limitations as cited by Kramer (1974). The care deals with only the immediate needs of the individual. Such needs as health teaching, health counseling, and discharge planning are not priority goals. Readmissions may result from the person's misunderstanding medication or self-care regimens.

The nurse in the bureaucratic model frequently feels pressured for time. Also, she often experiences feelings of role dissatisfaction and differences in ideals and reality in her nursing practice.

NURSING THEORY MODELS AND PRACTICE

Theoretical principles evolve from known laws. Laws precede theory. The theorist uses a system of laws that are translated into valid statements. The laws verify the occurrence of the events given the same conditions. An example is the law of the conservation of energy. All theories are derived from the established disciplines. Theory enables us to put ideas together. It gives us an organized body of concepts and facts. Any time you ask a question and have a possible answer, you are theorizing.

There are a number of different levels of theory. Examples of some kinds of theories follow.

1. Speculative—a hunch not based in knowledge
2. Activity—opinionated, not based in facts
3. Mathematical—number theory
4. Scientific—observable and tested facts
5. Philosophical—a search for man's place in relationship to the world

Some nurses may ask, "Why do I have to know nursing theory? I went to nursing school and learned all there was to know about nursing." Without theory, there is no possibility for growth in nursing. It is a vicious cycle. The nurse knows everything there is to know in nursing; there is nothing new in nursing to learn; therefore, the status quo is maintained, and it is a no-growth situation.

Nursing theory allows us to develop a network of theoretical statements from which models for nursing practice can be constructed. Nursing theories, models, and practice are all interrelated (Fig. 3-1). They have self-organizing capacities; that is, models flow from theories and are translated into options for practice. Thus, nursing theory becomes a springboard for prescribing and guiding practical activity in relation to nursing practice. As cited earlier, it is our position that Florence Nightingale posed the first nursing theory that grounded a nurse's practice in knowledge. Nursing theory equals a field of study; nursing models equal a framework for translating that field of

study; and nursing practice equals applying theory in the practice setting. The organizing capacities of theory, model, and practice permit opportunities for making corrections. For example, a model may be inappropriate for practice and have to be sent back to the theorist for verification, modification, or abandonment.

Nursing is striving to achieve the scientific level of theory. Scientific theory is based on observable evidence, and is tested and validated by the practicing nurse and the nurse researcher. These documented nursing facts then become part of the proven facts basic to professional nursing. A very simple but important example of this is pulse measurement. Traditionally, the pulse was counted for 1 full minute. Nursing research has documented that there is a far higher level of ac-

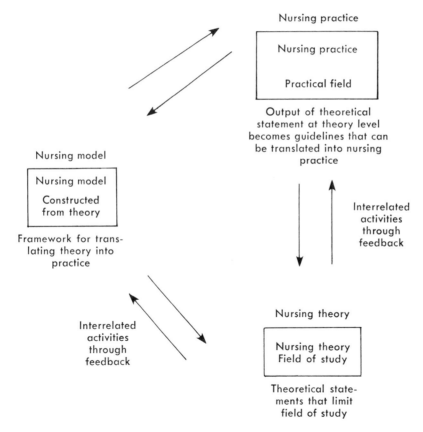

Arrows: Input of one is equal to output of the other.

Fig. 3-1. The theory-model-practice continuum.

curacy if the pulse is counted for 15 seconds and multiplied by four, except in the case of an irregular heartbeat, when a full minute is necessary for accuracy.

Why use theory?

Above and beyond the admirable goal of increasing nursing knowledge is the very mundane goal of meeting federal guidelines in health agencies. Medicare and Medicaid regulations mandate documentation of nursing practice. The nurse must be able to describe, explain, and predict nursing practice. Nursing theory enables the nurse to describe her practice. When her practice is grounded in knowledge, she is not just a good nurse, but one who can predict the outcome of her care. By stating the model of nursing she uses, she is stating the baseline of her care. Competency-based practice, nursing accountability, and decision making are products of practice based in knowledge. The nursing process is a model for practice that permits the nurse to help the client progress from where he is to the highest level of health possible. Nursing theory gives us a frame of reference and a stable vocabulary for nursing researchers. Nursing theories are derived from theories in the established disciplines.

Current theory review

Nightingale's original nursing theory is based on the manipulation of the environment to foster health maintenance. Most nursing theories today concur with her perspective. These spin-offs of the Nightingale theory are refined and brought up to date by using facts from the biological and social sciences. We must remember that Nightingale did not have the advantage of our scientific knowledge. Even germ theory was in its infancy in her day. Considering the state of the art and the sciences, she had very accurate insight into the world about her.

Roy adaptation theory. The Roy adaptation model developed by Sister Callista Roy had its beginning in 1964. Since that time, it has been further developed and refined as a framework for nursing practice, nursing education, and nursing research.

Basic to this theory are the beliefs that humans as biopsychosocial beings are in a constant state of interaction with their environment. To cope with this changing environment, they must use innate and acquired skills. At some point they must use their adaptive mechanisms to return to health from a state of illness. The success of people's adaptation attempts depend on the stimuli within their immediate situation. Beliefs, attitudes, and personal traits are the residual assets of the client; they help him adapt to the presenting situation. If the residual assets are greater than the stress of the presenting stimuli, then adaptation can occur. If the stress of the presenting stimuli is greater than the level of the residual assets, adaptation does not occur.

There are four ways to achieve adaptation: through physiological needs, self-concept, role function, and interdependence relations (Table 3-1).

People adapt according to their physiological needs, meeting their basic body requirements of oxygen, water, and food. Self-concept relates to the person's good feelings about himself. When he sees himself as a worthwhile person, he is able to relate to others in a positive way. The nurse can help the person feel better about himself. For example, the nurse makes sure that the older adult has accessible facilities for meeting personal hygiene needs. Proper hygiene and grooming foster a positive self-concept.

The performance of duties as prescribed by society are called role functions. Retirement is a role function of almost every older adult upon reaching the age of 65. When the industrial nurse initiates retirement planning discussions with a group of workers, she is helping them mobilize their adaptation abilities.

Interdependence relations involve the ways an individual seeks help, attention, and affection. The nurse who is admitting a client to a nursing home understands that the person's usual ways of seeking affection, attention, and help no longer are available to him. His needs remain. The nurse must foster adaptation abilities if the person is going to make the transition successfully.

The nurse who subscribes to the Roy adaptation model can answer the question, "What kind of nursing do you do?" She is more than a "good" nurse who renders "total patient care." With the brief outline of the four aspects of the Roy model, she describes her attention to her client's physical, social, and psychological needs.

Table 3-1. Example of Roy's adaptation model

Mode of adaptation	Adaptation occurs
Physiological needs	Thirsty → take a drink
Self-concept	Body image and mobility threatened because of loss of limb → acceptance and use of prosthesis
Role function	Retirement → change of life-style adjusting to increased leisure time
Interdependence relations	Separation because of admission to a nursing home → participate in activities, make friends in the nursing home

The nurse focuses all her energies on assisting the client's adaptation in his physiological needs, his self-concept, his role function, and his interdependence relations through health and illness. She utilizes the nursing process in assessing the client's behavioral responses to stimuli within his environment, and in establishing a nursing diagnosis. She plans nursing care to achieve the client's health goal. She acts as a change agent to manipulate the client's environment while carrying out nursing interventions. She evaluates the client's success in adaptation, which is the achievement of the goal of nursing care. Each component of the nursing process and the problem-solving process is followed in the Roy adaptation model. Roy cautions us that the model's assumptions about humans' adaptation require further validation. Research is now underway in masters' and doctorate nursing programs to test the adaptation model.

Rogers' holistic model. In 1970, Martha Rogers from New York University published a book discussing the theoretical basis of nursing. She perceives humans as holistic beings. That is, people and their environment are a unified whole involved in a continuous exchange of matter and energy. Life processes are tied in with space and time. Because humans are unified with their environment, the nurse strives to strike a balance. This balance is the difference between ease and disease. The research projects based on the Rogers model seek in-depth information regarding humans' perception of space and time at various stages of life development.

Rogers seeks to uncover new information about humans. Conclusions drawn from studies on body space and time and their effect on body image should yield knowledge regarding adult territoriality and other mental health concepts. The data from this research expand the options in health planning for every individual. The goal is to develop patterns of being in harmony with the environmental changes instead of in conflict with them.

Five basic assumptions underlying Rogers' unitary man*

1. Man is a unified whole possessing his own integrity and manifesting characteristics that are more than and different from the sum of parts.
2. Man and environment are continuously exchanging matter and energy with one another.
3. The life process evolves irreversibly and unidirectionally along the space-time continuum.
4. Pattern and organization identify man and reflect his innovative wholeness.
5. Man is characterized by the capacity for abstraction and imagery, language and thought, sensation and emotion.

The Roy and Rogers theories address research, education, and practice for nursing of all age groups. Gunter is developing theory specific to the older adult.

Gunter's gerontics. Laurie Gunter distinguishes some terms related to the older adult. She describes the term *geriatrics* as the study of medical treatments of old age and disease, and *gerontology* as the study of the aging process in people.

Missing from these definitions is the health promotional component, which she has called *gerontics*,

. . . wherein nurses assist the aged to understand the aging process, to separate the effects of aging from disease, to control the aging process through use of hygienic practices and life styles which promote health, vigor, and attractiveness into old age, and to prevent some of the pathogenic conditions which accompany aging when the principles of healthful living are disregarded.†

Nurses caring for the older adult can easily identify with the theory of gerontics. It relates to

---

*From Rogers, M.: Theoretical basis of nursing, Philadelphia, 1978, F. A. Davis Co.

†Gunter, L.: Education for gerontic nursing, New York, 1979, Springer Publishing Co., Inc.

the health focus of Nightingale and is a positive, energetic approach to the health maintenance of the older adult. Gunter is calling for more research in nursing and special education for the care of the older adult.

Some areas she suggests that need study are (1) the milieu of nursing units in institutional facilities and (2) the exploration of personnel characteristics such as attitudes and educational preparation as they affect client care. Gunter also stresses the need for the refinement of nursing service delivery across cultural and socioeconomic groups.

In the area of nursing education, she has defined a number of educational preparations in the care of the older adult. They range from the aide level in institutions to the doctoral level of teachers and researchers in gerontic nursing.

Future of theory development in nursing care of older adults

There is likely to be far more theory development in the care of the older adult in the years to come. More master's and doctoral level programs are addressing the specific needs of the older adult. Nursing associations have passed resolutions to encourage the study of the older adult as a specific curriculum component. Nursing journals are including more articles related to older adult topics. Some federal money is available to assist nurses in research and curriculum development.

LIFE-STYLE MODELS FOR OLDER ADULTS

Life-style models of the older adult are as useful to the nurse as nursing models are in her practice. Both types of models give her a blueprint for viewing common patterns of living for the older adult.

Since it is estimated that 5 percent of the older adult population are in nursing homes and other institutions, the remaining 95 percent are living in the community. The community models include the family model, the retirement model, and the self-care model. The nursing home model as a lifestyle will be addressed separately. The family model will be viewed from the older adults' perspective. The Bureau of the Census defines the family as a group of two or more persons related by marriage, blood, or adoption who reside together. This definition reflects a sociological view of a system that is charged with transmitting cultural norms and practicing standard social roles of various generations of parents and children.

Rollins and Feldman see the family as having eight stages:
1. Establishment
2. New parents
3. Preschool children
4. School-age children
5. Adolescent children
6. Launching center
7. Postparental family
8. Aging family

If the older adult has completed the developmental tasks of each of the preceding family stages, his attention is now on the final two stages: postparental and aging family.

Postparental family

The older adult is usually in the postparental or aging family stage. During this period of life, there are many developmental tasks for the older adult to successfully master. Success must be based on the accomplishment of the preceding family stages. Individuals who are unmarried still achieve a good deal of task accomplishment through alternate family activities. For example, unmarried aunts and uncles often serve as valuable support persons to the children in extended families. Volunteer work and church work are other means of accomplishment for successful completion of generativity work of this stage. The postparental family develops after the last child has left home for college, work, marriage, or to be on his own. It is a time of relatively high productivity and economic independence. Studies reflect that the postparental and aging family report satisfactory to high degrees of marital happiness. The relatively low divorce rate at these times reflects a process of selection of durable marriages. Usually, if a divorce occurs, it happens in the launching stage or before.

One major social event in the older adult's life is the additional role of grandparenting. Neugarten and Weinstein state that most grandparents find their new role comfortable, satisfying, and rewarding. The role enables the grandparents to have a feeling of biological renewal, biological continuity, and emotional self-fulfillment. They feel young again, see their family line carried on and feel that they can be more generous with their grandchildren than they were with their own children. The grandparents tend to be more indulgent with their grandchildren, allowing them to do many things their own children were not permitted to do and then returning their grandchildren to the parents for discipline.

The postparental stage allows the couple more time to renew old friendships and engage in new friendships. This is the time of life when the memorable vacation is planned and executed (Fig. 3-2). The cross-country motor trip, the cruise, or European trip to trace family roots is taken. Some families have more than one vacation of a lifetime; others have none, depending on the initiative, health status of either mate, and economic circumstances. With or without a vacation trip, the older adult couple find themselves alone at a developmental stage that lends itself to renewing, enriching, and expanding the intimacy in their marriage. Intimacy now means full and complete emotional rapport, based on mutual trust and respect. Time is budgeted for shared activities and experiences, such as talking about one's deepest fears, longings, and occupations, and going shopping, out to eat, or to a movie together.

The couple mutually support each other as they

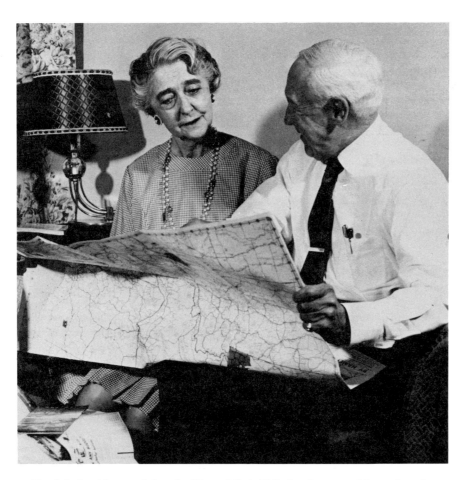

Fig. 3-2. An older couple has the "time of their life" planning a special vacation trip.

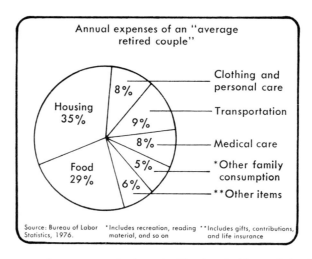

Fig. 3-3. Annual expenses of an average retired couple. (Reprinted with permission from AIM's guide to financial security, Washington, D.C., 1978, Action for Independent Maturity. Division of American Association of Retired Persons.)

Table 3-2. How much will you need in retirement?*

	Step 1: Current expenses	Step 2: Est. retirement expenses	Step 3: Projection for inflation
Food	_____	_____	Multiply the total from Step 2 by the
Housing	_____	_____	appropriate inflation factor from
Transportation	_____	_____	the Inflation Impact Table below.
Clothing	_____	_____	For example, if you are five years
Medical	_____	_____	from retirement, you'll use Infla-
Savings and Investments	_____	_____	tion Factor 1.3382 to learn how
Life Insurance	_____	_____	much you'll actually need that first
Other	_____	_____	retirement year. After that, project
	_____	_____	for five years into retirement and
TOTAL	_____	_____	make any other projections you

think are necessary.

Your first retirement year: _____

Five years after retirement: _____

Further projections: _____

Inflation impact table (*Compounded at 6% per year*)

End of year	Inflation factor	End of year	Inflation factor	End of year	Inflation factor*
1	1.0600	11	1.8983	21	3.3996
2	1.1236	12	2.0122	22	3.6035
3	1.1910	13	2.1329	23	3.8197
4	1.2625	14	2.2609	24	4.0489
5	1.3382	15	2.3966	25	4.2919
6	1.4185	16	2.5404	26	4.5494
7	1.5036	17	2.6928	27	4.8223
8	1.5938	18	2.8543	28	5.1117
9	1.6895	19	3.0256	29	5.4184
10	1.7908	20	3.2071	30	5.7435

*Authors' note: Adjust upward for increasing inflation.

Table 3-3. Earning money through savings*

How $50 invested each month and compounded semi-annually will grow.

Year	4½%	5%	6%
1	$ 614.50	$ 616.50	$ 619.50
2	1,257.50	1,264.00	1,277.00
3	1,929.50	1,944.00	1,974.50
4	2,632.00	2,659.00	2,714.50
5	3,336.50	3,410.00	3,499.50
6	4,134.50	4,199.00	4,332.00
7	4,937.00	5,028.00	5,215.50
8	5,776.50	5,899.00	6,152.00
9	6,654.50	6,814.00	7,147.50
10	7,572.00	7,775.00	8,202.00

*Reprinted with permission from AIM's guide to financial security, Washington, DC, 1978, Action for Independent Maturity (Division of American Association of Retired Persons).

develop their plan for retirement. This vital phase of life requires the older adult couple to draw upon previously acquired knowledge and skills for adjustment. The new stage of life offers fresh opportunities for self-fulfillment and happiness. Financial experts recommend that individuals start planning for retirement financial security between 45 and 50 years of age (Fig. 3-3). The major cause of "retirement failure" is simply lack of planning to avoid the hazards and pitfalls. The identified pitfalls follow.

1. Lack of a sound financial program that takes inflation into account
2. Hasty decisions regarding housing and relocation
3. Lack of interests and activities
4. Confusing retirement with aging
5. Failure to anticipate adjustments in roles and attitudes
6. Delay in planning ahead

Tables 3-2 and 3-3 are useful for planning retirement financial security.

However, retirement often causes difficulties for the wife who is not used to having her husband underfoot. The husband now seems to be the expert in the wife's domain and supervises all her household activities. Many wives dislike having their husbands in the home 24 hours a day and having to prepare three meals. Some wives rebel, and friction arises within the family. Each partner

needs personal time and recreational activities, preferably outside the home. Friends and other retired couples serve as social outlets and a source of social diversion.

Another development stage for the postparental family is coping with aging parents. The middle-aged family today is more likely to have a living parent than earlier in the century. A 65-year-old couple may have 85-year-old parents. Kin networks, however, are decreased because the postparental parent has raised fewer children and so has fewer options and resources than did his own parents. It is predicted that if the current fertility rate continues to fall, we will achieve zero population growth. Some sources state that if zero population occurs, society at large will have to provide the resources and support now supplied by the family. Society would then assume some of the responsibilities of the family, such as housing, recreation, health care, and income maintenance for the postparental family.

The postparental family may be likened to the age group of the young-old that ranges from 55 to 74 years of age. It may be distinguished from the aging family in that it has more social opportunities and is likely to be in better physical condition than the aging family. The most significant task of the postparental family is adjustment to retirement.

Aging family

The aging family (75 and older) is past the retirement stage and is now facing possible changes in health status.

The aging family must make a decision whether to maintain the family home or move into a smaller home or apartment. Often these decisions are determined by the economic status of the couple. House maintenance can be costly as well as physically demanding; therefore, life-styles may have to be altered. Household routines are also adjusted in view of changed social, occupational, and family roles. The aging couple should use each other as a mutual support system. The grief involved with the loss of a spouse is another common difficulty in the life of the aging family.

Communication lines must be maintained with family members, children, grandchildren, and even great-grandchildren. The brothers and sisters of the aging couple can themselves be aging and require economic and physical assistance. Overall, the aging couple is supported by maintaining a network of friends and by finding a purpose and enjoyment in life. As adults, the aging couple seeks to remain independent, and this goal should be respected.

The energy and stamina with which the family addresses these tasks will be influenced by cultural, social, and psychological variables—not to mention past experiences and health status.

There are any number of structural forms a family may take. For example, a family may be a couple—husband and wife with no relatives—a nuclear family, or a multigenerational extended family. No matter what the structure, there are certain health tasks required of a family:

1. Recognize health deviation
2. Seek appropriate health care
3. Consider actions for health and nonhealth crises
4. Care for sick, disabled, and dependent members
5. Support health maintenance behaviors
6. Utilize services of community and health agencies

CULTURAL INFLUENCES ON FAMILY LIFE

The heterogeneous mix of ethnic origins in the United States makes the subject of cultural influences on the aging person quite complex. The vast topic of ethnicity is now becoming a specialized area of study in itself. This introduction to cultural influences on family life comprises an overview of black and Asian-American families. The black population was selected because it comprises 90 percent of the nonwhite population and is found throughout all sections of the United States. The Asian-Americans have traditionally settled on the West Coast and Hawaii and are the least studied minority group. Birren (1977) predicted that Filipinos will comprise the largest group of Asian-Americans.

This book does not attempt to address all the cultural factors that contribute to aging. Instead, several cultural studies that yield insight into the area of ethnicity are cited and used as the organizing framework.

A research study is undertaken to answer specific questions, and care must be taken to prevent premature assumptions about ethnicity, since it is one variable, and not a cause, of aging. Also, with time the research may need refinement because the answers found in the study are no longer satisfactory. However, there is agreement that culture does influence the life-style of the older adult. Even though the black and Asian population residing in America are minorities, their family structure, coping mechanisms, and religious customs affect the older adult's attitudes and life-style.

Black family

One historical, cultural event for the black family was the crisis of the movement of the black people from their African origins to the Americas of the sixteenth and seventeenth centuries. Social structures were fragmented as families were wrenched apart and tribal roots demolished. Blacks have not had a uniform experience because such factors as geographical living situations, positions, and duties on the plantation determined the options available to the black family. The effects of slavery on the family were many:

1. They were dislocated from Africa into an alien culture.
2. They came from many different tribes, so their languages, cultures, and traditions did not serve to unify them in the United States.
3. Their family ties were destroyed, and often no black females were available to the black men to establish relationships.
4. They did not have the ordinary processes of enculturation that were available to other immigrant groups.

Over a period of 4 centuries, millions of Africans who had been free, independent human beings found themselves sold as chattel. Today the black family has certain basic similarities with all families in America. Black families differ in that they have a unique historical heritage and have experienced the sequellae of a postslavery status.

Population family characteristics. The United States Bureau of the Census, 1977, records the social consequences of the black historical past as demonstrated in the fact that:

1. Thirty-six percent of black persons 65 years of

age and over fall below the poverty level, compared with 14 percent of older adult whites.

2. Only 10 percent of black males and 13 percent of black females 65 years of age have attained a high school education.

3. Forty-eight percent of black older adults live in the inner city, and very few own their homes.

Kent (1971) reports that 29 percent of blacks of all ages live in poor housing, compared with 8 percent of whites of all ages. It is posited that the percentages of black and white older adults living in poor housing are comparable. Jackson (1971) found that black older adults living in the rural South seek their families first, even in illness. In the Southern City, however, the older adult black is more likely to turn to the hospital or church for help. The effects of rural versus urban life-styles on American blacks and longevity have been studied and compared. Rural black men survive women, but urban black women survive men. The urban black family relationship between mother-daughter-grandmother promotes a positive support bonding to the black older adult mother, no matter what her social class. Rubenstein (1972) reports that both black and white single older adult women score higher on a measure of morale than do single men.

Within the black culture, the extended family in most instances takes precedence over the nuclear family. Sometimes several generations live together. In the black family, the older adult is respected by the younger generations. The grandmother is the family pivot.

All other family members depend on her and turn to her for emotional support. Her knowledge and experience are valued, and she contributes much in the way of assistance with household chores, advice, child care and rearing. Children and the older adult are held in esteem in the black family. Grandmothers and great-grandmothers function as family historians, prescribers of folk medicine or home remedies, and translators of black culture. There is an especially strong bond between the grandchildren and grandparents. When the grandparents who live alone require help during times of illness, often the grandchild is sent to live with the grandparents or to stay with them after school. Even grandparents in an extended family receive the extra help and support needed from the grandchildren. Contrary to belief, the black family is not necessarily matriarchal. The husband is respected as head of the household. The older adult husband and wife have worked together as a team to hold the family together, to raise their children, educate them, and provide social, economic, religious, and emotional support.

Black older adults are no strangers to stress. They are genetic survivors of centuries of stressful situations and survivors of several decades of personal conditioning through physically and psychologically coping with a stressful environment. Their defense mechanisms are well established, and their religious beliefs support them through trying times.

Ethnic perceptions. In 1977, a Southern California study compared black, Mexican-American, and white persons' perceptions of health status, aging, and life expectancy at 10-year intervals, starting at 45 and ending with 75 years of age. At every age level, the black individual progressively increased his percentages for perceived poor health as compared with the white individual at the same age. For example, 27 percent of black older adults aged 65 to 75 see themselves as having poor health, contrasted to 4 percent of white older adults of the same age.

Blacks have a perception of themselves as old at age 65, 5 years younger than whites, who perceive themselves as old at age 70. However, on a national level, Jackson (1970) reports that blacks view themselves as old at a younger age than whites because of a disadvantaged economic and social life-style. Seventy percent of blacks age 75 participating in the study predicted they would live 10 years more. According to Birren (1977), 60-year-old blacks are inclined to have equal or better life expectancies than whites. According to U.S. Dept. of Health, Education, and Welfare (1972), nonwhites' life expectancy is the same as whites at age 70, and past age 70 nonwhites surpass whites in longevity. The United States Bureau of Census reported in 1979 that 8% of black Americans are over the age of 65, compared with 12% of the white population. As age increases, it appears that the survival of the fittest principle is operating. Blacks expressed a lower life satisfaction in old age than whites. Middle-aged blacks 45 to 54 revealed greater sadness and worry than older adult blacks.

The family was identified by Jackson (1970) as the social network for providing assistance and group interaction for the black older adult. Participation as a family member and kin relationships are more important for the black than for the white older adult. The Southern California study found blacks had more relationships than whites. The void in kin relationships of whites was compensated for by establishing more friendship relations with neighbors and acquaintances than blacks did. Rubenstein (1972) reports that fewer blacks than whites participate in membership in structured organizations such as clubs and fraternities. Other studies conducted in 1968, 1970, and 1973 document that blacks participate at a higher political organizational level than whites. Therefore, the black continues this function of his citizenship role. Antunes and Gaitz (1975) identify four areas in which black older adults interact at a higher level than whites: (1) voting, (2) church activities, (3) clubs, and (4) political activities. Church affiliations and religion are a significant factor in the black older adults' lives. Hirsh (1968) found that older adult blacks received more emotional support from their church memberships, which were established in independent, personable, religious institutions, than white older adults. Participation in church activities enables the older adult to continue many of his previous social roles.

The church meets the spiritual, educational, social, psychological, emotional, and recreational requirements of the black older adult. The church and its religious activities supply the older adult with a network of support systems that is an extension of the family. It also enables him to participate in a community activity. Religion provides the older adult with an acceptable outlet to freely express himself and helps him cope with the anxiety and stresses of daily living.

Bible devotions, or thoughts for the day, accompanied by daily prayer and weekly prayer meetings, help him face each day and solve his problems. For those who can no longer read the small print of the Bible, there are favorite radio or television religious services. The clergy are pillars of the community and knowledgeable individuals. Their services are sought in crises, and their advice is requested in solving problems. Most churches have organized senior citizens groups and sponsor activities such as day trips, vacations, parties, dances, special instructions in arts and crafts, health screening, hot lunches, and meals on wheels.

All researchers agree that the area of ethnicity needs further study. Research designs and instruments need to measure attitudes and behavior, not only demographic data, to present a comprehensive study of ethnic aging in the United States. Furthermore, there is agreement among researchers that the minority population is heterogeneous and can no longer be viewed as homogeneous.

Asian-Americans

The 1971 White House Conference on Aging recognized the Asian-American as one of the most underprivileged minority groups. As an example, during 1969 to 1971, the federal government allocated no monies for this minority group. The ethnic cultures that comprise at least 1 percent of the population are Chinese, Japanese, Filipino, Korean, Samoan, and are called Asian-Americans. Asian-Americans are lumped together as one people; however, they need to be viewed as separate groups, because each has its own language, customs, heritage, and unique history of immigration to the United States. Asian-Americans are a heterogeneous group that needs help in making their concerns known.

Immigration to the United States. Most Asian-Americans found their way to the United States as laborers. The Chinese men arrived at the end of the nineteenth century. Wives and families remained in China, and single men were not permitted to intermarry. Most men planned to return to their native China, but world wars and communist infiltration prevented their return. Today, the aftereffects are seen in the unusual ratio of a larger number of older adult men than women. There are older adult men with no sons to care for them and assume the financial support that is expected in the Oriental culture.

Filipino men came alone to the United States, getting work as farm laborers. They were awarded citizenship for participating in World War II. In the midforties after the war, soldiers set out for a new life in America. Contact with family and friends gradually disappeared. Unlike the Chinese-Americans, the Filipino men were permitted to marry. Today, the war veterans are the reason that there are more older Filipino men than women.

The immigration policies permitted the Japanese-Americans to come to the United States in family units. The Japanese family foundation in the United States has been in effect longer than that of the Chinese-American and the Filipino-American. Perhaps the family as a support mechanism is a significant variable for the Japanese survival of loss of roles, jobs, and possessions during World War II. The family provided the strength needed to survive the camp life that the Japanese were subjected to during World War II. The White House Conference on Aging delegates recommended that the Japanese older adults be permitted to count the years spent in American concentration camps during World War II toward their Social Security benefits.

Population family characteristics. Mead (1967) found that older adult Chinese men are given the role of meditating, relaxing, and nobility. Some of the daily behaviors within this role include a diet free of meat, abstaining from sex, worshiping, meditating, and cultivating the mind. As Chinese women age, they move from a passive mastery to an active mastery. The retired husband turns over authority to his wife. She shares this family control and responsibility with her oldest son. The same occurs in the traditional Japanese family, where power is shared by the aging mother and oldest son. As women become older adults, they also become more assertive and extraverted in their behavior. De Beauvoir (1972) reports a dissolving of sex differences among the Oriental culture. Older adult Samoan women are permitted to say and do things they would never think of saying and doing at an earlier age. Patriarchal roles are readily transferred to the older adult woman who rules the household.

In the Asian-American culture, the older adult is considered wise from an accumulation of knowledge and life experiences. Children and other family members consult with older adults for advice because they possess a "house of knowledge." All young people extend this common courtesy to the older adult; however, they do not necessarily have to follow the advice. Because of this constant contact with people and the high esteem placed on the authority role, most older adults are very attuned to reality. On the other hand, the older adult is expected to behave as old. This includes dressing in dark colors and styles that portray the image of old.

The family structures within the Asian-American group provide the support systems and kin relationships needed by the older adult. Many sources have documented that research is required to identify the extent of the groups' needs and to build upon their existing support systems. The government has already cited the poverty level and the poor housing that exists within the city ethnic neighborhoods. One third of the group have never had a medical or dental examination. Lifestyles and health care usually fall far below minimal standards. Rarely are meaningful bilingual counseling, recreation and leisure activities, and ethnic food found at government-supported older adult centers.

Areas of statistics are missing for the Asian-American because many times these people are lumped into the category of nonwhite minority. Accurate data are also difficult to collect about the size of the group because of illegal entry into the United States. Life expectancy data are subsumed under black and nonwhite data and are nonexistent. Some demographic data for specific areas of the country are available, for example, the poverty level of the New York Chinese.

Each society dictates the script its members are to play along the developmental continuum. Some of the roles within the ethnic script have been mutated by the infiltration of Westernization, with its accompanying urbanization and technology. However, with the present-day emphasis on one's heritage and roots, there is a current trend to respect the cultural family system and all the support and services that it provides for the older adult.

SELECTED LIVING ARRANGEMENTS FOR THE OLDER ADULT

Changing living arrangements are involving persons of various age groups. The health professional caring for the older adult in agencies often gets a distorted view. Most older adults are not outside the family circle, but are rather very well cared for by their families. They are in their own houses or apartments close to family members. Frequent communications are possible through telephone or short car rides. Even though the older adult lives apart from other generations, they still serve all the purposes of the family: the biological, sociological, economic, and psychological. For the older adult, the biological bond is with the children and grandchildren. The sociological purpose is the cultural link between the generations. The basic purpose of the family changes because of longevity; the time span of older adulthood (age 68 to 100 years), of necessity, brings many diverse levels of contribution of the older adult to these areas.

Although great attention and publicity are focused on the needy older adult, many older adults serve as economic support for younger people. For example, older adults lend a son or daughter money to buy a new car or a down payment on a house. Psychological bonds provide for mutual support in difficult and happy times. The point is, members of the family are often mutually supportive.

Family living and institutional living have been traditionally the two models of living arrangements for the older adult. Fortunately, there are a number of new models evolving, so there are more choices available. Older adults can choose to live in:

1. A multigenerational household
2. Their own home or apartment within a multi-generational neighborhood or community
3. Their own home within a one-generational community
4. A government-sponsored (HUD) apartment
5. A mobile home
6. A domiciliary arrangement
7. Single-room occupancy (SRO) arrangement
8. Retirement community
9. Nursing home: institutional model

A multiple-generation household is a style of living in which the older adult lives with the second and third generation. In a multigenerational community, the older adults may own or rent their own apartments or houses and are surrounded by multigenerational families of various age groups. Often, their own family lives within the community itself or a short distance from it.

Government-sponsored living usually takes the style of a garden or high-rise apartment. Rents are usually based on ability to pay. Sometimes, the tenants are all older adults and sometimes they are not, depending on the zoning laws.

Frequently, the older person will buy a mobile home, travel with it, or live in a mobile home park.

A domiciliary arrangement, in which three or four nonrelated adults live together, differs from the boarding house in that health problems are monitored by the house owner.

The single-room occupancy (SRO) arrangement has had a long history. Initially, after World War II, when living accommodations were not plentiful for families, persons started living by themselves in hotels particularly adapted for individual living. Many men's clubs now offer similar arrangements. In 1976, the US Census Bureau reported a steady increase in the number of single persons since 1900. However, the SRO model is not practical for single older adults who are not independent in activities of daily living and are unable to care for themselves. Being unable to monitor their own needs and with no one available to help them, older adults can develop major health problems.

A retirement community is a new development in the long-term-care field that has become popular within the last decade. Retirement communities are for people over 65 who meet the resident criteria. Some of these criteria follow. The person is ambulatory and able to independently carry out activities of daily living even with a chronic disease. He uses good judgment in decision making, which enables him to function within the community without supervision. His independent functioning places him in the first level health maintenance category, which is discussed in depth in Chapter 4.

Retirement communities advertise a life-care retirement concept. Membership assures meal and housekeeping services, entertainment and stimulation by recreational and cultural activities, available transportation for shopping, interesting friends, 24-hour security, a health officer should a problem arise, and comprehensive health care when needed. The choice of living arrangements may be either a house or apartment that offers freedom from housework, maintenance, and repair. Members have complete freedom, privacy, and independence. They may entertain family and friends in their own residences or use entertainment areas of the community. Retirement communities may be profit or nonprofit. The older adult needs to investigate the cost of the membership and monthly charges for the services provided and weigh these against his current expenses and his financial security.

A nursing home model is the model for institutionalized care in which all living and recreational activities are provided in a hospital-like setting. Nursing homes are also referred to as long-term-care facilities (LTCF).

The words *custodial care* suggest a place to put someone for care and safekeeping. A few years back, nursing homes, or long-term-care facilities, were the places that provided this type of service. Often, custodial care offers too little nursing care or too much nursing care. The better nursing homes offer therapeutic care. They seek to preserve health, and offer restorative and rehabilitative care that is directed to maintaining a normal or optimum level of self-care and independence. These homes also offer milieu therapy that provides a social and cultural environment.

However, the type of care that any facility or agency provides depends on its philosophy and policies. The personnel have an awesome responsibility for implementing the philosophy and policies and providing the type of environment and programs that enable the older adult to live with dignity and function within his limitations.

The philosophy should describe the agency's purpose for existence, how it expects to achieve this purpose, and its beliefs about older adults. The philosophy gives guidelines for the agency's policies. For instance, if the agency believes that every older adult will become incontinent, it might have a policy that every client wear incontinent pants. Consequently, there would be no need of a policy for a bowel and bladder training program.

Policies are statements that emanate from the administrative level spelling out guidelines for specific behaviors that govern a course of action. Administration usually seeks information from all concerned—department heads, medical staff, personnel, clients, and families—for developing policies. These policies enable the agency to provide services in an orderly fashion and to manage groups of people. The larger the size of the agency, the more at risk the institution is to being formal and rigid in its schedules for activities and nursing care.

Some policies for long-term-care facilities are mandated by the federal and state governments in order to qualify as a provider of Medicare and Medicaid. Examples of these policies are the number of nursing hours in a day and the nursing staff per 8-hour shift, not to mention the number of hours between meals, the establishment of a utilization review committee, and a life safety code. Nursing care is the most important service rendered by the long-term-care facility. It is so important that the scope of nursing care determines the kind of facility, skilled or intermediate, and the Medicare/Medicaid reimbursement payments.

A long-term-care facility may provide various levels of nursing care that range from residential to intermediate to skilled nursing care. As an alternative, a facility may choose to deliver only one level of nursing care. In either case, the intermediate or skilled care facility may have a special area set aside for residential living where persons not requiring nursing care or supervision reside.

An intermediate facility will have a transfer agreement with a skilled nursing facility in case a client's condition changes and he requires comprehensive nursing care. In the event that this happens, a client and family should always have the option of approving the transfer facility or selecting another one themselves. The difference between the nursing care that intermediate and skilled care facilities provide may be found in Table 3-4.

Facilities may be operated as a profit-making (proprietary) or nonprofit (nonproprietary) enterprise. The facility ownership and management may be individual, a partnership, an association, or a corporation. Nonprofit facilities are usually managed by religious or fraternal groups.

The laws of the state in which the facility resides are followed for filing an application for a license to operate as either a profit-making or nonprofit intermediate or skilled care facility. The license specifies the type of facility, ownership, and the number of beds and care level authorized. A license is issued annually when the facility is in complete compliance with all applicable statutes and federal and state regulations. Allowances are made for facilities that are not in complete compliance. These allowances vary from state to state. For example, Pennsylvania can issue a provisional

Table 3-4. Levels of nursing care*

Skilled long-term-care facility	Intermediate care facility
Any premises in which nursing care and related medical or other health services are provided, for a period exceeding 24 hours, for two or more individuals, who are not relatives of the operator and not in need of hospitalization, but who because of age, illness, disease, injury, convalescence, or physical or mental infirmity need such care. High-intensity, comprehensive, planned care provided with maximum efficiency by a registered professional nurse in instances in which her judgment is required, or by a licensed practical nurse under professional nurse supervision.	A facility that provides nursing care and related medical or other personal health services on a regular basis to individuals who do not require a degree of care and treatment that a hospital or skilled nursing facility is designed to provide, or who because of mental or physical disabilities require the above services within the context of a planned program of care and administrative management, supervised on a continuous 24-hour basis in an institutional setting. Such an institution shall have at all times, on a continuous 24-hour basis, qualified and licensed personnel to carry out the policies and responsibilities outlined above. In addition, an intermediate care facility is not to be confused with a personal care home or a custodial institution. An intermediate care facility is instead a facility that is designed to play an active role in helping each of its residents achieve or maintain optimal function in all dimensions of physical, social, and psychological health.

*Department of Health Regulations, Division of Long-term Care; Commonwealth of Pennsylvania. Revised July 1979.

Table 3-5. Comparison of custodial and therapeutic care*

Characteristics of custodial model	Characteristics of therapeutic model
Chronic disease–oriented based on the medical model of treating a specific condition.	Wellness-oriented based on health maintenance; client assumes responsibility for own health.
Care is administered by means of a bureaucratic delivery system.	Care is administered within simulated community lifestyle.
Residency may be for an appreciable period of time.	Residency is directed to short-term and return to the community unless contraindicated.
Residency and living activities are limited to one building or group of buildings, a single unit and room.	Residency and living activities are extended to include the surrounding community.
Environment and space do not allow for the client's privacy.	Client's privacy is respected.
The environment is sterile, nonstimulating, and noninvolving.	The environment simulates that of a normal society.
Only the patient role is available, with a focus on illness.	Client's individual, member of society, and social roles are available, with a focus on wellness.
Activities are directed toward meeting only physical needs.	Activities are directed toward meeting social, psychological, and physical needs.
Personnel are task oriented.	Personnel focus on meeting the individual needs of the client.
Routines and time schedules control daily activities.	Personnel function in a broad capacity beyond specific job descriptions.
Delivery of care is fragmented and involves many levels of personnel.	The major components of community life are interwoven throughout the day, making life an integrated whole.

*Adapted from Milieu Therapy and Program Design, Institute of Gerontology at the University of Michigan, Ann Arbor.

Table 3-5. Comparison of custodial and therapeutic care—cont'd

Characteristics of custodial model	Characteristics of therapeutic model
Clients are categorized, for example, as admissions, ambulatory, complete care, and CVAs.	Clients are respected and addressed as individuals.
Maintaining self-dignity is not a high priority.	Maintain self-dignity and self-esteem as first priority.
Personal property handled and personal territory invaded by others without permission.	Individual territoriality and property are respected.
Efforts are directed to eliminate stress.	Stress is controlled, but not eliminated.
Personnel are pessimistic about the older adult.	Personnel become optimistic as they see the older adult begin to function again in normal ways.
Very little client input for establishing goals.	Clients establish their own realistic goals with assistance.

Historical development of nursing homes*

Europe, England

1. *6th century* BC—Institutions for care of the aged existed.
2. *1535*—Church of England, Italian Renaissance, Middle Ages—Legislation for the aged.
3. *1601 "Poor Law"*—England tax levy for the poor specified kind of care.
4. *1601 First almshouse*—Bristol, England, for sick, aged, and feeble.
5. Further legislation separated housing—the aged with the insane, alcoholic, drug addict, sick, and orphaned.

United States

1. *American colonies*—Implemented England's laws and the almshouse model of care for the aged.
2. *19th century*—Revolt against almshouse resulted in the building of hospitals and insane asylums to separate those conditions from the aged.
3. Almshouses become homes for the aged. Controlled by local and county governments; also known as poorhouses. Minimal operating budget required the aged to work on farms or do odd jobs for their keep. Staff inadequate for the care of the aged.
4. *1930*—Federal government passed legislation to phase out almshouses because of their unpopularity. Boarding houses emerged, offering room and board to the aged.
5. Nursing homes emerged—"Mom and Pop" type operations; county nursing homes run by federal and local governments; and religious homes. All provided custodial type care. By 1939 United States had 1200 nursing homes or similar facilities for the aged. Proprietary and nonproprietary homes developed their own organizations.
6. *1940*—Boarding houses started to provide nursing care along with room and board.
   1940 to present—Each state has its own historical development of boarding houses. Today, some states require a license to run a boarding house; others do not.
7. *1966*—Medicare and Medicaid implemented.
   1968—19,000 nursing homes representing 880,000 beds. It is quite possible that Medicare and Medicaid changed the custodial model to medical model to restorative model to 1981 therapeutic model. Today 26,000 nursing homes representing 1.2 million beds.
8. *1985*—"Additional beds in nursing homes will be needed for 246,400 older adults.
   2000—503,086 additional beds will be required."†

---

*Adapted from Ainsworth, T. H.: Quality assurance in long-term care, Germantown, Md., 1977, Aspen Systems Corp.
†Herzog, B. R.: Aging and income, New York, 1978, Human Science Press, p. 242.

license to facilities that substantially meet compliance and have taken action to correct deficiencies. The specified time permitted for provisional license is 6 months (it may be renewed no more than three times). The facility's license to operate is to be displayed within the facility in a readily accessible place for the public to see. The facility's deficiencies and plan of correction are on file with the state and are available to the public upon request. This information is important data for clients and families who are reviewing nursing homes. It can provide a barometer of the care given, which includes the strengths and weaknesses of the facility, before one makes a selection.

Health professionals who see the older adult in nursing homes must realize the complexity of the placement and its effect on the family. Often, the family spends years caring for the older adult with an infirmity. Only after great personal, economic, and psychological expense is the care of the older adult relinquished to an agency. The emotional and economic expense continues after admission to the nursing home. Psychologically, often the guilt is overwhelming for the family. One very helpful support mechanism for the family is a friends and family council. Some states, such as Pennsylvania, are requiring a friends and family council as a regulation for relicensure as a nursing home Medicare/Medicaid provider. More information regarding the Council's implementation and its activities is presented in Chapter 11.

SUMMARY

In this chapter, the nurse was introduced to nursing theory and models. The medical model, the Nightingale model, and the bureaucratic model of nursing practice were described and contrasted so the nurse may identify which model of care she uses for her nursing practice. A brief explanation of nursing theory and its use in nursing, the Roy adaptation theory, Martha Roger's unitary man, and Laurie Gunter's definition of gerontics were presented.

The nurse who works with the older adult in the community or long-term-care facility is not working alone. She is on the front lines, and behind her is a small but growing corps of theorists and researchers working to supply her with an armament of information for practice. These front-line nurses are critical persons in the application of these theories. By participating in the testing of these data, the clinical nurse can confirm or discard the theories. Without clinical nurses, theories are mere exercises in rhetoric. Without theories, clinical nursing is random activity.

The older adult was viewed as a member of a family in the postparental and aging stage. The most significant task for the postparental family is planning for retirement. Major pitfalls that lead to retirement failure were identified. The aging family has many crucial developmental stages and health tasks to address. Each family will address these tasks according to the influence of several variables, which include their cultural, social, psychological, and financial assets, as well as experiences. Black and Asian-American families were presented as selected examples of how cultural variables affect the developmental and health tasks of the older adult.

The existing options for living arrangements outside the family for the older adult were explored. It was noted that 95 percent of older adults live within the community, maintaining their own living quarters or living within a family structure. The institutional model for the remaining 5 percent was traced from its beginning in the sixth century BC to its present-day characteristics. Long-term care in the United States has advanced from a custodial care model to a therapeutic, restorative care model. Medicare, Medicaid and federal and state regulations have been the deciding force behind these advances in the nursing home industry. For example, the levels of nursing care are defined by the rules and regulations for intermediate and skilled facilities. There is no doubt that Medicare and Medicaid create much paperwork; however, the client is the one who will reap the benefit from the paperwork.

REFERENCES

Abdellah, F. G., Foerst, H. V., and Chow, R. K.: PACE: an approach to improving the care of the elderly, Am. J. Nurs. **79:**1109, June 1979.

Adler, S. S.: Anemia in the aged: causes and considerations, Geriatrics **35:**49, April 1980.

Antunes, G., and Gaitz, C. M.: Ethnicity and participation: a study of Mexican-Americans, blacks, and whites, Am. J. Sociol. **80:**1192, 1975.

Atchley, R. C.: The social forces in later life: an introduction to social gerontology, Belmont, Calif., 1972, Wadsworth Publishing Co., Inc.

Auckland, A.: Community nursing care study: Mr. Hogg—chairman, Nurs. Times **73:**703, 12 May 1977.

Austin, B. D.: We managed, Nurs. Times **74:**333, February 1978.

Belsjoe, H.: Retirement: why mandatory? why selective? Hosp. Prog. **59:**6, January 1978.

Bengtson, V. L., Dowd, J. J., Smith, D. H., and others: Modernization, modernity, and perceptions of aging: a cross-cultural study, J. Gerontol. **30:**688, 1975.

Beverley, E. V.: Organizations for seniors—what they stand for, what they offer, Geriatrics **31:**121, November 1976.

Birren, J. E., and others: Handbook of psychology of aging, New York, 1977, Van Nostrand Reinhold Co.

Bolton, C. R.: Humanistic instructional strategies and retirement education programming, Gerontologist **16:**550, December 1976.

Borzilleri, T. C.: The need for a separate consumer price index, Gerontologist **18:**230, June 1978.

Brenneis, C. B.: Developmental aspects of aging in women: a comparative study of dreams, Arch. Gen. Psychiatry **32:**429, April 1975.

Brown, R. J.: Gap exists between what is being done and what can be done about older workers' problems, Geriatrics **32:**38, October 1977.

Butler, R. N., Gertman, J. S., Overlander, D. L., and Schindler, L.: Self-care, self-help, and the elderly, Int. J. Aging Hum. Dev. **10**(1):95, 1979-1980.

Bynum, J. E., Cooper, B. L., and Acuff, F. G.: Retirement reorientation: senior adult education, J. Gerontol. **33:**253, March 1978.

Clark, F. L., and Dunne, A. C.: Aging in industry, Westport, Conn., 1955, Greenwood Press, Publishers.

Conner, K. A., Powers, E. A., and Bultena, G. L.: Social interaction and life satisfaction, an empirical assessment of later-life patterns, J. Gerontol. **34**(1):116, January 1979.

Craigmile, W. M., and others: Domiciliary care of the elderly, Nurs. Times Suppl. **74:**13, 2 February 1978.

Craven, R. F.: Primary health care: practice in a nursing home, Am. J. Nurs. **76:**1958, December 1976.

Daubenmire, M. J., and King, I. M.: Nursing process models: a systems approach, Nurs. Outlook **21:**512, August 1973.

Denham, M. J., and Wills, E. J.: A clinico-pathological survey of thyroid glands in old age, Gerontology **26**(3):160, 1980.

De Beauvoir, S.: The coming of age, New York, 1972, J. P. Putnam's Sons.

Dent, R. V.: Geriatric care in hospital, Nurs. Times **83:**1507, 29 September 1977.

Fischer, D. H.: Growing old in America, New York, 1977, Oxford University Press.

Foster grandparent program sparks life and learning. Hospitals **52:**28, 1 June 1978.

George, I. K., and others: Subjective adaptation to loss of the work role: a longitudinal study, J. Gerontol. **32:**456, July 1977.

Gunter, L.: Education for gerontic nursing, New York, 1979, Springer Publishing Co., Inc.

Gunter, L. M., and Miller, J. C.: Toward a nursing gerontology, Nurs. Res. **26:**208, May-June 1977.

Hardie, M.: The elderly: a challenge to nursing—10. Housing and the elderly, Nurs. Times **73:**1996, 22 December 1977.

Hardy, M. E.: Theories: components, development, evaluation, Nurs. Res. **23:**100, March-April 1974.

Haynes, S. G., McMichael, A. J., and Tyroler, H. A.: Survival after early and normal retirement, J. Gerontol. **33:**269, March 1978.

Heinz, H. G.: How to stop retirement from being one of the toughest jobs in America, Geriatrics **32:**32, January 1977.

Hirsh, C., and others: Homogeneity and heterogeneity among low income Negro and white aged. Paper presented at the Annual Gerontological Society Meetings, Denver, Colorado, 1968.

Ingman, S. R., Lawson, I. R., and Carboni, D.: Medical direction in long-term care, J. Am. Geriatr. Soc. **26:**157, April 1978.

Jackson, J. I.: Aged Negroes: their cultural departures from statistical stereotypes and rural-urban differences, Gerontologist **10:**140, 1970.

Jackson, J. J.: Sex and social class variations in black aged parent-adult-child relationships. Aging Hum. Dev. **2:**96, 1971.

Johnston, D. R.: The impact of waiving compulsory retirement, Hosp. Prog. **59:**58, June 1978.

Katz, M. M.: Behavioral change in the chronicity pattern of dementia in the institutional geriatric resident, J. Am. Geriatr. Soc. **24:**522, November 1976.

Kent, D.: The Negro aged, Gerontologist **11:**48, 1971.

Kimmel, D. C.: Adulthood and aging, New York, 1974, John Wiley & Sons, Inc.

King, I. M.: A conceptual frame of reference for nursing, Nurs. Res. **17:**27, January-February 1968.

Kramer, M.: Reality shock: why nurses leave nursing, St. Louis, 1974, The C. V. Mosby Co.

Kratz, C.: The elderly: a challenge to nursing—3. Old people and their families, Nurs. Times **73:**1719, 3 November 1977.

Kurtz, J. J., and Kyle, D. G.: Life satisfaction and the exercise of responsibility, Social Work **22:**323, July 1977.

Langston, J.: To be aging and well informed, Geriatrics **33:**18, July 1978.

Lazarus, I. W.: A program for the elderly at a private psychiatric hospital, Gerontologist **16:**125, April 1976.

Leader, M. A., and Neuwirth, E.: Clinical research and the non-institutional elderly: a model for subject recruitment, J. Am. Geriatr. Soc. **26:**27, January 1978.

Leinback, R. M.: The aging participants in an area planning effort, Gerontologist **17**(5 Part 1):453, October 1977.

Levine, M. E.: Holistic nursing, Nurs. Clin. North Am. **6:**253, June 1971.

Levine, M. E.: The four conservation principles of nursing. Nurs. Forum **6**(1):45, 1967.

Linn, M. W., and Hunter, K.: Perception of age in the elderly, J. Gerontol. **34:**46, January 1979.

Lowenthal, G., Jr, and Breitenbucher, R.: The geriatric nurse practitioner's value in a nursing home, Geriatrics **30**:87, November 1975.

MacKinnon, M.: Take one empty ward: an experiment in redeployment of resources, Nurs. Times **74**:437, 16 March 1978.

Markides, K. S., and Martin, H. W.: A causal model of life satisfaction among the elderly, J. Gerontol. **34**:86, January 1979.

McEver, D. H.: Ode to patient care, Am. J. Nurs. **79**:1083, June 1979.

McGlone, F. B., and Kick, E.: Health habits in relation to aging, J. Am. Geriatr. Soc. **26**:481, November 1978.

McIver, V.: Freedom to be: a new approach to quality care for the aged, Can. Nurse **74**:19, March 1978.

McKenzie, H.: Help for the single woman with elderly dependents, Nurs. Times **74**:292, 16 February 1978.

Mead, M.: Ethnological aspects of aging, Psychosomatics **8** (Supp.):33, 1967.

Meissner, J. E.: Assessing a geriatric patient's need for institutional care. Nursing 80 **10**:86, March 1980.

Morrison, M. H.: Planning for income adequacy in retirement: the expectations of current workers, Gerontologist **16**:538, December 1976.

Naus, P.: The elderly as prophets, Hosp. Prog. **59**:66, May 1978.

Neugarten, B. L., and Weinstein, K. K.: The changing American grandparent, J. Marriage and Family **22**:199, 1964.

Nightingale, F.: Notes on nursing: what it is, and what is is not, Philadelphia, 1946, J. B. Lippincott Co.

Noelker, L., and Harel, T.: Aged excluded from home health care: an interorganizational solution, Gerontologist **18**:37, February 1978.

Preretirement planning program says, "goodbye is not enough," Hospitals **51**:12, 1 March 1977.

Reisner, C.: Medical screening of old people accepted for residential care (letter), Lancet **2**:474, 26 August 1978.

Rogers, M.: The theoretical basis of nursing, Philadelphia, 1970, F. A. Davis, Co.

Rollins, B., and Feldman, H.: Marital satisfaction over the family life cycle, J. Marriage Family **32**:20, January 1970.

Roy, C.: Introduction to nursing: an adaptation model, Englewood Cliffs, N.J., 1976, Prentice-Hall, Inc.

Rubenstein, D.: An examination of social participation found among a national sample of black and white elderly, Aging Hum. Dev. **2**:172, 1971.

Rule, W. L.: Political alienation and voting attendance among the elderly generation, Gerontologist **17**(5 Pt. 1):400, October 77.

Schorr, T. M.: Yet another scandal (editorial), Am. J. Nurs. **77**:53, January 1977.

Seelbach, W. C.: Gender differences in expectations for filial responsibility. Gerontologist **17**(5 Pt. 1):421, October 1977.

Seelbach, W. C., and Sauer, W. J.: Filial responsibilities, expectations and morale among aged parents, Gerontologist **17**:492, December 1977.

Sherman, S. R., and Newman, E. S.: Foster-family care for the elderly in New York State, Gerontologist **17**:513, December 1977.

Simms, M. L., and Lindberg, B. J.: The nurse person developing perspectives for contemporary nursing, New York, 1978, Harper & Row, Publishers.

Sloane, L.: How do you plan financially for retirement? Am. J. Nurs. **77**:685, April 1977.

Smith, H. L., Discenza, R., and Saxberg, B. O.: Administering long-term care services: decision-making perspective, Gerontologist **18**:159, April 1978.

Snow, R. B., and Havighurst, R. J.: Life style types and patterns of retirement of educators, Gerontologist **17**:545, December 1977.

Struyk, R. J.: The housing expense burden of households headed by the elderly, Gerontologist **17**(5 Pt. 1):447, October 1977.

Tallmer, M.: Some factors in the education of older members of minority groups, J. Geriatr. Psychiatry **10**(1):89, 1977.

Teaff, J. D., Lawton, P., Nahemow, L., and Carlson, D.: Impact of age integration on the well-being of elderly tenants in public housing, J. Gerontol. **33**:126, January 1978.

Thurmott, P.: The elderly: a challenge to nursing—isolation and loneliness. Nurs. Times **73**:1884, 1 December 1977.

Tobin, S. S., and Lieberman, M. A.: Last home for the aged, Washington, 1976, Jossey-Bass Publishers.

Treas, J.: Family support systems for the aged: some social and demographic considerations, Gerontologist **17**:486, December 1977.

Tyberg, D. A.: Creating an intermediate care facility, Am. J. Nurs. **79**:1236, July 1979.

United States Bureau of the Census: Current population report series, P-23, No. 59. Demographic aspects, 1976.

United States Department of Health, Education, and Welfare: Vital statistics of the United States, Vol. II, Sec. 5, Life tables: 1972, Rockville, Md.

Vinick, B. H.: Remarriage in old age, J. Geriatr. Psychiatry **11**(1):75, 1978.

Williams, L. M.: A concept of loneliness in the elderly, J. Am. Geriatr. Soc. **26**:183, April 1978.

4 Achieving health and a high level of wellness

HEALTH MAINTENANCE

What is health? Complete physical and mental well-being is the description of health. Health is more than the absence of disease or infirmity. What is wellness? Wellness is the optimum in efficiency and health in body and mind, characterized by energy, vitality, and zest for life.

Given the stressors present in today's world, health at a 100 percent level is an ideal rather than a reality in most cases. In order to even approximate this high level of wellness, a three-level approach is used: health maintenance, health support during acute illness, and rehabilitation. There are a number of different definitions of health. This three-level approach, however, is most consistent with the aims of the nursing process. In addition, this particular definition is used because it is consistent with the overall goal for the older adult: achievement of optimum health.

The first level, health maintenance, encourages individuals to keep mentally and physically fit and as vigorous as possible. The goal is to have them enjoy life to the fullest, and health education is one important way of achieving this goal. This nurse-client teaching can occur in small groups, large groups, or on a one-to-one basis. The audience and topic to be covered determine the teaching strategy. Such topics as nutrition, personal hygiene, and exercise and safety can be covered. Immunization is another part of first-level health promotion. For the older adult, the immunization protection reduces vulnerability during those months when influenza viruses are epidemic. Care of the older adult with stabilized chronic illnesses is in the realm of first-level health maintenance. Older adults are encouraged to keep as mentally and physically fit as possible, thus maintaining normal social relations, and to elevate the quality of their lives even in the presence of limitations.

The second level of health maintenance is the process of detecting deviations from normal development and noting early signs of ill health. The goal is that, through early screening and prompt attention, abnormalities or illness can be prevented or lessened in severity. The nurse does this through routine health assessment. In addition, second-level health maintenance addresses the need of supporting all the body systems during acute illness.

The third level of health maintenance is the rehabilitation process. The goal is to restore individuals who have been ill or disabled to as full a range of activities of daily living (ADL) as possible.

The family or significant others need to be involved if any of the three levels of health promotion is to be successful and health maintenance obtained. Client goals must be understood and have the support of the family. The nurse mediates between the client and others seeking to elicit appropriate participation.

Advantages of health maintenance

The physiology of the maturing body remains stabilized and fully functioning as long as a state of health is maintained. The trauma of an illness, even a minor one, forces the body to draw upon its limited reserves, and dysfunction follows. It takes a much longer time for the body of an older adult to restabilize itself and recover from illness.

Body and mind cannot be separated. The mental consequences of an illness limit physical activities of older persons, producing a domino effect. When they do not feel well for one reason or another, they become less mobile, are exposed to fewer stimuli, and have a generalized feeling of lack of well-being. Dependency needs increase. The older adult, instead of reaching out to the world around him, becomes introspective, and this often leads to feelings of isolation and loneliness.

Health maintenance is a positive approach to life and well-being for the older adult. The number one assumption in health maintenance is that the individual is an active participant and assumes responsibility for his health and life-style. Health education provides him with information regarding his body functions and living habits. With this information, he can evaluate his life-style and make health support adjustments. For example, Mr. Nash, a 72-year-old retired school teacher, whose joints feel a little stiff in the morning, can learn that a slow to moderate walking pace can offer him many advantages. His joints will be looser, he will have better muscle tone, and it will provide for good venous return in the saphenous veins in his legs. Before getting this health information, Mr. Nash had believed that rest was the only thing he could do for the aches in his joints. Now Mr. Nash walks one block every morning to pick up his newspaper at the local store. The morning exercise has advantages to his mental status too. The stimuli provided include seeing people on the street, talking to the store clerk, and noting the weather. After his walk, Mr. Nash has a feeling of "having done something." The older adult's participation in life's activities need not be extensive to be satisfying. Mr. Nash has a feeling of accomplishment, and that is the important factor.

Older adults can be encouraged to participate in health assessment programs. Such programs are often organized as a part of massive screening projects for hypertension, glaucoma, and diabetes. These are sponsored by the national organizations set up for the specific disease. The American Heart Association, for instance, organizes National Heart Week, when hypertension screening is done nationwide. Many nurses from various districts of the American Nurse's Association contribute their time to health fairs and do diabetic and hypertensive screening. Every region of the National League for Nursing has a community action committee. The Southeastern region of Pennsylvania distributes booklets to older adults detailing services available to senior citizens. Workshops for long-term-care nursing personnel have been presented throughout the state.

Controversy surrounds the cost effectiveness of annual health checkups. Although the cost benefits may be in doubt, there is no question that the client's point of entry for the health assessment does provide a one-to-one tie-in with the health system. This gives the individual an opportunity to complete a simple self-assessment form to indicate any particular worries. The self-assessment form also covers the area of social health. Such topics as smoking habits, drinking patterns, nutrition, and home conditions might be part of the social self-assessment.

Concurrent with the self-assessment is the individual health assessment of the client done by the nurse. During this head-to-toe examination of the client, the nurse notes each body system and identifies that each system is or is not within the norms for the adult. Any deviations from the normal characteristics of the older adult are noted and referred to the physician. The nurse can develop the health teaching plan around the areas of concern of the client and her findings from the health assessment.

Rehabilitation, the third level of health maintenance, seeks to restore the client who has been ill or disabled to as full and independent a life as possible. In this case especially, the client is the individual plus his family or significant others. All of the client learning taking place in the rehabilitation regimen will be for naught if the family does not understand the client's independent function in activities of daily living.

Fundamental to the concept of rehabilitation is the acknowledgement that it is a team effort. The team members often include a speech therapist, physical and occupational therapist, physician, nurse, and psychologist.

The key to effective rehabilitation is the attitude of the professional staff. Support and enthusiasm affect the client's morale and cooperation in the most positive way. Realistic goal setting with the client and therapists fosters feelings of success when they are met both on the part of the professional and the client. Unrealistic goals, whether too high or too low in reaching the client's potential, can lead to discouragement and disillusionment.

NURSING RECORD

In order to see the client as an individual, a nursing record is developed. It is a systematic process to objectively measure the individual's world and where he is in this world. Dimensions of the client's level of physical health, ADL (activities of daily living), social participation, intellectual status, emotional status, and quality of role participation are included.

The client's nursing record contains:

1. The nursing history
2. Findings from the health assessment
3. Results of laborarory examinations
4. Findings and diagnoses of nursing consultants
5. Nursing and medical diagnoses
6. Nursing notes, progress notes from nurses, physician, and other sources.

There are many pupuses for a client's nursing record. This record helps the nurse:

1. Make a nursing diagnosis
2. Design a plan of care for the client
3. Have a written record for teaching nursing and for nursing research
4. Document care for legal purposes

The nursing record provides the nurse with baseline data regarding the client. This record becomes the standard of measurement for this client's progress. The nurse can legally document the success of nursing intervention when she knows where the client started, and what progress he has made as a result of the nursing care.

Nursing interview

The interview period is an excellent time for the establishment of rapport between the client and nurse. A comfortable, private, and nonthreatening climate should be established for the interview, ideally when the client is well, or at least not at the height of an acute illness. It is important to remember that the record is a legal document and the recorded facts are privileged communication that cannot be revealed without the written consent of the client. All entries into the record must be legible, signed, and dated. At a future time, any part of the nursing record can be used as evidence in a court of law.

As the client shares perceptions of his life, and the nurse attends closely to what he is saying, a mutual trusting relationship is fostered. The nurse assesses the client's ability to understand and respond to questions. This provides a level of prediction of the client's ability to understand and cooperate with the nursing care plan.

Data are collected from family and significant others. This information fills gaps left in areas the client finds painful. For example, a community health nurse interviewing a family learns that Mr. Clements has not completed all his grief work after the recent death of his wife of 40 years. His daughter reports to the nurse, "Dad has not been the same since Mom died. Mom used to make all the social arrangements; now Dad does not go out at all."

Auxiliary personnel often collect and report to the nurse important information as they do their work. The data collected from all sources are recorded by the nurse as a part of the client's record.

The data collection phase of the nursing process is ongoing. It is a tool in the hands of the nurse to be used selectively and appropriately. For instance, the nurse cannot expect to get all the information required in one interview. She addresses those parts of the tool that relate to the priority needs of the individual. Bombarding the client with 50 questions is frustrating for the nurse and the client.

The initial interview establishes rapport. The nurse pursues only one or two areas on the nursing history tool. The areas chosen depend on the immediate areas of concern to the client. Anybody, especially the older adult, has difficulty tolerating long interview periods. The nursing history is taken over a period of time. Data collection may take place over several days in an acute care setting, or over several weeks and months in a community or long-term-care setting. It can be done in a structured face-to-face interview, or in an informal caregiving setting.

For example, the nurse teaching about protein sources may lead into questions regarding budget available for food and other necessities. Depending on the budget, appropriate protein sources are listed. The nursing interview requires the nurse to use all of her senses, interpersonal and motor abilities, and concomitant, cognitive elements essential to a nurse-client relationship while carrying out the assessment process.

Subjective and objective data

Data collected fall into two levels, subjective and objective data. Objective data are those that can be measured. For instance, the extent of a rash, the vital signs, or a report from the client of his ability to walk three blocks a day or play nine holes of golf is objective data. A client's complaint of pain or loneliness is subjective data. This is significant information even though it cannot be measured on a clinical scale. How lonely is lonely? Pain threshold varies from individual to individual. A thermometer reading of 103° F indicates fever and a threat to health. Loneliness, on the other hand, cannot be measured with a clinical instrument but can be as damaging to the wellness of the person as a raging fever. So the nurse must obtain both levels of information. Nursing intervention may still be necessary even though an obvious disease process is not present. Objective data give the nurse cues regarding potential health threats from subjective perception areas. Both subjective and objective data are collected by the nurse. The nurse often collects subjective data before clinical evidence appears. The predyspneic agitation signs the nurse sees are subjective signals that there are physiological changes about to occur. Voice tone can supply subjective data. It often gives the cue to look for signs beyond what the client is saying to what his voice is conveying.

NURSING HEALTH HISTORY

There is a relatively standardized format for the nursing history with details varying only slightly from agency to agency. The following list is from the nursing process record (NPR), which is used for clients by nursing students at Rutgers the State University of New Jersey College of Nursing.

Reason for contact
Biographical data
Current health status
Health history
Family history
Social history
Mental and emotional status
Review of systems
Health examination

Data collection, the first component of the nursing process, has as its main element the nursing health history. The nurse, using a broad knowledge base about the older adult, assesses the information in the health history and establishes a nursing diagnosis. The nursing diagnosis completes the first phase of the nursing process, the data collection.

Reason for contact

The reason for contact is a statement made by the older adult in his own words giving his reasons for seeing the nurse at this time. It is one of the few opportunities for the client to have recorded his perceived priorities of needs. In the case of the older adult who is well, the reason for contact might be:

"My yearly check-up."
"I need some help in planning my meals."
"I want my blood pressure checked."

Direct statements of the client should be put in quotation marks. When the older adult is ill, the reason for contact is stated as the chief complaint (CC). The chief complaint is a statement about the health problem that brought the older adult to see the nurse. Included with the statement is a notation regarding the duration of the symptom. Some examples of chief complaints might be:

Headache and blurred vision for 2 days
Cough for 2 weeks that causes chest pain
Joint pains for 6 weeks

When a client presents to the nurse *several* reasons for coming, or chief complaints, with the client's help, the nurse may record them in a priority listing.

Biographical data

Biographical data are usually self-explanatory and collected in the initial contact. They identify the older adult as an individual and give the nurse a frame of reference about him. The importance of this aspect of the nursing health history is its accuracy. The nurse must determine the reliability of the informant and information given. It will give a clue for the need to redo the health history or supply additional information from family, friends, or other reliable sources. The nurse rates the informant and data as *excellent, fair,* or *poor,* and *reliable* and *inclusive* or *confusing* in certain areas.

The following information is included in the biographical section of the nursing health history:

1. Name
2. Address
3. Phone number

4. Social Security number
5. Date of birth and age (in years)
6. Country of origin and current citizenship
7. Religion/ethnic affiliation/language spoken
8. Gender
9. Marital status
10. Occupation/school
11. Formal education
12. Living arrangements
13. Name of person to be notified in case of emergency
    a. Address
    b. Phone number
    c. Informant/relationship to client
    d. Reliability of informant
14. Health insurance
15. Date of interview

CLIENT'S NAME: The client's full first, middle, and last names are recorded. This affords precise identification of the person, because many family names are common in certain geographical areas.

ADDRESS AND PHONE NUMBER: The address given should be the complete mailing address of the client. The older adult occasionally has a permanent address and a residential address. Ask the older adult where he receives his mail, and use this address for any correspondence. The phone number given should be the one that you may use to get in touch with the client.

SOCIAL SECURITY NUMBER: Most older adults carry their Social Security cards and Medicare cards with them. It is important that the numbers recorded are accurate on the agency forms for identification and reimbursement purposes.

DATE OF BIRTH: You may have to help the older adult calculate the year of his birth when he states his age.

COUNTRY OF ORIGIN/RELIGION/ETHNIC AFFILIATION/LANGUAGE: Knowledge of the older adult's religious and cultural identification provides the nurse with cues regarding cultural implications for care planning and intervention.

GENDER: Gender is usually obvious; however, in the case of intersexuality, have the client identify his gender preference.

MARITAL STATUS: The older adult identifies himself as single, married, divorced, a widow, or a widower.

OCCUPATION/SCHOOL: State if the client is retired, and include the former occupation. Since many older adults attend educational programs, ask if they are involved in anything such as this.

FORMAL EDUCATION: Lack of or limited formal education is often an area of embarrassment for the older adult. Instead of asking, "Have you gone to college or high school?" ask "How many years of formal education have you had?"

LIVING ARRANGEMENTS: A statement describing living accommodations is essential in collecting data to plan care for the older adult. The type of housing and with whom they reside are presented in a brief sentence, "Lives with 86-year-old sister, three-room apartment, second story walk-up."

NEXT OF KIN INFORMATION: Request the name, address, and phone number of the person to contact in case of an emergency. This person may be a relative or friend whom the nurse may contact if the need arises.

INFORMANT AND RELIABILITY: When the client himself is unable to give the information to the nurse, the data are obtained from another source. By stating the relationship and reliability of the informer, the nurse can ascertain what additional information must be obtained.

HEALTH INSURANCE: Knowledge of the type and kind of health insurance carried by the older adult permits the nurse to counsel the client on the extent of coverage. If necessary, the nurse can refer the client to social services.

DATE OF INTERVIEW: The date of the interview is important because it places the interview within a specific time frame.

Taking the biographical data often sets the tone for the interview. The question-and-answer format can lead the older adult to believe that the entire interview will be in this style. If the client gets this notion, he sits back, waits for the questions, and feels he is not supposed to give the information on his mind until he is specifically asked. Another method of collecting this kind of information is giving the client a biographical work sheet to fill in himself. The nurse can later transfer the information to the permanent record. Any difficulties in reading and writing are apparent and can be assessed by the nurse. If the client has difficulty understanding English or reading and writing, the nurse is available to assist him. Knowing whether or not the client is literate in English will affect the teaching strategy used as health education is planned.

Current health status

The nurse begins collecting data regarding current health status of the client by eliciting the client's perception of his health at the present time. This perception is contrasted with the significant other's perceptions of the client's health. Specific complaints are listed, with details noting the date and time of the onset, any special characteristics of the complaint, and associated symptoms. The nurse asks the client if there are any factors that influence the complaint and if activities alter the symptoms. The client describes any treatments being given, whether self-prescribed or by a health professional.

After discussing the client's immediate concerns, the nurse explores the client's daily activities and habits. A 24-hour dietary intake is done by the recall method. The client states the food and fluid intake for the previous day. With these data, the nurse can make a gross assessment of his nutritional status. Information is obtained regarding daily bowel and bladder functioning and personal hygiene practices. Specific alcohol, tobacco, and caffeine consumption is recorded. It is best to record the exact quantity rather than expressing the amount with adjectives.

Say	Do not say
Drinks eight cans of beer daily	Heavy drinker
Smokes six cigarettes daily	Light smoker
Drinks three cups coffee and six colas daily	Moderate caffeine intake

Adjectives are subjective conclusions. What constitutes heavy drinking to one person might be light drinking to another.

The nurse lists all medications taken by the client, both prescription and over-the-counter drugs and, if possible, the dosage and frequency. The client relates his recreation and exercise patterns. The activity and the frequency of participation are recorded. Sleeping patterns are reviewed next. The client describes any presleep rituals, customary bedtime, incidents of nocturnal awakenings, and usual hour of arising.

Because adult sexuality is a prerogative of the older adult, patters of sexual interest are explored. Data regarding the availability of a sexual partner, the frequency of intercourse, and the client's perception of satisfaction are discussed. When the nurse initiates the topic of client sexuality, she offers the client the option of addressing any areas of question regarding his sexual functionings as an older adult. Cultural mores and religious values frequently make the topic of sexuality a difficult area for the client to address by himself.

All persons are subject to the stresses of daily living. The older adult is no exception. How a person manages to deal with these stresses depends upon how he has learned to cope with his environment. These coping behaviors develop over the years and are called coping mechanisms. The client should describe how he handles various emotions and stress.

As the current health status assessment continues, the nurse has the client describe his activities during a typical day. This information draws a picture of the general patterns of living for this person as an individual and is called a daily profile.

Health history

The health history describes the client's health promotion and disease prevention practices. Such things as dental examinations, immunizations, and counseling practices are listed.

Developmental data are related in detail. Areas of focus include the physical, psychological, and social parameters of development appropriate for the older adult. Successes and limitations in achieving the developmental milestones of the older adult are noted under the sections of developmental stressors.

Significant past illnesses and hospitalizations are reviewed. Dates of occurrence and descriptions of the nature of the illness, listing specific symptoms and the course of illness, are noted. The nature of the treatment and the prescribing health professional are included. Because of the serious sequence of antibiotic use and blood transfusions, these topics are reviewed as an individual item. The client is also asked specifically if he has any allergies to inhalants, foods, drugs, insects, physical agents, contactants, or biological agents. Foreign travel is noted, naming the country traveled to and the dates of the visit(s).

Family history

The next area of data collection in the nursing history is the family history. A three-generational genogram is recorded (Fig. 4-1). This genogram is basically a diagram of the client's family tree.

A genogram offers the advantage of allowing many facts to be available at a glance rather than having to go through paragraphs of narrative descriptions.

A genogram can be extensive or brief, depending on how it is to be used. When a family is being assessed by a family or mental health counselor, the genogram includes complex information regarding family issues, relationships, and roles. This information helps the therapist identify areas of stress that lead to family dysfunction. When doing a genogram of an older adult, it is important to include communication patterns with other family members and to note the frequency and types of contact. Knowledge of which family members can be included in the client's plan of care enables the nurse to use all the assets the client has available. The client's parents are the first level, the client is the second level, and the client's children are the third level. Knowing the names, ages, sex, health status, occupations, and educational levels of the client's family helps the nurse view much of the scope of the client's family support systems as well as identify potential familial health threats. For example, a client whose mother and aunts have hypertension or breast cancer is in a special risk category and should have more frequent examinations and additional health teaching and counseling in these areas.

It is often useful to include a note regarding the client's pets on the genogram. Frequently the older adult has a pet as a source of companionship or for safety. To some older adults, a pet can be a significant family member.

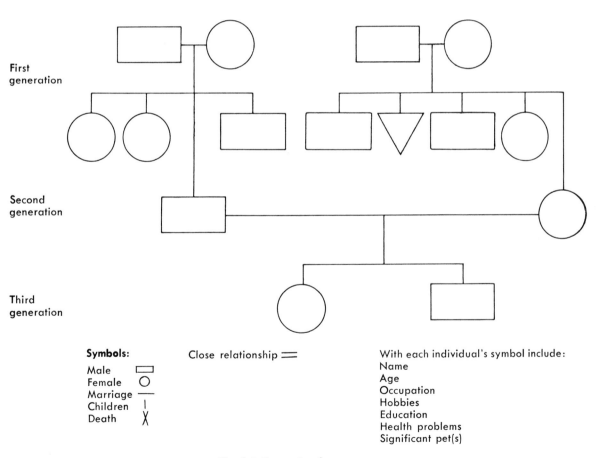

Fig. 4-1. Generational genogram.

Often a genogram will have symbols indicating special relationships and communication patterns within the family network. For example, an older man might socialize with a nephew or a son-in-law more often than with other members of the family. If there are persons who are of particular importance to the client, the nurse may include them in the options for the client as nursing plans are made. Mr. Paris is a 77-year-old man recovering from abdominal surgery, and after discharge from the hospital, will require a few weeks of convalescence. Upon discussing his discharge plans with Mr. Paris, the nurse notes that rather than his daughter's house, perhaps he might stay with his nephew (who is 60 years old, himself). Mr. Paris sees this plan as a good idea. Although he enjoys visiting with his daughter and her family, he tires easily with all the activity of her five children. The thought of staying with his nephew and playing cards and watching TV is much more appealing.

Social history

This area of social data collection is concerned with the community in which the client lives. It is a description of the general environment of the community and type of community (city, town, village, urban, suburban, rural). Since the political and economic systems within a community can set policy regarding recourse for the older adult, these are important items for the nurse to be aware of as she formulates a nursing plan. Such items as population density, environmental hazards, transportation facilities, and other community resources also help the nurse plan for the older adult. If the nurse knows what modes of transportation are available to the client, she can arrange clinic appointments accordingly. For example, some communities have senior citizen transport services on particular days of the week. Knowing this information makes it easy for the nurse to encourage the client to continue good follow-up care. Much information regarding the demographics of an area can be found in the census tracts, which are available at many public libraries. Since an agency often serves a specific geographical area, the nurse can know much about most of her clients' living situations by reading the census tracts. Also, it is useful for a nurse to drive around a community in which she

serves. A firsthand look at the housing available and the conditions of the streets and parks will make her quite aware of the reality of her clients' living situations.

The client's former or present occupation is noted. Since many older adults now attend school or college or avocational programs, the nurse should ask if they are currently attending any programs and to what year did they attend formal educational classes. Fig. 4-2 shows one couple who are in a college history course. Knowing a client's interests certainly enables the nurse to know the older adult as an individual.

The following is a suggested organization of sociological data.

A. Relationships with family and/or significant others
    1. Client's position in the family
    2. Persons with whom client lives
    3. Persons with whom client relates
    4. Recent family crises or changes
B. Environment
    1. Home
    2. Community
    3. Work
    4. Recent changes in environment
C. Occupational history
    1. Jobs held
    2. Satisfaction with present and past employment
    3. Current place of employment
D. Economic status and resources
    1. Source of income
    2. Perception of adequacy or inadequacy of income
    3. Effect of illness on economic status
E. Educational level
    1. Highest degree or grade attained
    2. Judgment of intellect relative to age
F. Daily profile
    1. Rest-activity patterns

Mental and emotional status

A note is always made regarding the client's perceptions of his own mental and emotional status. Is the client generally happy or sad? Take note of the words used to express emotional feelings.

The nursing health history interview is conducted in a style that permits the client to speak

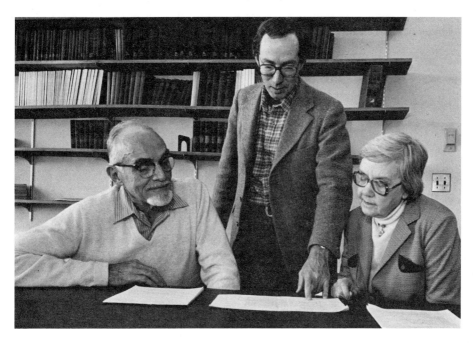

Fig. 4-2. William and Dorothy Crawford discuss aspects of "Family and Society in Europe and America" with Dr. Philip J. Greven, professor of history at Rutgers College. The Crawfords are among dozens of senior citizens auditing courses at Rutgers the State University of New Jersey.

about the various aspects of his life in his own words and in a subject order that is comfortable for him. The nurse listens to the client, and after he has told his story, goes back to cover any area that has not been touched upon. For example, a client may describe in detail his health history and his present health condition without mentioning his family situation. The nurse can then encourage him to discuss this area.

Review of systems (ROS)

The review of systems is designed to survey each body system and to help the client fill in any forgotten information that would be important to complete his record. By asking the client specific questions regarding organ functioning, the nurse helps the client jog his memory. There are a number of ways to do an ROS. The client can be given a printed list of signs and symptoms from each organ system and he checks off those aspects he finds that relate to himself. Care must be taken that the vocabulary used is appropriate for the reading

level and understanding of the older adult. This method has the advantage of not being tied to time restrictions. The client fills the form out at his leisure and brings it with him to the health interview. Another method of doing an ROS is to go through the list verbally with the client after the health interview and before the hands-on health examination. If the nurse is very familiar with all the items on the ROS, she can incorporate it as she does the health examination, reviewing the system as she reaches it in the examination.

The ROS gives the nurse an overview of the past and present health status of each of the client's systems. The nurse recognizes that the human body is composed of integrated subsystems, each of which has its own structure, composition, and function. In addition to the physical system, the person's social and psychological systems are included.

Only the client's positive responses are recorded. A positive response indicates the presence of abnormal signs, symptoms, or medical history. Negative responses are not recorded, simply to facilitate the procedure and eliminate a collection of negatives.

General
Usual state of health
Episodes of chills
Sweats
Episodes of weakness or malaise
Fatigue
Fever
Frequency of infections
Exercise tolerance
Recent and significant gain or loss of weight (if present, amount, time interval, and possible causes)
Usual maximum and minimum weight

Skin
Usual state of health
Previously diagnosed and treated disease
Color changes
Dryness
Ecchymoses
Lesions
Scaling
Masses
Odors
Petechiae
Pruritus
Temperature changes
Texture changes
Care habits

Hair
Texture changes
Unusual pattern of hair loss or growth
Use of dyes
Care regimen

Nails
Changes in appearance
Texture changes
Pitting, curvature
Health maintenance (usually not recorded unless there is a positive response to a symptom; if positive, pattern of bathing and use of soaps, creams, and so on)

Head and face
Usual state of health
Dizziness
Pain
Convulsive seizures
Past trauma

Syncope
Unusual or frequent headache

Eyes
Use of corrective or prosthetic devices
Blurred vision
Current vision, with corrective lenses if applicable
Cataracts
Changes in visual fields or vision
Diplopia
Excessive tearing
Glaucoma
Infections
Pain
Pattern of eye examinations (date of last refraction)
Photophobia
Pruritus
Unusual discharge or sensations

Ears
Usual state of health
Use of prosthetic devices
Discharge
Hearing acuity
Infections
Presence of excessive environmental noise
Tinnitus
Vertigo (subjective or objective)
Care habits, especially ear cleaning

Nose and sinuses
Usual state of health
Olfactory ability
Discharge (seasonal associations)
Epistaxis
Frequency of colds
Obstruction
Pain in infraorbital or sinus areas
Postnasal drip
Sinus infection
Sneezing (frequent or prolonged)
Increased nasal hair

Mouth and throat
Usual state of health
Use of prosthetic devices
Abscesses
Bleeding or swelling of gums
Dryness
Excessive salivation
Chewing and swallowing abilities
Hoarseness

Lesions
Odors
Sore throat
Voice changes
Pattern of dental care
Pattern of dental hygiene
Neck and nodes
Masses
Node enlargement
Pain with movement or palpation
Mobility limitations
Swelling
Tenderness
Breasts
Discharge
Masses
Pain
Nipple changes
Tenderness
Self-examination pattern
Gynecomastia
Respiratory and cardiovascular systems
Usual state of health
Past diagnosis of respiratory or cardiovascular
  system disease: pleurisy, bronchitis, tubercu-
  losis, pneumonia, asthma, respiratory infec-
  tions, emphysema
Cough
Cyanosis
Dyspnea (if present, amount of exertion pre-
  cipitating it)
Edema
Hemoptysis
Orthopnea (number of pillows needed to sleep
  comfortably)
Night sweats
Pain (exact location and radiation and effect of
  respiration)
Palpitations
Sputum
Stridor
Wheezing
Paroxysmal nocturnal dyspnea
Date of last roentgenogram or electrocardiogram
Hypertension
Intermittent claudication
Cold extremities
Phlebitis
Postural or permanent skin color changes
Rheumatic fever

Chorea
Syphilis
Diphtheria
Gastrointestinal system
Usual state of health
Appetite
Bowel habits
Previously diagnosed problems
Abdominal pain
Ascites
Change in stool color
Constipation
Diarrhea
Dysphagia
Eructations
Flatulence
Food idiosyncracies
Hematemesis
Hemorrhoids
Hernia
Indigestion
Infections
Jaundice
Nausea
Pruritus
Rectal bleeding
Rectal discomfort
Recent changes in habits
Thirst
Vomiting
Previous roentgenograms
Urinary system
Usual state of health
Past diagnosed problems
Usual patterns of urination
Anuria
Color
Change in stream
Dysuria
Enuresis
Flank pain
Frequency
Hematuria
Hesitancy of stream
Incontinence
Passage of stones or gravel
Nocturia
Oliguria
Polyguria
Pyuria

Urinary system—cont'd
Retention
Stress incontinence
Suprapubic pain
Urgency
Genital system—male
Usual health
Lesions
Impotence
Masses
Discharge
Pain
Prostate problems
Swelling
Genital system—female
Diagnosed problems
Lesions
Pruritus
Vaginal discharge
Frequency of Pap smear (date of last exam)
Menstrual history
Age at menarche
Age at menopause
Obstetrical history (for each pregnancy)
Prenatal course
Complications of pregnancy
Duration of pregnancy
Description of labor
Date of delivery
Type of delivery (vaginal, caesarean section)
Condition, sex, and weight of baby
Postpartum course
Place of prenatal care and hospitalization
Frequency of menses
Duration of flow
Amount of flow
Date of last menstrual period (LMP)
Dysmenorrhea
Menorrhagia
Metrorrhagia
Polymenorrhea
Amenorrhea
Dyspareunia
Genital system—both sexes
Ability to perform and enjoy satisfactory sexual
    intercourse
Infertility
Sterility
Veneral disease

Extremities and musculoskeletal system
Usual state of health
Past diagnosis of disease
Extremities
    Coldness
    Deformities
    Discoloration
    Edema
    Intermittent claudication
    Pain
    Thrombophlebitis
Muscles
    Cramping (day/night)
    Pain
    Weakness
    Wasting or atrophy
Bones and joints
    Stiffness
    Swelling
    Redness
    Heat
    Pain
    Limitation of movement
    Fractures
    Back pain
Central nervous system
Usual state of health
Past diagnosis of disease
Anxiety
General behavior change
Loss of consciousness
Mood change
Nervousness
Seizures
Speech
    Aphasia
    Dysarthria
Cognitive ability
    Changes in memory
    Disorientation
    Hallucinations
Motor
    Ataxia
    Imbalance
    Paralysis
    Paresis
    Tic
    Tremor
    Spasm

Sensory
  Pain
  Paresthesia (hyperesthesia, anesthesia)
  Sleep disturbances
Endocrine system
Usual state of health
Adult changes in size of head, hands, or feet
Diagnosis of diabetes or thyroid disease
Presence of secondary sex characteristics
Dryness of skin or hair
Exophthalmos
Goiter
Hair distribution
Hormone therapy
Hypoglycemia
Intolerance to heat or cold
Polydipsia
Polyuria
Polyphagia
Postural hypotension
Weakness
Hematopoietic (blood-forming) system
Usual state of health
Past diagnosis of disease
Anemia
Bleeding tendencies
Blood transfusion
Blood type
Bruising
Exposure to radiation
Lymphadenopathy

Health examination

The health examination differs from the review of systems in that it is a direct physical evaluation of each system. In the health examination, the nurse determines if each system is within the normal range of adequate functioning.

As the selected reading at the end of the chapter, Physical Assessment Skills: a Historical Perspective," describes, nurses have been doing health examinations since Florence Nightingale's time. The examination in its entirety is used in a health screening program or in parts as the nurse gives care in hospitals or long-term-care facilities. It is also useful for the community health nurse making home visits. She can make an initial assessment of her older adult client or note significant reportable changes in his condition.

Systematic health assessment courses are now being taught in schools of nursing as well as many continuing education programs. In addition, textbook sources offer the nurse complete presentation of health assessment skills.

The following pages present a health examination outline geared specifically for the older adult. It incorporates the normal physiological changes of aging and common characteristics of the older man and woman.

The examination begins with the general survey and then includes each part of the body systematically:
  Integumentary system
  Head and face
  Ears, nose, mouth, and throat
  Eyes
  Neck and thyroid
  Chest and lungs
  Breasts
  Heart and neck vessels
  Abdomen
  Male and female genitalia
  Muscles, bones, and joints
  Neurological system
  Psychosocial status

General survey

The *general survey* is an overall inspection of the client as the nurse first meets the client and is seated for the interview. The nurse notes the older adult's appearance, manner of dress, personal hygiene, body development, and posture. She notes the relationship of apparent weight and height proportions, apparent age, gait, and general body movements. As she listens to the client during the introduction, any obvious speech problems are noted. In the initial phase of the interview, the nurse notes the appropriateness of mood and mental state.

After explaining to the client what is included in the health examination, the nurse permits the client to have privacy while changing into the examination gown.

Vital signs

1. To document age-related height decrease in status, measure the person head to toe without shoes. Then measure fingertip to fingertip with

arms extended. The head-to-toe measurement should equal the fingertip measurement. Any difference in height indicates skeletal shrinkage.

NORMAL FINDINGS: Any skeletal reduction in skeletal height up to 1½ to 2 inches is normal.

2. Weight: Weigh the client.

3. Blood pressure: Postpone blood pressure until at least 10 minutes into the interview if the client is anxious. Choose a bladder cuff at least 20 percent wider than the diameter of the arm. Any smaller or wider will distort the reading.

NOTE: Increased blood pressure will be seen as an increased systolic rate, particularly after exercise. Pulse pressure should range from 30 to 50 mm Hg.

4. Temperature: May be febrile at 99° F (37.2° C).

NORMAL FINDINGS: The older adult can have low (95° F) early morning temperatures. Daily range: 95° to 100° F oral (35° to 37.8° C).

5. Pulse rate, apical and radial: Usually 50 to 100 beats/minute. Pulse deficit should be noted on all older adults.

NORMAL FINDINGS: Resting heart rate declines. This is reflected in decreased cardiac output.

6. Respiration rate: Slow and irregular rate; range 14 to 18/minute.

Integumentary system

1. Describe findings in assessing the skin. Inspect and palpate the skin, noting its color, edema, lesions, mobility, moisture, pigmentation, temperature, texture, thickness, turgor, and vascularity.

NORMAL FINDINGS: Skin is very slightly cooler and pale. Wrinkling is due to shrinkage of the dermis. Epidermis undergoes little structural change, appears thin, particularly over the backs of the hands. Age spots (senile lentigo) appear. Sebeceous and sweat glands are less active. Turgor is reduced; skin appears lax. Test skin at the iliac crest—it feels dry. Lesions appear: seborrheic, keratosis, irregular round or oval, brown, warty. Follow skin creases on the trunk and head and neck. Comedones (blackheads) appear. Small, round, red or brown cherry angiomas are found on the trunk. Senile telangiectasia is common. Vitiligo is a lack of pigment, local or generalized. Acrochordons, small, soft, flesh-colored skin tags, are found near the neck and axilla.

2. Describe findings in assessing the hair. Inspect and palpate the hair noting its color, distribution pattern, quantity, and quality (on scalp, pubic area, and other parts of body), texture (feels dry and appears fine), and luster.

NORMAL FINDINGS: The hair is gray and thinning; there is a loss of scalp hair. Pubic hair is thinned, with low luster.

3. Describe findings in assessing the fingernails and toenails. Inspect the nails noting thickness, color, contour, and consistency of nailbed.

4. Palpate the nails, noting their mobility.

NORMAL FINDINGS: The rate of nail growth is slower.

5. Describe findings in assessing the mucous membranes. Inspect the mucous membrane noting the state of hydration and the color.

Head and face

1. Describe findings in assessing the head.

NORMAL FINDINGS: Nasal and facial bones appear sharp and angular. The loss of outer eyebrows is not uncommon in women. Facial features may appear asymmetrical because of missing teeth or poorly fitting dentures.

2. Inspect and palpate the scalp noting the condition, lumps/lesions, and scars.

3. Inspect the general size and contour of skull. Note any lumps, deformities, or tenderness.

4. Palpate superficial temporal arteries for thickness, pulsations, or tenderness.

5. Note the client's facial features: expression, symmetry, size, movements, and position.

6. Note the presence and distribution of eyebrows.

NORMAL FINDINGS: The eyebrows in older men may be bushier than in younger men.

7. Observe the skin, noting its color, pigmentation, texture, thickness, hair distribution pattern, and lesions.

8. Describe the findings in assessing the sinuses. Note any tenderness, swelling, or redness.

9. Auscultate head and neck for bruits.

10. Describe findings in assessing client's complaints of hearing sounds in the head or neck.

Ears, nose, mouth, throat

1. Describe the findings in assessing auditory acuity. Test one ear at a time for soft, medium, and loud whisper, soft, medium, and loud voice, or watch ticking. Speak slowly, do not overlap

words. A stress situation is created when words come too fast to be processed by the central nervous system of the older adult. Use tuning forks for the frequencies of 512 Hz, 1024 Hz, and 2048 Hz, the essential range of speech. Report findings for each frequency bilaterally. Use 2048 Hz frequency test screens for high frequency loss; which is common in the older adult.

NORMAL FINDINGS: Hearing loss is gradual over the seventh, eighth, and ninth decades; it includes all frequencies. One fourth of all persons in the eighth decade have difficulty with fine discriminations. Pitch discrimination is less discrete.

2. Test for lateralization using the Weber test: The client may become confused when tone is perceived in the poorer ear, a result of vibratory, not sensory, stimulation.

3. Test for air and bone conduction using the Rinne Test. The opposite ear must be masked with another noise source of a gently moving finger.

4. Describe the findings in assessing the external ear. Inspect the auricle and surrounding tissue, noting deformities, skin lesions, or lumps.

NORMAL FINDINGS: The ears appear large in proportion to the face.

5. With the otoscope, describe the findings in assessing the inner ear. Inspect the canal for presence of wax (cerumen), discharge, foreign bodies, hair, and color of canal walls.

NORMAL FINDINGS: If hearing loss is age related, otoscope examination results should be normal. Cerumen is often the cause of hearing loss.

6. Identify landmarks: pars tensa, umbo, handle and short process of malleus, anterior and posterior folds, and pars flaccida.

7. Inspect the tympanum for color, luster, position of handle of malleus, arc of light, and lesions.

NORMAL FINDINGS: The tympanum may not have the pearly white color of a younger person. It often has a dull and retracted appearance bilaterally.

8. Describe findings in assessing the nose. Inspect the nose for shape, symmetry, inflammation, exudate, and flaring.

9. With the otoscope, inspect the lower portions of the nose, then tilt the head backward to visualize the upper portions. Note the color, hair, swelling, exudate, or bleeding of nasal mucosa; bleeding, exudate, perforation, or deviation of nasal septum;

inferior and middle turbinates, and color, swelling, exudate, or polyps of middle meatus.

10. Describe the findings in assessing the mouth and pharynx. Inspect the lips for color, symmetry, hydration, lumps, ulcers, cracking, dribble, and edema.

11. Palpate mandibular joint and have client open and close mouth to test for mobility and absence of crepitus and tenderness.

12. Note the general hygiene of the mouth. Inspect buccal mucosa for color, pigmentation, ulcers, and nodules.

13. Describe the findings in assessing the gums and teeth. Have the client remove dentures. Inspect the gums for inflammation, swelling, bleeding, retraction, and discoloration.

NORMAL FINDINGS: Gums recede, and more of the tooth is exposed.

14. Inspect the teeth for position, shape, caries, mobility, number, and malocclusion.

15. Inspect the hard palate for color, architecture, and lesions.

16. Describe the findings in assessing the tongue. Inspect the dorsum for color, papillae, smoothness, cracks, and coating.

NORMAL FINDINGS: Lateral papillae atrophy is common. Generalized papillae atrophy is abnormal.

17. Test the hypoglossal (twelfth) cranial nerve.

18. Inspect the tongue for size, symmetry, and movement. Observe for cyanosis under indirect light. Florescent light can give a blue hue to tongue. If the tongue and lips appear cyanotic, have the client breathe oxygen for 2 minutes. A color change confirms arterial hypoxemia.

19. Inspect under the surface of tongue and the floor of the mouth for coating, nodules, ulcerations, induration, swelling, and varicosities.

20. Palpate the Wharton ducts for swelling and abnormalities.

21. Observe the tongue in mouth at rest for movement.

22. Inspect the soft palate, the anterior and posterior pillars, the uvula, tonsils, and posterior pharynx, noting the color, symmetry, evidence of exudate, edema, ulceration, tonsillar enlargement, and thrush.

23. Palpate suspicious area for induration and tenderness.

24. Describe the findings in assessing the pharynx. Note the swallowing reflex and muscle con-

trol while observing the client drinking a small glass of water.

25. Test for vagus (tenth) cranial nerve. Note the number of swallows needed, if any fluid remains in mouth, and dribbling, and any coughing or sputtering.

26. Note any mouth odors.

Voice and speech

Report slurred sounds in speech pattern. "S" and "R" sounds are frequent, and early sounds are affected.

NORMAL FINDINGS: After 50, the female voice becomes more masculine, with a drop in fundamental frequency. After 60, voice fatigue, or "tired voice," is common after long conversations. After 80, voice frequency is significantly higher than at 65 to 79.

Eyes

1. Test visual acuity at least every 3 to 5 years. Test near vision. Have the client read newspaper print of various sizes. Use the Snellen eye chart. Give instructions slowly and clearly. A hurried pace distorts findings because the client is under stress. With the client at 20 feet, and using an eye shield, not a hand, to cover the eye, test both eyes with and without glasses if the client wears glasses. Reading glasses will cause blurring in distant vision. Note if bifocals are being worn. Record findings. Vision changes leading to more frequent change of lenses are suspicious. When the E on Snellen chart cannot be read, note (1) if hand movements at 12 inches from eye can be seen, or (2) if penlight beam on the eye can be perceived.

NORMAL FINDINGS: Presbyopia is common.

2. Test visual fields using the confrontation method with the client and nurse positioned correctly and the client instructed on the procedure. Test both eyes. Map out the visual field on a graph.

NORMAL FINDINGS: Peripheral vision diminishes. Gross visual field defects result from diabetic and hypertensive complications more than from age, per se.

3. Test pupillary reaction to light. Inspect for direct reaction and consensual reaction.

NOTE: A decrease in accommodation is progressive.

4. Test pupillary reaction to accommodation. Observe for pupillary constriction and convergence of the eyes.

NORMAL FINDINGS: The pupils should react quickly to light and accommodation.

5. Test the extraocular movement range in the six cardinal positions of gaze. Inspect for parallel movements in each direction, abnormal movements of eyes, relation of upper eyelid to globe in upward and downward gaze, and convergence.

NORMAL FINDINGS: The extraocular movement range should be same as in younger persons. Nystagmus is normal on lateral gaze.

6. Test the corneal light reflex. Perform the cover-uncover test. Describe the findings in assessing the eyes. Inspect the eyelids for position in relationship to eyeballs, edema, infection, color, lesions, and the ability to close completely.

NORMAL FINDINGS: The eyelids and surrounding skin become thin, wrinkled, and pigmented. Folds or bags appear under the eyes.

7. Inspect the eyelashes for distribution, condition, and direction of growth.

NORMAL FINDINGS: Ectropion and entropion are common and painful, but easily correctable.

8. Inspect the lacrimal apparatus for enlargement, swelling, and tearing.

NORMAL FINDINGS: Tearing increases; the eyes of older adults are particularly sensitive to wind, cold, and dust.

9. Palpate the nasolacrimal duct for tenderness and regurgitation of material through the puncta.

10. Inspect the conjunctiva and sclera for color, nodes, and swelling, which may be the first signs of disease.

NORMAL FINDINGS: The conjunctiva are thinner and more sensitive; subconjunctival hemorrhages are more frequent; the pain threshold in the eye is reduced. Small yellow papular growths called pinguiculae may appear nasally toward the limbus. Normally, few changes occur in the color of the sclera.

11. Inspect the cornea and lens for opacities and ulcers.

NORMAL FINDINGS: The light permeability of the lens and cornea decreases. The lens becomes progressively more dry and opaque. The age of onset varies widely. Every lens opacity is actually a cataract but is significant only when vision is impaired.

12. Test the corneal reflex. Inspect the iris for shape and coloration.

NORMAL FINDINGS: Arcus senilis is a white ring

around the outer margin of cornea depigmentation. Irregular pigmentation is common. Normal pigment is replaced by pale brown areas.

13. Inspect the pupils for size, shape, and equality of size. Do not dilate pupils; that could produce acute closed-angle glaucoma.

NORMAL FINDINGS: Gross irregularity is abnormal, but the pupils are smaller and more irregular than in younger persons.

14. With the ophthalmoscope, inspect the lens noting the red reflex and opacities.

NORMAL FINDINGS: Peripheral wedge-shaped opacities and cobweblike central opacities are common.

15. Inspect the vitreous body, noting transparency.

NOTE: Peripheral opacities do not interfere with vision to any great extent. Central opacities cause vision impairment and decreased light permeability of the vitreous humor.

16. Inspect the retina noting the size (disc diameter) shape, margin distinctness, and color of the optic disc; the disc/cup ratio; and the vessels—the number, direction, A:V ratio, light reflex, vessel crossing, vessel pattern, venous pulsations, fundus color, and macula color.

NORMAL FINDINGS: The optic disc is the same in older adults as in younger age groups. Minor irregularities of vessel size and tortuosity are common. Gross irregularities of the retinal vessels or macular changes are significant.

NOTE: Black pigmentation and hemorrhages around macula often indicate visual impairment.

17. Assess intraocular pressure. Palpate the eyeball to complete the tactile tension test. Use the tonometer test to assess intraocular pressure.

Neck and thyroid

1. Describe findings in assessing the neck. Inspect the neck for symmetry, masses, scars, swelling, muscle function, and stiffness.

2. Auscultate for bruits.

3. Identify the hyoid bone, thyroid cartilages, and trachea.

4. Inspect the trachea for deviation.

5. Inspect the neck for visible thyroid tissue; have the client swallow sips of water, and observe for bulging of thyroid tissue.

6. Palpate the thyroid, noting its size, shape, symmetry, tenderness, and nodules.

NOTE: The thyroid is not normally palpable; the isthmus may be palpable.

7. Auscultate the thyroid for bruits.

Lymphatics

1. Palpate the lymph nodes for location, size, delimitation, mobility, surface characteristics, consistency, and tenderness. Palpate nodes in each of major chains as the particular area of the body is being assessed.

NORMAL FINDINGS: Small firm mobile nodes in axilla and groin are not uncommon. All other areas should have nonpalpable nodes.

The breasts

1. Examine the female breasts, noting the size, shape, position, contour, appearance (color, thickening, edema, venous pattern), and skin retraction.

NORMAL FINDINGS: Breasts appear flaccid and drooping.

2. Inspect the nipples and areola noting their size, shape, direction in which they point, and any rashes, ulcerations, discharge, pigment change, erosions, crusting, scaling, nodules, and swelling.

NORMAL FINDINGS: The size and erection ability of nipples are diminished.

3. Palpate the breasts with the client's arms in the following four positions:

At side

Raised over head

Hands pressed against hips

Leaning forward

Palpate the breast systematically, noting consistency/elasticity of tissue, induration, tenderness, and nodules—their location, size, shape, consistency, delimitation, mobility, and tenderness.

NORMAL FINDINGS: Breast tissue is atrophied. Lumps are very easy to palpate. Fat tissue remains primarily in the lower quadrants. After age 70 any palpable mass not fat tissue is likely to be malignant. Most lesions occur in the upper quadrants. Alveolar ducts reduced in size.

4. Palpate each nipple and areola, noting the elasticity, discharge, nodules, and tenderness.

NOTE: Any nipple discharge should be sent to a lab for cytology study. Note the color, amount, and consistency. Nipple and areolar areas are particular cancer sites in the older woman.

Be particularly sensitive to a client's sense of modesty. A woman in her seventies is very much a product of Victorian modesty. An examination gown worn backwards (that is, with the opening in the front) offers the client a feeling of being covered while the breasts are being examined. She can keep her underpants on until it is time for the pelvic exam. These coverings will help keep her warm during the examination also.

5. Examine the male breast. Distinguish between fat pads and mammary tissue.

NOTE: If breast cancer is to occur in a male, it most often occurs after age 65.

Chest and lungs

1. Identify major anatomical landmarks of the thorax: the suprasternal notch, sternal angle, second rib, second interspace, seventh cervical and first thoracic vertebrae, midsternal line, midclavicular lines, midaxillary lines, intraclavicular space, sixth rib at the midclavicular line, and eighth rib at the midaxillary line. Note the trachea, left main bronchus, and right main bronchus anteriorly and posteriorly.

NOTE: Important landmarks should be identified in the presence of kyphoscoliosis.

2. Examine the posterior chest first, noting posture, contour, general development, anteroposterior diameter, lateral diameter, profile, deformities of the thorax slope of the ribs, retraction of interspaces during inspiration, local lag, respiratory movement, and rate and rhythm of breathing.

NORMAL FINDINGS: Anterioposterior diameter increases with age.

NOTE: Kyphosis is progressive. It is additionally permanent when combined with osteoporosis in older women. Also, calcification of the costal cartilages can cause reduced mobility of the ribs.

3. Palpate the posterior chest for tenderness, masses, sinus tracts, crepitation, edema, respiratory excursion (range and symmetry), and vocal or tactile fremitus (compare symmetrical areas using one hand). Identify, describe, and localize any areas of increased or decreased fremitus; palpate chest expansion; and estimate the level of the diaphragm on each side.

4. Percuss the posterior chest for areas of abnormal percussion sounds; locate and describe them. Percuss diaphragmatic excursion.

NOTE: Poor muscle tone might decrease respiratory excursion.

5. Auscultate the posterior chest for air flow through the tracheobronchial tree; the presence of fluid, mucus, or obstruction in the passages; the condition of the surrounding lungs and pleural space; quality, intensity, and duration of breath sounds; and adventitious (abnormal) breath sounds. Identify, describe, and locate any abnormality.

NORMAL FINDINGS: Breath sounds may be distant as a result of kyphosis. Observe the client for light-headedness during the deep breathing portion of examination. Hyperresonance may be auscultated as a result of progressive, age-related, emphysemic changes. However, blood gases do not show the increased serum CO_2 and bicarbonate found in pathological emphysema.

6. Examine and inspect the anterior chest for posture, contour, general development, pattern of respiration, shape, width of costal angle, retraction of interspaces or supraclavicular fossae during inspiration, bulging during expiration, use of normally quiet accessory muscles of breathing on inspiration and abdominal muscles on expiration, local lag or impairment of respiratory movement, rate and rhythm of breathing, increased length in expiration, and the presence of spontaneous coughing or sputum. Ask the client to cough and note the strength of the cough. Note any spontaneous cough or sputum production. They often become so routine that the client fails to mention them in the history.

7. Palpate the anterior chest for areas of tenderness, edema, masses, crepitation, respiratory excursion, and vocal or tactile fremitus.

NOTE: A weak or absent cough ability places the client in great risk of respiratory infection. A combination of an increasingly rigid chest wall, decreased muscle strength, and few respiratory cilia decreases the propulsive action of the cough in the older adult. This in turn greatly increases the risk of mechanical or infectious respiratory problems. Any sputum should be thin and clear.

8. Percuss the anterior chest for areas of abnormal percussion; note, describe, and locate any abnormal area; identify the area of liver dullness; and identify the area of gastric tympany.

9. Auscultate the anterior chest for quality of breath sounds, intensity of breath sounds, duration of breath sounds, and adventitious sounds.

Heart and neck vessels

1. Inspect and palpate the heart, rating precordial size, pulsations, symmetry, thrills, vibrations of valve closure, heaves, and retractions.

2. Palpate the apical impulse, noting the point of maximal impulse (PMI), its location, diameter, amplitude, and duration.

NOTE: The PMI is normally at the midclavicular line at the fifth intercostal space. It may be displaced with kyphoscoliosis or thoracic cage deformation. The PMI should be palpated as less than 2 cm. A larger palpable PMI indicates hypertrophy. The PMI should be synchronous with the carotid impulse.

3. Identify the left cardiac border, and percuss it, moving medially at the third, fourth, and fifth intercostal spaces.

4. Percuss the heart, the outline of left border of cardiac dullness at the third, fourth, and fifth interspaces, then measure the distance between the border of dullness and the midsternal line in centimeters.

NORMAL FINDINGS: It is normally 7 to 10 cm.

5. Auscultate the apical pulse for 1 full minute. Note the rate and rhythm; S_3 gallops are abnormal and are heard best at the apex on expiration; S_4 or atrial gallops can be functional or indicate pathological conditions.

6. Auscultate the heart, identifying the first and second heart sounds and the heart rate and rhythm.

7. Auscultate the aortic, pulmonic, third left interspace (Erb's point), tricuspid, and mitral areas systematically. At each auscultatory area, listen to the first and second heart sounds for intensity and splitting (extra sounds in systole or diastole), noting the timing, intensity, and pitch. Note also systolic or diastolic murmurs: their timing, location, radiation, intensity, pitch, and quality.

NORMAL FINDINGS: A soft systolic ejection murmur can be heard at the apex in 60 percent of older adults, a result of sclerotic changes in the aortic valve. Diastolic murmurs are always abnormal.

8. Inspect and palpate jugular veins for pressure and pulse waves. Identify the highest point at which pulsations of the internal jugular vein can be seen. Palpate the external jugular vein bilaterally. Observe the jugular venous pulsations, noting amplitude and timing.

9. Examine the neck for carotid artery pulsations, noting amplitude, contour, quality, rate, and rhythm. Auscultate for bruits.

NOTE: When the client is sitting, jugular venous pulsations should not be visible. At a 45-degree elevation of the trunk, jugular venous pulse should be no more than 1 to 2 cm above the manubrium. When venous pressure is markedly elevated, the neck vein distension can be up to the jaw. Measure the vertical distance between this point and the sternal angle.

10. Palpate all major pulse sites: temporal, carotid, radial, brachial, femoral, popliteal, dorsal, and posterior tibial. They should be present and of equal rate, quality, volume, and amplitude.

Abdomen

1. Drape a towel over the genitals to provide privacy, and inspect the skin of the abdomen, noting scars, striae, dilated veins, rashes, lesions, distributions of hair, signs of dehydration, and pigmentation.

NORMAL FINDINGS: The abdominal wall appears slack and thin.

2. Inspect the umbilicus, noting contour, location, inflammation, and hernia.

3. Inspect the abdomen, noting contour, shape, edema, symmetry, visible bowel loops, masses, hernias, pulsations, venous patterns, and movement—respiratory or peristaltic. Check hernia-prone areas: the midline, umbilicus, and surgical scars at the inguinal ligaments.

4. Auscultate the abdomen systematically in each quadrant, including the inguinal region, noting bowel sounds, bruits, and friction rubs.

NORMAL FINDINGS: Men are abdominal breathers more than are women. Bowel sounds occur every 5 to 15 seconds; the normal range is 5 to 34 per minute.

5. Percuss the abdomen lightly in each of the four quadrants, noting tympany, dullness, presence of fluid, organ enlargement, abdominal tenderness or pain, muscular resistance, and superficial organs and masses.

6. Percuss gastric tympany.

7. Percuss splenic dullness, noting the level of the inferior splenic border.

8. Palpate the abdomen systematically and lightly, including inguinal areas, noting muscular

resistance, abdominal tenderness or pain, and superficial organs and masses. Use light palpation to examine hernias found upon inspection.

NORMAL FINDINGS: Frequently abdominal muscles feel flabby and thin; abdomen feels soft, not elastic.

NOTE: The presence of good muscle tone aids in the processes of urinating and defecating.

9. Palpate the abdomen systematically using deep palpation, noting abdominal organs; masses, further noting their location, size, shape, consistency, tenderness, pulsations, and mobility; tenderness or pain (including rebound); and area of rectum and sigmoid for fecal material, which has the consistency of a boggy, round, soft mass.

10. Palpate the liver, noting the border of the liver and any tenderness.

NORMAL FINDINGS: Normal liver dimensions are 4 to 8 cm at the midsternal line.

11. Percuss the border of liver dullness at the midsternal line and the midclavicular line (6 to 12 cm).

NOTE: The lower border of the liver should not be more than 3 cm below the costal margin.

12. Palpate the right kidney, noting size, contour, and any tenderness.

NOTE: The thin abdomen permits palpation of the lower pole of the right kidney 4 cm above the right iliac crest at the midinguinal line.

13. Palpate the left kidney.

NOTE: The left kidney is not normally palpable.

14. Palpate the spleen.

NOTE: It must be enlarged three times normal size in order to be palpated.

15. Palpate the aorta, noting aortic pulsation.

NORMAL FINDINGS: The normal aorta is 2.5 to 4 cm wide.

16. Auscultate for bruits, and always include screening for abdominal aneurysm.

NORMAL FINDINGS: Most older adults have overt symptoms.

Male genitalia

1. Describe findings in assessing the male genitalia. Inspect the penis skin and prepuce glans and urethral meatus, noting their location and any ulcers, scars, nodules, discharge, edema, and lesions.

2. Palpate the penis, noting size, contour, inflammation, tenderness, induration, scarring, masses, and shaft induration.

3. Inspect the scrotum, noting size, consistency, masses, contents, contour, nodules, inflammation, ulcers, and swelling.

NORMAL FINDINGS: Seminal vesicles decrease in weight.

4. Palpate each testis and epididymis, noting size, shape, consistency, and tenderness.

5. Palpate the spermatic cord, vas deferens, epididymis, and superficial inguinal ring, noting any nodules and swelling.

6. Inspect inguinal and femoral areas, noting bulges and weakness of the internal ring.

7. Palpate the external inguinal ring, noting any herniating mass.

8. Describe findings in assessing the anus and rectum of a male client. Inspect sacrococcygeal and perianal areas, noting any lumps, inflammation, rashes, or excoriation.

9. Inspect the anus, noting any lesions.

10. Palpate the anus, noting the sphincter and any tenderness, irregularities, or nodules.

11. Palpate the rectal wall systematically, noting any nodules and irregularities.

12. Describe findings in assessing the prostate in the male client. Palpate the prostate, noting the size, shape, consistency, and any nodules or tenderness.

NORMAL FINDINGS: At age 40 to 50, the prostate shows slight irregularity in epithelium thickness. At age 50 to 60, there is muscle atrophy leading to fibrosis, also decreased elasticity and hypertrophy.

13. Have the client describe urine stream initiation and flow. Impaired stream indicates urethral obstruction.

14. Inspect fecal material, noting any occult blood.

Female genitalia

1. Describe findings in assessing the female genitalia. Inspect external genitalia: the labia minora, the clitoris, the urethral orifice, the introitus, Skene glands, and Bartholin glands, noting signs of inflammation, ulceration, discharge, swelling, nodules, lesions, plaques, lacerations, varicosities, and masses.

NORMAL FINDINGS: During early postmenopausal years, the labia become thin and the pubic hair sparse. The vulva becomes markedly atrophic during later years because of loss of subcutaneous fat of the labia majora and minora and the clitoris.

2. Assess the support of the vaginal outlet. Have the client strain down, and note if there is any loss of urine.

3. Using a speculum, inspect the cervix, noting the color, position, and any lacerations, ulcers, nodules, masses, discharge, bleeding, erosions, and polyps. Immerse the speculum in warm water before inserting. This provides lubrication without altering the Pap smear specimen.

4. Obtain a specimen for a Papanicolaou smear. Prepare the plates. Take three specimens: (1) an endocervical swab, (2) a cervical scrape, and (3) a vaginal pool.

5. Inspect the vaginal mucosa, noting the color and any inflammation, discharge, ulcers, or masses.

NORMAL FINDINGS: The vaginal wall appears paper thin, and the canal is shortened up to half its previous length.

Perform a bimanual examination.

6. Palpate the vagina, noting nodularity, tenderness, the state of relaxation, bulging of anterior or posterior walls, firmness, and induration.

7. Palpate the cervix and fornix, noting the position, shape, consistency, regularity, mobility, and tenderness.

NOTE: The mean age of menopause is 50 to 51 years.

8. Palpate the uterus, noting the size, shape, position, contour, consistency, mobility, and any tenderness or masses.

9. Palpate the cul-de-sac, noting any bulging, tenderness, or masses.

10. Palpate the ovaries and adnexa bilaterally, noting the size, shape, consistency, mobility, and any tenderness or masses.

NORMAL FINDINGS: The ovaries should be less than 5 cm across and regular in shape. The fallopian tubes feel smaller than in younger women.

11. Palpate the posterior uterus and rectum, noting any tenderness, masses, or stool (note the amount and consistency of stool).

NOTE: Ninety percent of all older adults have a bowel movement at least once a day.

12. Describe findings in assessing the anus and

rectum of a female client, noting the presence of occult blood.

Muscles, bones and joints

1. Describe findings in assessing the musculoskeletal system. Inspect the client's ability to perform activities of daily living. Observe posture, noting the cervical curve, thoracic curve, and lumbar curve.

NORMAL FINDINGS: Muscle mass decreases; muscle strength is not lost in the same proportion.

2. Inspect and palpate muscles and joints at rest and during range of motion (ROM), noting the ROM, strength, condition of surrounding tissues, and any heat, swelling, pain, or crepitation.

NORMAL FINDINGS: Narrowing of the joint spaces occurs.

NOTE: Kyphosis is a common exaggerated posterior curve. Have the client seated on a table to do ROM exam. Do each joint separately.

3. Systematically inspect and palpate muscles and bones of the head and neck, shoulders, arms, elbows, hands and wrists, spine, knees, and feet and ankles.

NOTE: Lipping of the joint edges of fingers is normal. Lipping at the femoral head causes pain and immobility.

4. Perform special maneuvers for carpal tunnel syndrome, stability of the knee, torn meniscus, herniated lumbar disc, and sacroiliac pain.

NORMAL FINDINGS: Slight knee flexion on standing is commonly seen in the older adult. This affects the posture on standing both at the knee and at the hip.

Neurological system

1. Describe findings in assessing the neurological system. The neurological examination will be brief or extensive, depending on the signs exhibited by the client. Complete assessment of the neurological system includes assessment of motor and sensory system function, reflexes, cranial nerve function, cerebellum function, and cerebral function.

2. Inspect the client, noting sensation on the arms, trunk, and legs, including pain, temperature, light touch, vibration, position, discriminative sensation, stereognosis, number identification, two-point discrimination, point localization,

extinction, sensation, and kinesthetic sense.

NORMAL FINDINGS: The threshold for skin response to pain lowers after age 60. Light touch on the palm and thumb normally is diminished.

3. Inspect muscles of the limbs and trunk, noting atrophy, fasciculations, involuntary movements, abnormal position, muscle tone, and proprioception.

4. Test muscle strength of the arms, elbows, wrist, fingers, trunk, diaphragm, hip, knee, ankle, and feet.

5. Assess coordination testing using rapid rhythmic alternating movements and point-to-point testing.

6. Test the cranial nerves: the olfactory, optic, oculomotor, trochlear, abducens, trigeminal (motor, sensory, and corneal reflex), facial, acoustic, glossopharyngeal, vagus, spinal accessory, and hypoglossal.

7. Perform the following screening tests for proprioceptor and cerebellum functions: note gait, assess balance and coordination, and perform the Romberg test, finger-to-nose test, heel-to-shin test, and alternating action test.

8. Percuss superficial and deep tendon reflexes for absent, diminished, or hyperactive reflexes, including biceps, triceps, supinator, abdominal, cremasteric, knee, ankle, and plantar reflexes.

NORMAL FINDINGS: Deep tendon reflexes are more difficult to elicit in the older adult. Ankle reflexes are often absent.

Psychosocial status

1. Assess the client's mood, thought processes, memory, orientation, and calculation ability. Describe findings regarding appearance and behavior. Observe the client's posture, motor behavior, dress, grooming, personal hygiene, facial expression, speech (quality, quantity, and organization), manner, mood, relation to environment, intellectual performance, and judgment.

NOTE: Use interviewing skills to elicit the client's mood.

2. Observe the client's description of the health history, including the coherency and relevance of thought processes, thought content, and perceptions (illusions or hallucinations).

3. Describe findings regarding cognitive functions. Test for attention and concentration, including digit span and serials, memory (remote and recent), information, vocabulary, abstract reasoning, similarities, judgment, sensory perception, coordination, and orientation to time, place, and function.

SUMMARY

Health is not only the absence of disease, but the optimum state of efficiency and well-being both in mind and body. Through the use of the nursing process, health maintenance is encouraged, health is supported during acute illness, and rehabilitation is instituted to restore the fullest range of daily living that is feasible. Health maintenance conserves the older adult's physiological assets and limits dysfunction.

The nursing record enables the nurse to compile an individualized nursing data base for the client that both documents nursing intervention and serves as a standard or measurement of the client's progress. The data base is collected during the nursing interview, a time for establishing a working rapport with the client. All data on the client's record are privileged information and constitute part of the legal document.

Data are categorized as subjective and objective. Subjective data, although considered significant, cannot be measured on a clinical scale. Objective data can be measured clinically.

The nursing health history explores the client's reason for contacting the nurse, biographical data, and current health status. The client's personal and family histories, as well as his social history, are then reviewed. During the interview, the nurse assesses the client's mental and emotional status and does a review of systems with the client. The final aspect of the nursing health history is the health examination. This examination is a direct physical evaluation of each body system to determine if it is within the normal limits of healthful function. The characteristic alterations in physiology that accompany normal aging are seen as changes in the body system. However, the body of the older adult tolerates these changes and remains functional. Knowledge of the parameters of health of each system of the older adult enables the nurse to assess the client's selected body systems or total body system and plan nursing intervention accordingly.

REFERENCES

Benedict, R. C.: Making the health care system responsive to the needs of the elderly, Aging (295-296):25, May-June 1979.

Best, P.: The elderly: a challenge to nursing—13. Health promotion for the elderly, Nurs. Times **74**:111, 19 January 1974.

Brink, T. L.: Geriatric rigidity and its psychotherapeutic implications, J. Am. Geriatr. Soc. **26**:274, June 1978.

Burger, D.: Breast self-examination, Am. J. Nurs. **79**:1088, June 1979.

Caird, F. I., and Judge, T. G.: Assessment of the elderly patient, Kent, England, 1977, Pitman Medical.

Conner, K. A., Powers, E. A., and Bultena, G. L.: Social interaction and life satisfaction: an empirical assessment of late-life patterns, J. Gerontol. **34**:116, January 1979.

Craven, R. F.: Primary health care: practice in a nursing home, Am. J. Nurs. **76**:1958, December 1976.

Diekelmann, N.: Staying well while growing old: preretirement counseling, Am. J. Nurs. **78**:1337, August 1978.

Frisgen, I., and others: How much sense is there in an attempt to resuscitate an aged person? Gerontology **24**(1):37, 1978.

Galinsky, D., Herschkoren, H., Kaplan, M., and Alyagon, R.: The need for a new approach to neglected elderly patients, Geriatrics **33**:103, January 1978.

Geboes, K., Hellemans, J., and Bossaert, H.: Is the elderly patient accurately diagnosed? Geriatrics **34**:91, May 1979.

Gelfand, D. E.: Ethnicity, aging and mental health, Int. J. Aging Hum. Dev. **10**(3):289, 1979-80.

Gruber, H. W.: Geriatrics-physician attitudes and medical school training, J. Am. Geriatr. Soc. **25**:494, November 1977.

Hardie, M.: The elderly: a challenge to nursing—10. Housing and the elderly, Nurs. Times **73**:1996, December 1977.

Harris, R.: Graduate training in geriatrics: new dimensions and trends, Aging (295-296):28, May-June 1979.

Harrison, J. F.: Geriatrics in medicine: both sides of the fence, Lancet **1**:866, 22 April 1978.

Holtzman, J. M., Berman, H., and Ham, R.: Health and early retirement decisions, J. Am. Geriatr. Soc. **28**:23, January 1980.

Jordheim, A.: Old age in Norway—a time to look forward to, Geriatr. Nurs. **1**:46, May-June 1980.

Kelly, J. T., Hanson, R. G., Garetz, F. K., and others: What the family physician should know about treating elderly patients. Part 2, Geriatrics **32**:79, October 1977.

Leinbach, R. M.: The aging participants in an area planning effort, Gerontologist **17**(5 Pt. 1):453, October 1977.

Levine, M. E.: Adaptation and assessment: a rationale for nursing intervention, Am. J. Nurs. **66**:2450, November 1966.

Mauksch, I.: Old age in the U.S.—a time to wait, Geriatr. Nurs. **1**:42, May-June 1980.

McGlone, F. B., and Kick, E.: Health habits in relation to aging, J. Am. Geriatr. Soc. **26**:481, November 1978.

Malasanos, L., Barkauskas, V., and Stoltenberg-Allen, K.: Health assessment, ed. 2, St. Louis, 1981, The C. V. Mosby Co.

Meador, R.: Old age in Denmark—a time to enjoy, Geriatr. Nurs. **1**:48, May-June 1980.

Medical screening of old people accepted for medical care (letter), Lancet **2**:422, 19 August 1978.

Medical screening of old people (letter), Lancet **2**:532, 2 September 1978.

Metress, J., and Kart, C.: A system for observing the potential nutritional risks of elderly people living at home, J. Geriatr. Psychiatry **11**(1):67, 1978.

Mullins, A. C., and Barstow, R. E.: Care for the caretakers, Am. J. Nurs. **79**:1425, August 1979.

Patter, J. J.: Training objectives of a well-developed geriatrics program, J. Am. Geriatr. Soc. **26**:167, April 1978.

Peppers, L. G.: Patterns of leisure and adjustment to retirement, Gerontologist **16**:441, October 1976.

Reisner, C.: Medical screening of old people accepted for residential care (letter), Lancet **2**:474, 26 August 1978.

Richmond, J. B., and others: Health promotion and disease prevention in old age, Aging (295-296):11, May-June 1979.

Ridley, J. C., Bachrach, C. A., and Dawson, D. A.: Recall and reliability of interview data from older women, J. Gerontol. **34**:99, January 1979.

Roy, S. A.: Factors which affect the economics of a geriatric private practice, J. Am. Geriatr. Soc. **25**:502, November 1977.

Roy, S. A.: The role of medical societies in the care of the aging patient, J. Am. Geriatr. Soc. **25**:500, November 1977.

Sandler, R. B.: Comment: the physician and the competitive market: a gerontologist's viewpoint, Gerontologist **17**:560, December 1977.

Schaeffer, L. D., and others: Making compassionate programs work efficiently, Aging (295-296):21, May-June 1979.

Sheppard, H. L.: Toward an industrial gerontology, Cambridge, Mass., 1970, Schenkman Publishing Co., Inc.

Silver, C. P.: Tests for assessment of mental function, Age Ageing Suppl.:12, 1978.

Spangler, R.: Small Business Administration program keeps retired executives active, Geriatrics **33**:21, March 1978.

Stare, F. J.: Three score and ten plus more, J. Am. Geriatr. Soc. **25**:529, December 1977.

Steel, K.: Continuing education in geriatrics, J. Am. Geriatr. Soc. **25**:492, November 1977.

Stoll, R. I.: Guidelines for spiritual assessment, Am. J. Nurs. **79**:1574, September 1979.

Stuart, M. R., and Mackey, K. J.: Mobile center links providers with isolated senior citizens, Hospitals **52**:101, 1 January 1978.

Wales, J. B., and Treybig, D. L.: Recent legislative trends toward protection of human subjects: implications for gerontologists, Gerontologist **18**:244, June 1978.

Weiner, M. B., and Weinstock, C. S.: Group progress of community elderly as measured by tape recordings, group tempo and group evaluation, Int. J. Aging Hum. Dev. **10**(2):177, 1979-80.

Weinstock, F. J.: Ophthalmologic aspects of geriatric care, Geriatrics **33**:33, July 1978.

Whitehouse, R.: Forms that facilitate patient teaching, Am. J. Nurs. **79**:1227, July 1979.

Wood, V.: Age-appropriate behavior for older people, Gerontologist **11**:74, 1971.

World Health Organization: Constitution of the World Health Organization, Chronicle World Health Organization **1**(1 and 2):29, 1947.

Wright, W. B.: How to investigate an old person, Lancet **2**:419, 19 August 1978.

Zwezey, R. L., and others: Evaluation and treatment, Geriatrics **34**:56, January 1979.

SELECTED READING

Physical assessment skills: a historical perspective

Virginia M. Fitzsimons □ **Louise P. Gallagher**

The nurse's use of physical assessment skills for health maintenance and health promotion indicates a new, expanded role for the profession. Or does it? A look at the historical development of physical assessment skills by the nursing profession discloses that these skills have been an integral part of nursing since the time of Florence Nightingale. For many years, nursing has been aware that physical assessment skills are indispensable as a tool for data collection. Nurses have developed, refined, and availed themselves of these methods in much the same manner as have physicians.

INSTRUMENTS USED FOR PHYSICAL ASSESSMENT

The narrow view of nurses adopted by the medical profession has made it difficult to precisely define the function of nursing. Moreover, physicians have always jealously guarded the right to use medical tools, displaying a characteristic reluctance to hand them over to nurses.

In the early 1930s, simple instruments of measure such as the clinical thermometer and the sphygmomanometer were considered exotic, and their use was regarded as being beyond the scope of nursing skills. In a graduation address given in 1931 to nurses at the Massachusetts General Hospital, a physician, referring to the clinical thermometer, stated, "At the beginning of nursing in the Massachusetts General Hospital there was a regulation that no nurse was to handle that 'instrument

Reprinted from Nursing Forum **17**(4): 344, 1978.

of precision.'" The belief was that the thermometer "had to be used by a properly qualified medical man." (Cabot, 1931) However, no one today would question the use of a thermometer by a nurse in the course of collecting data regarding the patient. Taking the temperature is standard procedure for the nurse to follow, and is quite expected on the part of the patient.

About the same time Massachusetts General was struggling with the mighty problem of whether a thermometer was too intricate an implement for general use, nurses in the Kentucky Frontier Nursing Service were using the blood pressure cuff and stethoscope as part of their routine method for assessing a patient's condition. Furthermore, in an effort to screen for toxemia of pregnancy, they did urine checks and took blood pressures on all prenatal women. Although the use of a sphygmomanometer was considered avant garde in the thirties and raised some eyebrows, the prenatal program was such a success that one physician was heard to say, "Someday all nurses shall take blood pressure readings even though it is costly." (Lester, 1931)

Today, the ophthalmoscope is the precision instrument whose use by nurses is under question, and the issue is whether nursing should consider incorporating the instrument into its repertoire of tools for health screening. Use of the ophthalmoscope would allow the nurse to collect more refined data about the cardiovascular system of the eye, and evidence of the systemic status of the cardiovascular system, instead of

gathering data only on the gross cardiovascular system.

THE CARDINAL TOOLS OF PHYSICAL ASSESSMENT

In the days of Florence Nightingale, the nurse had to rely on her natural senses alone, commonly using the skills of inspection and palpation. These skills were developed as a result of teachings by Nightingale, which focused on the importance of patient assessment by means of such naturally given aids as sight and touch as essential in fulfilling the nurse's role.

Through techniques of observation, the nurse collected data about the patient's condition, and implemented the patient's care accordingly. Then, as now, the nurse considered not only the disease process and treatment regimen, but also the patient's physical responses to the environment. The nurse realized the importance of observing the face and body for changes in color, temperature, muscle strength, use of limbs, body output, and degrees of nutrition and hydration. (Nightingale, p. 116)

Stressing that precision was needed to collect data, Nightingale stated, "the most important practical lesson that can be given to nurses is to teach them what to observe [and] how to observe. . . ." (p. 105)

To accomplish this objective, Nightingale taught the skill of palpation to measure pulse rate and quality, emphasizing that the nurse was responsible for gaining proficiency to ensure accuracy in decision making. Up-to-date treatment of Nightingale's time also included the use of palpation and inspection in the care of the puerperal woman. The nurse was responsible for palpating the fundus and observing the woman's responses to the stresses of delivery. The surgical nurse routinely observed patients' respiratory patterns and inspected dressings.

DOCUMENTATION OF THE USE OF ASSESSMENT TOOLS

Nursing journals are filled with examples of accepted nursing practice, which include the use of independent inspection, palpation, and auscultation in the everyday role of the nurse.

In 1901, the *American Journal of Nursing* recorded that palpation was used by the nurse as a method of gastrointestinal therapy. The nurse massaged the GI tract to increase peristaltic actions, and promoted bowel evacuation. To begin the procedure, the nurse identified the fundus of the stomach and the area of the pylorus. The complete length of the intestine was palpated and manipulated, including the cecum and the colon. An assessment of the results was then made by the nurse, and the treatment was repeated prn. (Williams, 1901) In that same year, a doctor made the following observation in the *American Journal of Nursing,* "It is the duty of the nurse . . . to examine the eyes of the new-born baby each day during the lying-in period (for the signs of Blenorrhea Neonatorum)." Included in the inspection was the cornea, conjunctiva, and lacrimal sacs. As one doctor observed, "Without the good nurse the doctor is powerless in these cases, and her responsibility is even greater than his, because upon her . . . care really depends the sight of a fellow creature" (Wescott, 1901).

In 1901, the *American Journal of Nursing* examined the role of the nurse in testing the function of the eighth cranial nerve in patients. Early detection of defects was stressed, and while the technology of

testing auditory acuity was primitive, the nurse was expected to take a measure of auditory function. (Kerr, 1901).

Other evidence substantiates the role of the nurse as a recognized part of the health care team, both in maintaining and promoting health. During the early 1900s, contagious diseases posed major health threats to the population of New York City. In a concerted effort to stop the spread of the contagion, 141 nurses were employed by the city to work within the school system. (Kerr, 1901) Following the first school examination at the beginning of the term by the medical inspector, it became the nurse's responsibility to examine the children at specific intervals. The nurse's inspection included the eyes, hair, skin, mouth, and throat. Furthermore, the nurse's role as health maintainer and health teacher extended not merely to the school child, but to the family and the community at large.

Although given an early start in New York City, school health supervision continued to be regarded as a new phenomenon into the 1920s. The health team was employed by the city or school board. While the initial physical examination was not part of the nurse's role, she was responsible for subsequent in-class inspections, "for the detection of communicable diseases and physical defects." (Hiscock, 1923) In some cities, it was the nurse's responsibility to find physical defects in children in grades two and three, while the physician was responsible for physical examination of children in grades one and four. "In Detroit the examination is made every three months by the nurse, who especially examines the throat, skin and head of the pupil," Hiscock reports. The same source noted that the nurse was responsible for examining the children in all grades in Omaha and Des Moines. In eleven of the smaller cities, examinations were made either every other year or

three times during the school years.

These accounts leave no doubt that the school nurse used her assessment skills of inspection extensively at regular intervals, especially during those times when certain diseases were prevalent. Furthermore, no longer were inspections confined to external body surfaces. Included in the exam was the assessment of internal structures such as the pharynx. It became standard practice for a school board to require a certificate, signed by the school nurse, as a condition for re-admission for any child who had contracted a communicable disease, Hiscock states.

By 1938, physical assessment as a component of health maintenance was an integral part of the health program at the Lincoln School in New York City. The nurse screened for visual and auditory acuity, appraising the function of the second and eighth cranial nerves. Today, this procedure is recognized as an important component of the neurologic examination. (Axelson, 1938)

In the classroom, the nurse did health inspections and teaching. She was responsible for the screening for communicable disease via ear, nose, and throat inspections in school-age children. By the 1940s, even colleges were relying on the nurse to screen students and give health consultations.

There is evidence of parallel developments in the field of public health nursing during the first part of the century. In 1912, the public health nurse was making routine inspections of the home. As reported in the *American Journal of Public Health,* MacNutt (1913) proposed the term "health nurse" in an address before the American Public Health Association, since the function of the board of health nurse was the "positive promotion of health."

In the 1930s, rural public health nursing flourished, affording the nurse recognition as the vital force on the health team. Her role included casefinding, and carrying out prevention programs against typhoid, malaria, diphtheria, and other communicable diseases. Using her physical assessment skills, she conducted integumentary and ear, nose, and throat examinations. The nurse was the primary person to reach out to the community, acting as health care liaison among the people, the physician, and the sanitary engineer. (Marriner, 1931) In addition, the nurse carried a full caseload of women for prenatal and perinatal care, Lester reports (1931), adding that for a majority of these women, prenatal and perinatal care was previously unknown.

The public health nurse did urine testing, took blood pressure measurements, and conducted abdominal examinations. Skilled in physical assessment techniques, she was the patient's major contact with the health care system. The nurse understood the necessity of adapting skills to the particular psychological and sociological concepts of the community. Often, the public health nurse's system of assessment included conferences with patients to encourage them to participate in their own care, Lester notes. Complex cases were presented on nursing rounds, so that learning experiences could be shared with colleagues. As a professional practitioner with a developed sense of autonomy and accountability, the public health nurse cared for virtually all the health needs of patients.

It should be noted that the greatest progress in freeing the nurse to fulfill her potential as a health care practitioner occurred in poor inner city areas, or in such special services as the Frontier Nursing Service or the rural Red Cross. (Lester, 1931) The Red Cross nurse was analagous to the Frontier Nurse in that she created rural outposts and ran public health nursing centers. According to Ames (1928), "When

the patient cannot go the Outpost, the nurse goes to the patient. Where the physician is too far away to be available, the judgment of the nurse is called upon to an extraordinary extent." Ames continues, "Last year (1928), 3,088 patients received over 30,000 days of attention of the Red Cross nurses. Seven hundred and forty-three babies were born, most of whose mothers would have gone unattended. Both preventive and curative work are done." (p. 121)

In the poverty areas of the cities, immigrant groups accepted the nurse more readily than the physician. (Noble, 1923) Clinics became quite common. As early as 1923, the *American Journal of Public Health* documented that the nurse midwives' use of the tools of inspection, palpation, and auscultation were essential to the delivery of prenatal services. If the woman did not come to the clinic, the nurse went to the patient's home to check her urine and auscultate her blood pressure. (Ames, 1928) In this manner, nurses performed both a preventive and curative role as they attended their patients.

During that same year, the state of Pennsylvania, with the object of keeping "well babies well," opened clinics for children. After the initial visit with the physician, according to Noble, the child was seen by the nurse for "weighing and visé." All state centers were run by the nurse, who saw the baby on all return visits to the clinic, and also made home visits. In an effort to reduce the rate of infant mortality, nurses assumed the responsibility of initiating campaigns to improve sanitary conditions. These efforts were focused primarily on the home and children, stressing clean water and the necessity of milk in the diet. (Noble, 1923)

In more recent times, industry as well as health care institutions have shown a greater recognition of the

value of using the nurse as the initial performer in the health care schema.

In 1953, the telephone firm of Bell Canada began using nurses to do initial health reviews for their employees, orienting the program to maintain and promote health. Included in the plan were the taking of a complete history and physical examination. Initially, nurses examined only female patients, but by 1968, all applicants were referred to the nurse. (Bewes and Baillie, 1969)

A study to explore and evaluate the effect of introducing a public health nurse to work in association with a physician was conducted by Montefiore Hospital in New York City between 1963 and 1967. The nurse in obstetrics was to determine fetal position, weight gain, fetal heart sounds, as well as to give anticipatory guidance and handle medical and emotional problems. In pediatrics, the nurse, in addition to taking routine measurements, was to give anticipatory guidance, discuss problems with the mothers, conduct a physical examination, and check the children's developmental milestones. The results of this study indicated that patients were satisfied with the care they received from these nurses. In fact, a majority preferred the combined nurse-physician approach to being seen just by a physician. (Ford, 1966)

The Harvard Community Health Plan, originating in the 1960s, provided another study in which nurses could use their skills in a group practice organization. (Bates, 1972) Nurses were able to manage 70 to 80 percent of the patients they saw in this setting. According to the plan, nurses were used at the point of first contact with the patient and throughout the entire process. Nurses received all telephone calls from adult medical patients seeking appointments; took a preliminary history and decided on a course of treatment; requested laboratory tests, made diagnoses, and had input into management decisions; were active in the triage process, interviewing patients and making physical and psychosocial assessments. The attitude of the nursing staff was summed up by one member who stated, "What we're doing is not really new. We've been doing it in public health for years." (Bates, 1972)

CONCLUSION

Nursing has made, and will continue to make, critical contributions to the viability of the health care system through the use of physical assessment skills. Florence Nightingale called the nurse a "health conservationist," convinced that the primary focus of nursing was health maintenance and health promotion. That focus has not changed. The perspective of history shows us that physical assessment skills have been a traditional tool of the nurse for many decades, aiding in the competent fulfillment of responsibility by the professional practitioner.

REFERENCES

Ames, Miriam, "Public Health Nursing," *American Journal of Public Health,* 18(1):121, 1928.

Axelson, Alfhild, "Health in a Progressive School," *American Journal of Nursing,* 38(7):516-519, 1938.

Bates, Barbara, "Nursing in a Health Maintenance Organization: Report on the Harvard Community Health Plan," *American Journal of Public Health,* 62(7):991-994, 1972.

Bewes, D. C. and J. H. Baillie, "Preplacement Health Screening by Nurses," *American Journal of Public Health,* 59(12):2178-2184, 1969.

Cabot, Richard, "What is Worthwhile in Nursing," *American Journal of Nursing,* 31(3):279, 1931.

Ford, Patricia A., Seacat Milvoy, and George Silver, "The Relative Roles of the Public Health Nurse and the Physician in Prenatal and Infant Supervision," *American Journal of Public Health,* 56(7):1097-1103, 1966.

Hiscock, Ira V., "School Health Supervision," *American Journal of Public Health,* 13(4):259-269, 1923.

Kerr, Anna W., "School Nursing in New York City," *American Journal of Nursing,* 10(2):106-108, 1901.

Lester, Betty, "The Experience of a Midwifery Supervisor in the Kentucky Hills," *American Journal of Nursing,* 31(5):573-577, 1931.

MacNutt, J. Scott, "The Board of Health Nurse: What She Can Do for the Public Welfare in a Small City," *American Journal of Public Health,* 3(3):344-350, 1913.

Marriner, Jessie L., "Rural Public Health Nursing: A Vocational Study of Interest to Student Nurses," *American Journal of Nursing,* 31(1):45-52, 1931.

Nightingale, Florence, *Notes on Nursing What It Is and What It Is Not,* Unabridged replication of first American edition, Dover Publications, London, 1969.

Noble, Mary Riggs, "Child Health Work In Pennsylvania," *American Journal of Public Health,* 13(9)756-759, 1923.

Wescott, Cassius D., "The Management of Blenorrhoea Neonatorum with Especial Reference to the Duties of the Nurse," *American Journal of Nursing,* 1(9)635-639, 1901.

Williams, Kate W., "Massage for Constipation," *American Journal of Nursing,* 1(10):713-715, 1901.

5 Nursing diagnosis

A diagnosis is a careful examination and analysis of the facts in an attempt to explain something. Not every decision the nurse makes in clinical practice is a nursing diagnosis. The nursing diagnosis merely summarizes assessment findings. The nurse makes many decisions during the collection of data, judgments regarding which areas should be explored, which findings are significant enough to be recorded, and what additional information is imperative. The outcome of these decisions or judgments will be seen in the record as data relating to the individual client. These data are summarized as a nursing diagnosis.

The ideas behind nursing diagnosis have been used in nursing for years. The nurse might be more familiar with the terms *total patient care* or *caring for the whole person.* The concept underlying all these terms is one that offers care to the client, recognizing him as an individual person with particular needs.

The nursing diagnosis system is a refinement of the total patient care approach. By specifically naming (the diagnosis) the ways in which we give the patient complete care, we are stating how we are giving him individualized attention. When a nurse first uses *nursing diagnosis,* the words might seem awkward and new. They do not have a familiar ring of the vocabulary she learned in nursing school. By using nursing diagnosis in the client's record and in conversations with other nurses, this new term loses its unfamiliar sound, and the nurse soon feels more comfortable in using it.

Mrs. Clark is being admitted to the hospital for some elective surgery. The nurse who does the admitting nursing health history has a good knowledge base regarding the physiology of the older adult. She knows that older adults, especially over the age of 70, often have limitations in musculoskeletal functioning. She decides to review Mrs.

Clark's range-of-motion abilities as a part of her assessment to determine if she has an actual or potential limitation. It is the nurse's judgment that this is an important area of nursing concern because she understands the implications of immobility for the client, particularly after surgery. A quick review of Mrs. Clark's upper and lower extremities reveals full range of motion. The client, however, describes in detail how difficult it is for her to get going in the morning because of joint stiffness, pain, and resulting limited mobility. The nurse makes a decision on which findings are significant enough to be recorded. This nurse decided that early morning mobility limitations must be a part of her client's nursing data. In addition, she decided to seek out more data pertaining to how her client normally responds to this stiffness and pain. Does she take aspirin or other types of medication, or does she apply heat or do exercise? In other words, what is the client's usual response to this situation, and is relief obtained? In addition, given these nursing signs and symptoms, she knows that she must inspect and palpate the client's joints for evidence of swelling, heat, crepitus, and pain. The assessment approach identifies the client as an individual because it examines more than just the organ system that is malfunctioning. The nurse is exploring for potential health threats. Mrs. Clark will be required to ambulate quickly after her surgery, and now the nurse can accommodate her particular limitations in her planning. Without these data, Mrs. Clark is just the umbilical hernia in room 429. The nurse decided to pursue the special needs of this older adult, and her nursing diagnosis reflects the scope of her practice. The nursing diagnosis recorded on Mrs. Clark's chart were:

1. Alterations in morning comfort levels
2. Potential immobility hazard
3. Fear concerning the surgery

The nurse has diagnosed three health threats for this client, two actual and one potential. As the nurse continues to interview Mrs. Clark, more diagnoses may be made, perhaps related to the impending surgery. Certainly in the preoperative period, Mrs. Clark will have the need for additional nursing interventions, and the nursing diagnoses will reflect the progressive changes in her condition. As the nurse learns more about the client, the diagnoses will be revised. Skill is developed when the nurse uses the nursing diagnosis routinely for planning care. In fact, her diagnoses will become more specific.

For example, the diagnosis "Fear and anxiety concerning the surgical procedure" might be stated as "Fear and anxiety of possibly dying during surgery." The nursing diagnosis helps the nurse clarify her statements and thus enables her to focus on areas she knows she has to investigate. When she can state the exact nature of the client's fear, she has documented the psychological dimension of nursing care. She has not merely given "emotional support" in a general way, but has used the first step in the nursing process to systematically identify her client's needs. The nursing diagnosis has summarized her data collection activities.

DIFFERENCE BETWEEN NURSING PROCEDURE AND NURSING DIAGNOSIS

A procedure is a standardized way of doing something, usually set down in specific steps to accomplish a particular activity. No decisions are required; each step is completed, and that is it. For example, bedmaking is a procedure, and the steps in making a bed can be recited by rote by any nurse or nurse's aide. Every agency has a nursing procedure manual. The purposes and specific instructions for equipment needed and steps involved in order of activity are spelled out; even how to chart the procedure is dictated. Having procedure manuals in an agency is useful because it provides for a certain uniformity of activity. Also, time and motion studies usually have been done to assure that the approved procedure is the most time efficient and safest way of doing the activity. Procedures relate to the how to's of client care. Functioning on a procedural level exclusively limits the nurse's opportunities

for making decisions related to individualizing client care.

A diagnosis, on the other hand, is the process of deciding the nature of a situation by examination. The facts are analyzed and understood, and a conclusion or an opinion is stated. It has at the base of action a full thinking and analyzing process. Nursing diagnosis states the *why* of care chosen for this particular client.

SUMMARIZING THE DATA COLLECTED

Nursing diagnosis is the final step in the data collection phase of the nursing process; it summarizes all the information obtained about the client. Both medical and nursing diagnosis use the client's data base as the source of information needed for the diagnosis. A medical diagnosis identifies disease pathological conditions by their presenting signs and symptoms. The nursing diagnosis identifies the client's needs for delivery of basic nursing care. Nursing diagnosis (1) recognizes the health problems the nurse will address, (2) evaluates the effects of signs and symptoms on the client's coping and adaptation mechanisms that lead to his response to actual or potential health problems, and (3) helps the nurse intervene appropriately to alter the life-style or adjust the signs and symptoms so that the client is no longer threatened. The nursing diagnosis completes the assessment component and begins the care planning of the nursing process.

Nursing diagnosis has been with us for 25 years; however, nurses are just beginning to be comfortable using it. The more we read about nursing diagnosis in the literature and the more we test it in clinical practice, the more nurses can contribute to refining a nursing diagnostic classification system. Nursing terminology will be developed to such a finite standard that we will be able to communicate the nature of nursing practice rather than nursing procedure. For instance, a client with a nursing diagnosis of malnutrition in Pennsylvania should require similar nursing intervention to a client in New Mexico with the same diagnosis. Nursing is in the initial stage of developing a dictionary of nursing nomenclature that lists the signs and symptoms for each identified nursing diagnosis. Among the pioneers in this major undertaking are Gebbie, Lavin, and Campbell. Thirty-four tentative nursing diagnoses were the outcome of the First National Conference on the Classification of Nursing Diagnosis, codirected by Gebbie and Lavin in 1973.

In 1978, Campbell set forth a comprehensive approach to nursing diagnosis. She expanded the original 34 diagnoses to an extensive list of diagnoses covering all areas of nursing practice and nursing intervention.

Medicine started its taxonomy with five nonrelated, nonextensive categories of medical diagnoses. It has taken medicine over 300 years to develop and standardize their International Classification of Disease and the Systematized Nomenclature of Pathology. Gebbie predicts that we can use the experience of other disciplines to shorten the standardization procedure for our diagnoses, but cautions us that it may take more than 30 years.

VALUE OF NURSING DIAGNOSIS

When a nurse wants to communicate her unique and independent function as a nurse, to reflect the accuracy of her assessment data, and to give clear direction for her subsequent nursing intervention, the most effective communications tool is a nursing diagnosis. Nursing diagnosis gives nursing a common frame of reference for communicating with nurse colleagues and other members of the health care team. The nursing diagnosis gives direction for nursing orders and goals of nursing care. It summarizes nursing knowledge and expands and upgrades nursing research.

Nursing's contribution to the health care team can be readily identified in concrete terms. Third party payers such as Blue Cross, Medicare, and Medicaid require specific information regarding nursing intervention. Nursing diagnosis will help establish nursing intervention protocols that can be translated into computer language for storage and retrieval. By describing the care given in a precise statement, it becomes much easier to identify nursing costs and the exact services nursing performs. Until now, nursing costs have been lumped together with other agency departments such as housekeeping and dietetics. When it comes time to review the annual budget or to bill Medicare, Medicaid, or Blue Cross, it is very difficult to zero in on what nursing expenses actually are. In order to get paid for services rendered, nurses must be able to state their services and the exact cost that should be reimbursed. Right now, nurses do many things for which they do not get paid because they cannot state their activities in the computer language spoken by the large government agencies and insurance companies. Unless nurses can document nursing care succinctly on insurance forms and budget lines, they will not be fully paid for their services.

DEVELOPMENT OF A NURSING TAXONOMY

A taxonomy is a classification system. It can apply to almost any area of thought that can be put into list form. The Yellow Pages section of a telephone directory is an example of a basic taxonomy. Common elements are listed together. The listing of elements must have some order and purpose; this is the basic principle in developing a taxonomy. The order for the Yellow Pages is the alphabetical listing. The purpose is to help the telephone user locate the telephone number and provider of the service that he is seeking. In the Yellow Pages under "A" are listed *Accountants, certified public,* then those accountants that specialize in specific services, such as business accountants and tax accountants. The next listing is *accountant and bookkeeping machines,* then several pages later *accountant and bookkeeping supplies.* The point is, a taxonomy's order makes it most useful. It can be distinguished from a random list with no order or purpose.

We unconsciously use taxonomies in our everyday encounters. An example of a taxonomy in nursing service is the hierarchical order of nursing personnel:

Director of Nursing
Associate Director of Nursing
Assistant Director of Nursing
Supervisor or Patient Care Coordinator
Head nurse or charge nurse
Registered professional nurse
Staff nurse
Licensed practical nurse
Nursing assistant or nurse's aide
Orderly

The order and purpose is for leadership responsibilities, administrative channel of command, job descriptions, status, promotional levels, and the use of nursing service personnel.

If you are looking for a restaurant, you would

look up restaurants in the telephone book, and then proceed to find an Italian, Greek, or Mexican restaurant. That is a classification or taxonomy of restaurants. Medicine has a taxonomy also, and the general categories are heart disease, respiratory disease, and the subgroups are angina, congestive heart failure, or emphysema. Nursing is compiling a taxonomy or list of nursing diagnoses. These identify actions unique to nursing in a precise and concise form. We have been able to state how we do things by procedures, but not what we do. Going back to the restaurant example, consider the menu in an Italian restaurant, which states what the chef offers for dinner, veal piccata or chicken parmesan. This menu or list (taxonomy) does not say how the chef cooked these dishes. It mentions only what is offered. The how of cooking the dishes can be found in a cookbook. A cookbook is a type of procedure manual that lists the how to's of cooking. Nurses are developing a menu of the care they give and stating it as the nursing diagnoses. How they do it can be found in a procedure manual. Of course, the how to is much more inclusive than a procedure manual because the nurse utilizes a scientific rationale drawn from her broad knowledge base of the biopsychosocial sciences and nursing sciences. Other resources may be used, such as reference books, nursing literature, research, and clinical nurse specialists.

Simply stated, the nursing diagnosis gives the nurse direction on what areas must be included in the care plan for a client, and a nursing taxonomy is one source offering a complete selection of nursing diagnoses.

LEVELS OF NURSING DIAGNOSES

The complexity of client's health needs will be reflected in the number of nursing diagnoses. According to Gebbie and Lavin,* the nurse may look for a client's response to her nursing diagnosis on any one of five levels:

Level 1: None. Patient shows no evidence of a problem and is able to handle and meet needs.

Level 2: Minimal. Patient shows some evidence of a problem, primarily related to knowledge or anticipation of a problem.

Level 3: Moderate. Patient can handle problems with supervision or minimal assistance.

Level 4: Severe. Patient is dependent; problem is acute and probably reversible.

Level 5: Very severe. Patient is dependent; problem is long term and probably not reversible.

CLINICAL APPLICATION OF NURSING DIAGNOSIS

Initiating nursing diagnosis terms into an agency's record system requires a team effort. Each level of nurse in that agency, from staff nurse on up to the top nursing administrator should agree that it is useful. In-service programs help the nurse learn its basics and set up goals for implementation. Because all personnel have the mutual interest and goal of providing quality health care, communication lines must be kept open between nursing and other service areas. For example, consultation with the medical records department can provide nursing service with information on indexing nursing diagnosis within the agency's filing system. Upon a client's discharge, the nursing diagnoses are coded and filed. Periodic reviews are then made of the nursing diagnoses. Charts having the same categories of diagnoses and similar patterns of client behavior are examined. These are then compared with the subsequent nursing plans and intervention. Client responses to nursing intervention are summarized. This style of investigation was done in the medical field when physicians were developing a taxonomy of medical diagnoses. For example, many charts were examined before a pattern specifically for appendicitis was identified. Now, when a person has an elevated white blood cell count over 10,000, rebound tenderness at McBurney's point, and low-grade fever, appendicitis is suspected. As nursing diagnoses are summarized, information is cross-checked, and a finite list of tested diagnoses emerges.

NURSING DIAGNOSIS AS STANDARD OF CARE

The American Nurses' Association states as a part of its purpose that it is responsible for representing the practitioner's measures of nursing practice. Nurses, through the American Nurses' Association, have described competency in nursing practice and evaluation of the quality of nursing

---

*Gebbie, K. M., and Lavin, M. A.: Classification of nursing diagnoses, St. Louis, 1975, The C. V. Mosby Co., p. 50.

service as a basic responsibility to the public. These attributes of competency and quality of care must be measured in some way. A standard refers to ordinary or typical expectations for care. The ruler used to measure competency and quality is the ANA Standards for Gerontological Nursing Practice.*

Standard I

Data are systematically and continuously collected about the health status of the older adult. The data are accessible, communicated, and recorded.

*Published by and reprinted with permission of the American Nurses' Association, Kansas City, Mo.

Standard II

Nursing diagnoses are derived from the identified normal responses of the individual to aging and the data collected about the health status of the older adult.

Chapter 3 presents the health assessment norms and normal characteristics for the older adult and discusses a systematic approach to data gathering. These activities constitute Standard I of the American Nurses' Association Standards of Gerontological Nursing Practice. All the assessment factors are used to identify normal patterns of aging before deviations that require nursing interventions are recognized. Standard II of the ANA Standards of Gerontological Nursing Practice

Nursing process: Data collection component

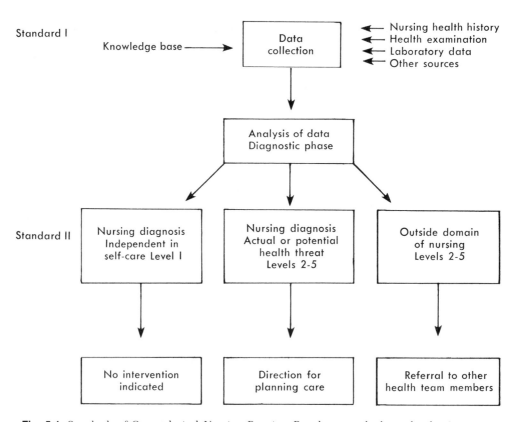

Fig. 5-1. Standards of Gerontological Nursing Practice. Based on standards set by the American Nurses' Association and Gebbie and Lavin's levels of nursing diagnosis.

addresses the need to state the nursing diagnosis as a summary of the data collected in the health interview, the health assessment, and other sources of client information.

Fig. 5-1 diagrams Standards I and II as a flowchart. This flowchart is applicable in the care of clients who are well, acutely ill, or in a stabilized state of a chronic dysfunction. The following case study presents an operational description of the nursing process flowchart through the first and second ANA Standards of Gerontological Nursing Practice.

SAMPLE CASE STUDY—NURSING PROCESS
DATA COLLECTION
ANA Standard I: Health assessment
Health history

A. Reason for contact: Health checkup
B. Biographical data
   1. Name: M. R.
   2. Address: 40 Conger Street.
   3. Phone: 567-1234.
   4. Social Security No.
   5. Date of birth and age: 9/8/16 (age 65).
   6. Sex: Female.
   7. Marital status: 39 years married.
   8. Occupation: Housewife.
   9. Educational status: High school graduate.
  10. Religion: Roman Catholic.
  11. Ethnicity: Italian American.
  12. Language spoken: English.
  13. Informant's relationship: self.
  14. Reliability of informant: good.
  15. Health facility and personnel.
    a. Usual facility: doctor's office.
    b. Dr. J., MD affiliated with hospital.
  16. Facility's address and phone.
    a. Office: N.J.
    b. Hospital: N.J.
  17. Health insurance: BlueCross/Blue Shield.
  18. Date of interview: 10/11/79.
C. Current health status
   1. Client's perception of health: "I think I'm not in excellent health and I'm not in poor health—I'm in between." Client also states, "I know I have certain health problems, but they are under control."
   2. Significant others' perception of health: "I believe my husband and children feel that I need guidance concerning health needs. For example, my youngest son, Kenny, is always telling me what I should and should not eat. My family thinks that their health status is very good."

3. Specific complaints.
  a. Hiatus hernia.
   (1) Onset: Six years ago.
   (2) Complaints: Indigestion and burning sensation in sternal area after eating a large meal or spicy food, pain in back, pain under left breast.
   (3) Symptoms: Sour taste in mouth.
   (4) Diagnosis: Client felt fear; she contacted physician because she thought she was having a heart attack the first time symptoms were experienced.
   (5) Treatment: Client must not eat spicy foods; small frequent feedings; Digel whenever symptoms occur; must not lie down after meals or wear constricting garments.
   (6) Outcome: Treatment very effective. Client states that the hiatus hernia has not bothered her since diagnosis and treatment.
  b. Hypertension.
   (1) Onset: Seven years ago.
   (2) Complaints: None.
   (3) Symptoms: None.
   (4) Diagnosis: Physical checkup revealed hypertension.
   (5) Treatment: Low salt consumption, switch to low tar and nicotine cigarettes (Vantage), take medication (see D-5), try to avoid stress, adequate intake of potassium (one banana) daily.
   (6) Outcome: Physical checkup (every 4 months) has indicated that hypertension has been under control since diagnosis and treatment.
  c. Umbilical hernia.
   (1) Onset: One year ago.
   (2) Complaints: Slight pain in umbilical area upon stressful activity.
   (3) Symptoms: Bulge in umbilical area.
   (4) Diagnosis: Client walked into the end of a table, felt pain, and on self-examination noticed a slight bulge in umbilical area.
   (5) Treatment: Client must always wear a girdle, unable to bowl for a year (able to bowl provided a constrictive binder is worn). Client must lose approx 50 pounds so a corrective operation can be performed without added risk.
   (6) Outcome: Treatment is not complete; an operation is needed.
  d. High blood cholesterol.
   (1) Onset: One month.
   (2) Complaints: None.

(3) Symptoms: None.

(4) Diagnosis: Blood test.

(5) Treatment: Restrictive diet.

(6) Outcome: Unknown to date.

D. Personal health history/daily habits

1. Diet (low cholesterol)—24-hour food log.

   Breakfast: One cup of coffee with skim milk and artificial sweetener, toast with margarine, 4 ounces of orange juice.

   Lunch: Turkey sandwich on rye with lettuce and tomato, banana, tea with skim milk, artificial sweetener.

   Dinner: Boiled chicken (no skin) and escarole.

   Snack: Two graham crackers with peanut butter.

2. Elimination: Bowel movement every 2 days—large, formed brown stool. Urinates about six times a day, clear amber urine. Client reports no complaints in this area.

3. Personal hygiene: Client's overall appearance is clean and neat; showers and washes hair every other day (once a day in summer); brushes teeth three times a day.

4. Smokes low tar and nicotine cigarettes, one pack a day. Drinks about once a week when her husband takes her out, two glasses of white wine; drinks tea during the day.

5. Medications: Hydrochlorothiazide, 50 mg daily PO.

6. Recreation and exercise: Client walks every day. She walks to the stores (about five blocks). Considers housework exercise. Knits sweaters and afghans.

7. Sleep patterns: Client feels she has normal sleep patterns. She sleeps 7 to 8 hours per night. No periods of wakefulness. She doesn't take naps.

8. Sex: Client still functions sexually three times a week with husband. LMP 7/65. No untoward menopausal complaints. On days when intercourse is not performed, client states that she experiences sexual gratification through kissing and touching. She states, "sex is important, but not vital."

9. Coping mechanisms: Screaming, slamming doors, and cleaning the house.

10. Daily profile: Cleans and puts the house in order, shops, sews, goes to bingo, occasionally watches TV, socializes (telephone), cooks.

E. Past health history

1. Promotive and preventive practices.

   a. Client states that she has a physical examination every 6 months. Visits the dentist once a year.

   b. Only immunization client can recall is vaccination against smallpox.

c. Never received any counseling.

2. Developmental data.

   a. No physical deformities. Menarche at age 17. At first, her cycle was irregular. In the client's opinion late menstruation revealed improper function of her reproductive system. She believed these improper functions led to an (actual) ovarian cyst.

   b. Client says she did well in English, spelling, and math, but she did poorly in the sciences. She felt sciences were boys' subjects. Client was a responsible individual during her adolescence; she helped in her father's grocery store.

   c. Client stated she had many friends at school and had good rapport with friends. Client began dating at age 20.

   d. Client's father was disciplinarian. He verbally and physically abused the family. He did not accept makeup on young girls or dating before the age of 20. Client says she lived in constant fear. Example of punishment: The client had her hand placed on a hot stove for eating a piece of candy taken from the store. She was once struck on the head with a flashlight because of missing her curfew. Her mother was her protector. She was her mother's confidante. Client stated that she did not hate her father; she loved him but did not feel remorse when he died.

3. Past illness, injuries, hospitalization, surgery.

   a. Car accident at age 41.

      (1) Description: Head went through the windshield.

      (2) Symptoms: Cut on forehead, 16 sutures required to close.

      (3) Hospital stay: Outpatient.

      (4) Treatment: X-ray studies, wound bandaged.

      (5) Treatment center: Staten Island Hospital.

      (6) Outcome: Scar on forehead.

   b. In 1941, client's flannel nightgown caught on fire, first and second degree burns.

      (1) Description: Client was 7 months pregnant with first child. She turned her back to the stove. The area between her elbow and shoulder caught fire. Client rushed into the shower.

      (2) Symptoms: Burns and pain.

      (3) Hospital stay: Hospitalized for approx 2 weeks.

      (4) Treatment: Medications and bandages.

      (5) Treatment center: Hospital.

      (6) Outcome: Scar on back.

   c. Unilateral oophorectomy, 1955.

      (1) Description: Large ovarian cyst.

(2) Symptoms: Severe pain in pelvic area.

(3) Hospital stay: Hospitalization approx 10 days.

(4) Treatment: Removal of ovary.

(5) Treatment center: Hospital

(6) Outcome: One functioning ovary intact.

d. Cystocele, 1972.

(1) Description: Prolapsed bladder.

(2) Symptoms: Stress incontinence.

(3) Hospital stay: Hospitalization approx 10 days.

(4) Treatment: Plastic surgery.

(5) Treatment center: Hospital

(6) Outcome: Favorable; no recurring symptoms.

e. Allergies: None.

f. Foreign travel: None.

F. Family history

1. Composition of family: Refer to genogram (Fig. 5-2).

2. Health history of family members: Refer to genogram (Fig. 5-2).

G. Social history

1. Environment.

a. Housing and physical facilities: The client and her husband own a house in the downtown section of their city. The house is walking distance to a park, public transportation (buses), a supermarket, a bank, a church, a post office, family restaurants, a bridge to Staten Island,

grammar schools, employment agency, and other minor shops.

b. Description of community: Upper middle class residential section of urban city; streets are tree lined. The homes are kept clean and painted and lawns manicured. She describes her neighbors as friendly. It is a small city; everyone seems to either be related or know each other because of social contact or their children attending the same schools and houses of worship.

(1) Ranked relatively crime-free, the city is considered residential.

(2) Urban residential.

(3) Politics: Client is active in Democratic party, and political affairs (voting, fundraising dinners).

(4) Economics: Class of workers

Private wage and salary workers	25,323
Government workers	4,376
Self-employed	1,300
Local government workers	2,704

(5) Population: Over 50,000

(6) Environment: The physical environment is clean and orderly. Pollution from local chemical industry and mass transit system is considered high.

(7) The city has one hospital with 299 beds. General merchandise stores, 14; eating and drinking places, 178; gasoline service sta-

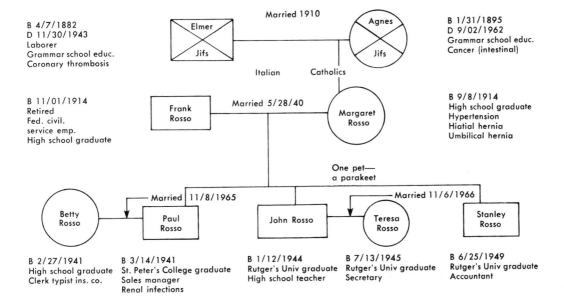

Fig. 5-2. Case study genogram.

tions, 47; home furnishing and equipment stores, 29; building and hardware supply dealers, 16; apparel and accessory stores, 68; drug and proprietary stores, 18.

(8) Transportation: Most families own an automobile. The city has three major bus lines, three companies that provide taxi service, and two private ambulance services.

2. Relationships outside the family: The client is socially active. She participates in charity dinners, shops with friends, participates in church activities (bingo, bus rides, carnivals, chance and raffle selling) and is associated with the Knights of Columbus through husband's affiliation.

3. Occupation/school: Client completed high school education. She worked for a few years as a secretary (small office), got married, and started a family.

Health examination

BP: 168/86
TPR: 98.2—88—26
WT: 160¾ lbs.
HT: 5'4"
GENERAL: M. R. is an alert, well-developed, slightly obese, white woman in no apparent distress.
SKIN: Pale, good turgor, warm, no lesions or excoriations.
HAIR: Normal distribution and consistency. Head and pubic hair gray.
NAILS: No deformities or clubbing. Evidence of nail biting. Nail beds pink, good blanching.
HEAD: Symmetrical, normocephalic.
FACE: Symmetry of nasolabial folds, no muscle weakness, no tics. Appropriate facial expression. Sense of touch, temperature, and pain intact.
EYES: Normal distribution of eyebrows and lashes. Ocular tension not tested. Conjuctiva clear. Sclera white. Pupils equal, round, and reacting to light and accommodation (PERRLA). No corneal defects. Snellen 20/90 OD, 20/100 OS, 20/70 OU. Color intact for red-green. Visual fields normal. Extraocular movements intact. Red reflex present. Fundi normal.
EARS: Whisper test normal left ear at 2 feet; right ear not heard. Weber: air conduction greater than bone conduction bilaterally. Large amount of dark brown cerumen in right canal. No masses or lesions. Tympanic membrane normal left ear; not visible right ear.
NOSE: Patent bilaterally. Mucosa pink. Smell intact for coffee and vinegar.
MOUTH: Mucosa and gingiva pink. No masses, lesions. Full upper and lower dentures. Taste positive for sweet, sour, bitter, and salty.

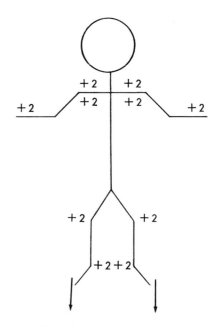

Fig. 5-3. Deep tendon reflexes.

PHARYNX: Mucosa pink, no lesions, uvula rises with "ah." Gag reflex intact.
NECK: Thyroid not palpable. Trachea midline. Lymph nodes not palpable.
CHEST: Contour normal. Thoracic expansion equal. AP diameter 1:2. Vocal fremitus normal bilaterally. No adventitious sounds. Resonant throughout.
BREASTS: Left slightly larger than right. Nipple position normal. No masses or discharge.
HEART: Neck veins not distended at 90-degree angle. No heaves or lifts. Apical impulse regular at fifth left intercostal space at midclavicular line. Sounds normal. No splits, murmurs, or gallops.
ABDOMEN: Flat, no lesions, tenderness, masses, or visible pulsations. Bowel sounds normal in each quadrant. Liver borders 11 cm at midclavicular line. Right and left kidneys nonpalpable. Spleen purcussed at sixth to tenth intercostal space at midaxillary line.
BACK: Slight kyphosis, no costovertebral angle tenderness.
EXTREMITIES: Full ROM. Normal gait; muscle and grip strength normal. All pulses palpable and equal.
GENITALIA: Pubic hair scanty. No labial swelling. No masses or lesions. Normal clitoris. Vagina pale, mucosa intact. No lesions or masses. Uterus posterior, average size, regular shape and mobile. Cervix compatible with multipara. No erosions or discharge. Tubes, ovaries, normal for age. Pap smear to laboratory.

NEUROLOGICAL:

CEREBRAL: Alert and cooperative. Oriented to time and place. Appropriate affect.

CRANIAL NERVES: Within normal limits.

CEREBELLAR FUNCTION: Finger/finger/nose, circle-eight and heel-to-shin coordination intact. Gait normal. Romberg test negative.

MOTOR FUNCTION: No tremors or weakness.

SENSORY FUNCTION: Touch, vibration, pain, heat, and cold intact.

DEEP TENDON REFLEXES: See Fig. 5-3.

ANA Standard II: Nursing diagnosis

Insufficient knowledge regarding breast self-examination.

Insufficient knowledge regarding effects of medication regimen.

Diminished auditory acuity right ear. Refer to ENT physician.

Excessive caloric intake.

SUMMARY

A nursing diagnosis is a summary of the assessment findings. It is a way of itemizing aspects of individualized care from a nursing framework.

A nursing diagnosis is not a nursing procedure. The nursing diagnosis states the area of client care to be addressed, whereas the nursing procedure delineates the specific steps needed to carry out the care itself.

Nursing diagnoses provide nursing with a unified nursing language that can be used in communications for developing client care plans, in research, and for third-party reimbursement of nursing care.

The vocabulary of nursing diagnosis has been evolving over the last 25 years. These diagnoses are being classified in a nursing diagnosis taxonomy, which classifies various areas of nursing concerns. When the process of nursing diagnosis is being introduced into any agency, it is most useful if (1) in-service programs are available to the nurses, (2) agency stationery is designed to record the diagnoses, and (3) if time is available to the staff to learn and use the system. The American Nurses' Association has stated that nursing diagnosis is an essential element in the evaluation of nursing care.

REFERENCES

Campbell, C.: Nursing diagnosis and intervention, New York, 1978, John Wiley & Sons.

Gordon, M., and Sweeney, M. A.: Methodological problems and issues in identifying and standardizing nursing diagnoses, Adv. Nurs. Sci. **2:**1, October 1979.

Gordon, M., Sweeney, M. A., and McKeehan, K.: Nursing diagnosis: looking at its use in the clinical area, Am. J. Nurs. **80:**672, April 1980.

Henderson, B.: Nursing diagnosis: theory and practice, 1978, Practice Oriented Theory, Part I, Aspen Systems Corp., p. 75.

Jones, P. E.: A terminology for nursing diagnoses, Adv. Nurs. Sci. **2:**65, October 1979.

Kritek, P. B.: Commentary: the development of nursing diagnosis and theory, Adv. Nurs. Sci. **2:**73, October 1979.

Matthews, C. A., and Gaul, G. L.: Nursing diagnosis from the perspective of concept attainment and critical thinking, Adv. Nurs. Sci. **2:**17, October 1979.

McCloskey, J.: Nurse's orders: the next professional breakthrough? R.N. **43:**99, February 1980.

Orr, J. G.: Care of the elderly patient in hospital, Nurs. Times **73:**1028, 7 July 1977.

Price, M.: Nursing diagnosis: making a concept come alive, Am. J. Nurs. **80:**668, April 1980.

Roberts, I.: Should geriatric nursing be a specialty? Nurs. Times **73:**1566, 6 October 1977.

SELECTED READING

Classifying nursing diagnoses

Kristine Gebbie ☐ **Mary Ann Lavin**

Use of the term diagnosis is gaining acceptance as the logical end product of nursing assessment. Inclusion of the term in recently revised nurse practice acts and related bills reflects this acceptance not only by nurses but also by the public. And nursing diagnosis has been included in the generic Standards of Nursing Practice developed by the American Nurses' Association.

Perhaps we have hesitated to use "diagnosis" because so many of us automatically preface it with the adjective "medical" in our effort to be very clear that we practice nursing, not medicine.

While diagnosis may be a troublesome term to some of us, we must make it our own. And we must determine what legitimate nursing diagnoses are, their signs and symptoms or characteristics, and what

Copyright © 1974, American Journal of Nursing Co. Reproduced, with permission, from the American Journal of Nursing, February, Vol. 74 No. 2.
Ms. Gebbie (B.S., St. Olaf College, Northfield, Minnesota; M.N., University of California at Los Angeles) is assistant professor of nursing at St. Louis University School of Nursing and Allied Health Professions, St. Louis, Mo. She is project director of the graduate program for nursing in distributive care settings. **Ms. Lavin** (St. John's Hospital School of Nursing, St. Louis, Mo.; B.S.N., M.S., St. Louis University) is a graduate student at Harvard School of Public Health. She was an assistant professor of nursing at St. Louis University. Ms. Gebbie and Ms. Lavin were co-directors of the First National Conference on the Classification of Nursing Diagnoses held at St. Louis, Mo., University, October 1-5, 1973.

interventions are specific to them.

While a standard classification system is no panacea for nursing's ills, it should, indeed, make many ordinary tasks much easier and aid us in focusing directly on those things which are essential to developing our contribution to overall health care. The level of our research can also be raised through the use of a standard nomenclature to communicate the content of our practice rather than the forms in which it is carried out.

DEVELOPING A SYSTEM

The first step in developing a classification is to identify all those things which nurses locate or diagnose in patients. This means nothing less than describing the entire domain of nursing. This does not mean the identification of all of the tasks performed by nurses or of all the things nurses have ever done in any situation or under any circumstances. It is the identification of those patient problems or concerns most frequently identified by nurses, problems which are usually identified by nurses before they are recognized by other health care workers, and problems which are amenable to some intervention which is available in the present or potential scope of nursing practice.

The second step is to reach some agreement about consistent nomenclature which can be used to describe the domain of nursing as identified in step one. For nurses to collaborate effectively, even within one health care setting, much less across organizational and geographic boundaries, we must know what we

are all saying. Terms should be sufficiently well defined so that if a nurse from one setting says she cares mostly for patients with "x" nursing diagnosis, another nurse in another setting knows at once the problem she is referring to or can go to a recognized dictionary of nursing nomenclature for a concise description of the cardinal signs and symptoms. Hypothetically, this terminology or nomenclature can be expanded readily from diagnosis to intervention, for interventions should be diagnosis specific, rather than symptomatic. If we are communicating more directly about the diagnoses we treat, we should be able to be clearer about the treatments we actually apply or provide.

The third step in the classification process is the grouping of identified diagnoses (the labels) into classes and subclasses so that patterns and relationships among them can emerge. This process may involve the division of some labeled diagnoses into two or more distinct entities, and the merger of what first appeared to be different conditions under one label. In this process much of the work already done on philosophies and conceptual frameworks for nursing may be of help. Also, the study and labeling of the diagnoses may reveal some more appropriate classification system than those attempted by deductive processes.

The final step in the process is the substitution of numbers or equivalent abbreviations for terminology, so that data related to the various diagnoses can be manipulated more readily by machine or hand. Substitution of computer language for the usual diary-type of nursing notations does not assist in the manipulation of data—it merely compresses the amount of space needed to store data. If we can reach the stage where coding of the diagnostic entities and related interventions is possible, we will be able to use computerized data retrieval systems to gain access to multiple cases of a given problem or multiple instances in which a given intervention was used, and the process of nursing research should be speeded.

GROUND RULES

The First National Conference on Classification of Nursing Diagnoses, though only a beginning, was a significant beginning. Four "instant old proverbs" emerged from the planning process and served as a partial guide to participants.

1. We won't satisfy everyone, but we must be intelligible to many. There is no way that the beginning phase of a work project such as the classification of nursing diagnoses can make all practicing nurses perfectly happy. However, even the beginning work must be in a form and language which can be used by and be intelligible to the majority of nurses. Only then will it serve as a springboard for the continuing development of the nomenclature and classification.

2. If it comes to a pinch of time and energy in the initial stages of work, detail must be sacrificed for comprehensiveness. If the material developed is broad enough so that almost every practicing nurse can see that it has meaning for the diagnosis of problems she encounters in her daily practice, there will follow multiple opportunities to test the labels and develop the details. If only a small portion of the domain of nursing is covered in detail, and the rest ignored, few will be stimulated to continue the work.

3. We must not reject existing material for new merely for its newness, but we cannot wed ourselves too rigidly to the present merely to encourage rapid acceptance. There is no point or merit in reinventing the wheel. If available materials or terms will serve our purpose, we should use them. It is always tempting to do something all over again just so the world will know it is really ours. However, if we really can't agree that the old terms serve our purpose, we should articulate new ones, because it is hazardous to attempt to bend an already existing concept. We may lose the meaning we wanted as we try to keep others comfortable with our language.

Tentative list of nursing diagnoses

Alterations in faith
Altered relationships with self and others
Altered self-concept
Anxiety
Body fluids, depletion of
Bowel function, irregular
Cognitive, functioning, alteration in the level of
Comfort level, alterations in
Confusion (disorientation)
Deprivation
Digestion, impairment of
Family's adjustment to illness, impairment of
Family process, inadequate
Fear
Grieving
Lack of understanding
Level of consciousness, alterations in
Malnutrition
Manipulation
Mobility, impaired
Motor incoordination
Non-compliance
Pain
Regulatory function of the skin, impairment of
Respiration, impairment of
Respiratory distress
Self-care activities, altered ability to perform
Sensory disturbances
Skin integrity, impairment of
Sleep/rest pattern, ineffective
Susceptibility to hazards
Thought process, impaired
Urinary elimination, impairment of
Verbal communication, impairment of

The more nurses who become familiar with the preliminary list of nursing diagnoses and begin testing them, the more opportunities we will have to quickly develop a sound, comprehensive system of classifying nursing diagnoses. The initial classification of medical diagnoses, which listed causes of death, was done over 300 years ago, and consisted of five categories which were neither comprehensive nor logically consistent with one another. It has taken the intervening 300 years to reach the sophisticated level of the International Classification of Disease and the Systematized Nomenclature of Pathology. The improved state of communication and our potential ability to learn from other disciplines should shorten our developmental time to considerably less than 300 years, but it will take many more years than 3, or even 30.

The concepts developed must be tested formally. This can occur in research centers, in practice settings of all kinds, and in education settings. This involves the commitment, not only of the individual nurse, but of the nursing organization in the specific locale. Administrators, directors, and supervisors can be instrumental in the beginning of testing projects in their institutions.

PRELIMINARY DIAGNOSES

Because the conference participants could not agree on any one classification scheme for the diagnoses they identified, the diagnoses were listed alphabetically. Obviously, then, the order in which a diagnosis appears says nothing about its frequency of occurrence, importance for patient welfare, or relationship with those diagnoses which precede and follow it. The 34 diagnoses on which the group reached some consensus are listed in the preceding section.

Some of these labels may mean something to you, others may be so much Greek. Even if the clinical situation labeled by any of these diagnoses is identifiable, no diagnostic label makes real sense unless it is accompanied by a list of characteristics. By characteristics, we mean the signs or symptoms actually present in a person who has the diagnosis in question. This is not the same as assessment parameters, which serve as guidelines in selecting what to observe in order to determine whether or not the pertinent characteristics are present. If a characteristic or "urinary elimination, impairment of" is "output below 500 cc in 24 hours," the assessment parameter can be listed as "urinary output." The diagnostician must know the specific characteristics of a given diagnosis before making a judgment about the patient's condition.

For some of the identified diagnoses, no specific characteristics were listed. The participants could only agree that the problem was in the domain of nursing. To clarify this, we will compare the present levels of sophistication of the first three diagnoses: alterations in faith, altered self-concept, and anxiety.

Alterations in faith has three subdiagnoses: alterations in faith in one's self, alterations in faith in others, and alterations in faith in God. These can be further modified by two other concepts which were considered fairly significant in describing a diagnostic category: its etiology, whether anatomical, physiological, psychological, or environmental; and its duration, whether chronic, intermittent, acute, or potential. Some characteristics noted for this diagnosis were obstacles to responding in a love relationship to man and God, recognition of sinfulness, acceptance of one's self, and acceptance of others' needs for a relationship with God.

As you can see, these are not behavioral signs, nor are they necessarily symptoms which a person might describe himself as having. But even with this lack of clarity regarding the characteristics of this diagnosis, a sufficient proportion of those attending the conference believed that it was appropriate to be concerned about the patient's faith, at least in himself, and so the diagnostic label stands until further testing validates its inclusion and yields more specific diagnostic criteria, or leads to the exclusion of the category from the classification system.

Initial testing of this diagnosis would be anecdotal. Someone could collect records of any patients about whom a nurse says, "He's just lost faith," or "He seems to have given up." A list of the common characteristics from these records could be developed, and this list of signs and symptoms could then become the basis of a wider case-finding effort. Or, perhaps, no commonalities would be found and we might learn that its diagnosis is meaningless and leads nowhere in the clinical situation.

Altered self-concept has four subdiagnoses: altered body image, depersonalization, identity conflict, and role disturbance. Again, each of these may have any of the four etiologies and any of the four durations. For example, an altered body image of anatomical etiology and chronic duration might be the diagnosis of a person who had lost a limb one year prior to contact with the diagnosing nurse and had not yet incorporated the loss into the image of himself. An altered body image of environmental etiology and acute duration might be the diagnosis of a patient forced to wear translucent goggles during a diagnostic procedure.

While no discrete characteristics were identified for all of these sub-sub cases, the subdiagnosis of altered body image is fairly well defined as being characterized by negative verbalization about the body, expressions of grief over the loss of a body part or function, nonverbal behavior (such as not looking at the body part, not touching the body part, hiding or overexposing the body part, purposeless activity, change in eye contact, change in hygiene), general reactions of poor comprehension of facts and explanations, changes in total self-concept (sexual roles, productive roles, and so on), and use of nonpersonal pronouns. Some of these characteristics also seem to apply to other subdiagnostic categories. We must, then, work to discover which are the general signs or symptoms which lead one to the general diagnosis of altered self-concept, and which are the finer distinguishing marks that enable one to apply one of the subdiagnostic labels. Work on clarifying this diagnosis could reach a more sophisticated level much more rapidly than work on that of alteration in faith.

The third diagnostic label is anxiety. Here, the conference participants drew on well-recognized portions of nursing literature and selected subdiagnoses in line with the four types of anxiety identified and studied by Hildegard Peplau[1]. These subcategories of anxiety are each described by discrete characteristics. If the patient's reason for concern or anxiety is not identifiable, the general diagnosis of anxiety is made and then a subcategory is selected, based on the following:

Mild anxiety: increased learning ability, alertness to environment, increased awareness of detail, increase in goal-directed behavior, restlessness.

Moderate anxiety: narrowing perceptual field, attention to detail, muscle tension, perspiration, needing help to focus problem-solving.

Severe anxiety: very narrow perceptual focus or scattering of attention, inability to relate parts to whole, trembling, nausea, headache, feeling of dread, rapid pulse.

Panic: distortion of reality, extremely narrow focus, difficulty verbalizing feeling, bizarre behavior, dilated pupils, increased pulse, ashen color.

As with all diagnoses, these may be modified by their etiology. Anatomical etiology did not seem probable, though some might want to research this. Examples of physiological, psychological, and environmental etiologies can be identified readily. The duration of an anxiety state can also be identified as chronic, intermittent, acute (situational), or potential. Research on this diagnosis might begin with the identification of all interventions ever used in conjunction with the diagnosis and move to the determination of which interventions yielded the most success in a given subdiagnostic situation.

Clearly, diagnostic development is an evolutionary process. An example of this can be drawn from the biography, *The Doctors Mayo*(2). Having decided that *bellyache* was appropriate to the domain of medicine, someone began keeping records of all cases of bellyache. In reviewing these cases, someone observed the major distinction: some people had a fever and some did not. This process of making distinctions continued, coupled with distinctions in intervention. For example, surgery prior to or following the onset of abdominal rigidity led to the eventual identification of acute appendicitis as discrete from the generic acute peritonitis to which it sometimes leads.

The process of inclusion and exclusion of diagnostic terms involves decisions. At present there is no statement of the criteria for inclusion or exclusion though some might be inferred. Some labels were proposed which are not developed well enough for us to decide whether they should be included or eliminated. These diagnoses were depression, developmental lag, jaundice, sexuality problems, stress, and suicide potential. Several other labels were discussed, accepted as preliminary, and then discarded. Dependent personality

and drug dependence, for example were identified and then discarded.

Dependent personality was eliminated because of the experiences other disciplines have had in attempting to label so-called personality types and the extreme difficulty of making the labels sensible and useful. Drug dependence was discarded because we had decided not to duplicate previous efforts, and the various types of chemical dependency are well categorized in the Standard Diagnostic and Statistical Manual of Psychiatry. There is no prohibition against using a label from another field if we use it with the characteristics and accuracy usually expected and it says what we want it to say.

We may well come to similar decisions regarding other diagnoses on the preliminary list. We may also subsequently decide to include labels which were eliminated or not considered during this first conference. That is for nurses to determine collectively.

FIRST STEPS

How can nurses everywhere take part in this? How does one begin? A simple method of primary data collection, which can be used almost immediately and can develop into sophisticated research designs, involves the cards used in medical records departments to cross-index medical diagnoses and procedures. When a patient is discharged from the facility, the face sheet of his record is numerically coded by the physician's discharge diagnoses and procedures. A card like this is prepared for each one of hundreds of medical diagnoses and procedures. The record number of each chart which was coded by that procedure or diagnosis is entered on the appropriate card. It is then possible to retrieve the last 100 cases of X or all examples of Y performed in an institution in 1971.

The card can be modified for nurs-

ing use. One nurse, a ward nursing staff, or the entire staff of an agency, could decide to keep records on one or more of the diagnoses on the preliminary list. Each time a nurse diagnosed a patient as having the problem in question, whether she used the characteristics listed in the preliminary manual or just said "I know that's what he has," she would enter the patient's name, age, record number, her own name, and other cross-referencing data, such as concurrent medical diagnoses or other nursing diagnoses also present, on the card for that diagnosis. Then, when sufficient cases are identified, the indicated records can be retrieved and studied to see if people were consistent in applying the label, if the chief criteria are readily identified, if our notes reflect what we say we saw, and how we intervened. If cards were kept for all the diagnoses and an attempt made to diagnose all patients, it would also be possible to review all the cards after a given time to determine the morbidity rate for each diagnosis so that attention could be focused on those which seemed to occur most often.

This approach is relatively simple and many people could be involved, even though only one or two people might do the final data analysis. Also, these cards are standard from institution to institution and duplicate copies of completed cards could be sent to a central data collection point. This would permit regional or national study of one or more diagnoses.

In their collective consciousness, nurses have a wealth of data about nursing. Together, we can develop a standard nomenclature of nursing diagnoses.

REFERENCES

1. Peplau, H. E. Interpersonal relations in nursing, New York, G. P. Putnam's Sons, 1952.
2. Clapesattle, Helen. The Doctors Mayo, 2d ed, Minneapolis, University of Minnesota Press, 1954.

Why nursing diagnosis?

June S. Rothberg

Nursing diagnosis is a term which, in recent years, has been used with ever increasing frequency and often with little accuracy. For various reasons, the term can be an emotion-laden or frightening concept to nurses and to other health personnel. Before discussing what a nursing diagnosis is, let us review what it is not. It is not a medical diagnosis made by nurses. It is not a psychiatric diagnosis made by nurses. It is not a socioeconomic diagnosis made by nurses.

In making a nursing diagnosis, the professional nurse may utilize specific information from the diagnoses which other qualified persons have made. However, she will add to this information her own independent observations to form an evaluation which is uniquely nursing.

In 1961, Abdellah stated, "We must face up to the responsibility that making a nursing diagnosis is an independent function of the professional nurse."[1] I believe that for far too long a time we in nursing have abdicated this responsibility.

As a starting point, in broad and very general terms, a nursing diagnosis may be thought of as an evaluation by nurses of those factors affecting the patient which will influence his recovery. These factors may include intrinsic dimensions such as physical condition or emotional state, and, also, external influences such as economic problems. All nurses, I am certain, know of a patient whose physical progress was impeded be-

cause he was frantic over bills or who couldn't be discharged because he was unable to walk up three flights of stairs. Some of these factors will need to be referred to appropriate disciplines for action. Some are directly the responsibility of nursing.

It is precisely in the area of interdisciplinary functions and relations, that difficulties in patient care arise. There is considerable overlap at the boundaries of each profession's practice. Instead of leading to increased cooperation and communication for the benefit of the individual and all society, this overlap has led to the reverse. The various disciplines are warily watching their own vested interests—guarding their particular prerogatives and preserves. Lest I be misunderstood, I mean nursing, too.

In the past 15 years, there has been a tremendous increase in the number of persons working in the health arena. The 1960 census indicated that in a 10-year span, the health field has risen from seventh to third place among major United States industries in terms of numbers of persons employed[2]. This was six years ago! Not only are numbers increasing but as knowledge expands and is intensified, becoming more advanced and more highly technical, new specialties are proliferating. In my own field of rehabilitation, there are physical, occupational, and recreational therapists, vocational and rehabilitation counselors, and prosthetists to mention only a few of the occupational specialists. It is now possible for a person to obtain a professional degree (a bachelor of science) in orthotics, the newest specialty field.

With the impetus given by recent health and social legislation which is directed toward the preparation of health workers to meet the needs of our continually burgeoning and aging population, there will be an ever larger number of persons working in health fields.

We may expect ever greater fragmentation of services than current and anticipated growth warrants unless each and all of us become completely aware of a single overriding fact—the common denominator in health or disease is the individual man. It is not an institution—not a doctor—not a nurse—not any other health worker. It is the human being who needs to be kept well and treated when sick. Without awareness and understanding of this central fact, health care and particularly nursing care has neither direction nor meaning.

The challenge to us today is to furnish the kind of health care people need, when and where they need it. To do this, we must bring the patient into the foreground. There is no one idea having greater importance for nursing than that of viewing the patient as a person. It is only when the patient is so viewed, as a person, that care is provided to him according to his needs in an appropriate, continuous, and dynamic pattern which is sometimes described as comprehensive care. Nursing diagnosis makes it possible to provide such care.

One hears much today about meeting total needs of patients. This is a reaction to a practice which has concentrated primarily on two areas: routine physical care concerned with fundamental physiologic processes such as nutrition and elimination, and highly technical complex aspects of nursing. We have emphasized the physical and the technical while ignoring or not understanding the perceptions, the responses, the social, and psychologic needs of people. To further complicate the picture, we have so fragmented our services that the basic physical care of patients has been relegated to increasingly less well-prepared personnel and we have taken to our professional bosom those highly complex and often painful procedures which were formerly the province of the physician.

All too frequently, we have centered on the medical diagnosis, the psychiatric or other diagnosis. We have carried out medically prescribed orders, briskly and efficiently applied some highly routine or ritualized procedures, and considered the whole process nursing, while neatly ignoring the patients' perceptions, feelings, and individual problems.

As a reminder of the hazard, encountered when we concentrate on physical diagnosis as the sole determining factor in planning nursing care, consider the following. The patient in bed 13 has a gastric neoplasm, the one in bed 32 has a viral pneumonia, and the one in bed 20 has a cerebral aneurysm. What do we know about these three persons? Only their medical diagnoses! The person in each bed could be any combination of either half of the following: a man or a woman, 35 years old or 75, ill for years with a chronic disease or sick for the first time in his life, a valued and loved family member or a socially isolated person living without family or friends, destitute or financially secure.

It is the combination of such factors plus many others which will strongly influence the particular patient's progress and recovery. These characteristics exert this influence because they are the resources—physical, emotional, social, and eco-nomic—which the person can call upon to overcome his illness. Nursing diagnosis is the process which identifies the patient's resources and deficits, thus indicating his needs for nursing assistance.

Historically, patient care has been considered the core of all nursing activity regardless of the setting in which it was performed or the type of nursing function required. Modern nursing extends over the broad spectrum of health services and encompasses promotion of health, prevention of illness, as well as care of patients and their families. In order to administer patient care, the nurse must identify the individual's needs for nursing services. Ever since nursing was first performed, the nurse, by a process either wholly or partially conscious, looked at the patient and determined on the basis of intuition, experience, rote learning, knowledge, or in some cases ignorance, which nursing acts were needed to relieve his distress.

What must the nurse know about the patient? This is the central question in determining, in a professionally responsible manner, the patient's requirements for nursing services. What must she understand of the intrinsic processes (physical, physiologic, emotional), occurring within him? What must she know of the extrinsic factors (sociologic, economic) surrounding him, and the influence these exert upon him? How well does he manage himself in relation to the stresses he faces? What probable results can she expect from her nursing? When the nurse is able to answer these questions accurately, she is ready to provide appropriate comprehensive nursing.

Answering these questions in a clearly ordered, reasoned manner, based on scientific fact, requires the establishment of a nursing diagnosis and nursing therapy. Nursing diagnosis is an evaluation within the framework of current knowledge, of the patient's condition as a person including physical, physiologic, and behavioral aspects.

Let us examine the key word of this definition: *evaluation.* An evaluation is a process, implying a continuing operation. There are many kinds of evaluations which go on all the time, continually influencing our choice of actions. Some are not conscious evaluations but are implicit or intuitive. At this moment, you are evaluating what you read. As I write, I am subconsciously evaluating your possible response to my words. But neither of us is sharply aware of this evaluation process as it goes on—it is almost automatic.

However, these kinds of evaluations—intuitive, implicit, and automatic—are not what is required in making a nursing diagnosis. It is definitive, clearly focused, and completely conscious evaluation which is necessary for our decision making about patients. In order to be of help to ourselves and especially to others, we must practice evaluation in an explicit manner as a consciously planned activity. It may be practiced informally. However, it frequently is carried out within the framework of a formal evaluation instrument.

What is it we are evaluating? We are determining the patient's condition—the relative state of health or ill health in physical, functional (or physiologic), and behavioral areas. We are looking for both strengths and weaknesses in these areas and for both overt and covert problems.

How are we evaluating? We are consciously and systematically observing physical signs and activities, physiologic indications and reports, and observing social and interpersonal behavior. The interpretation of observations is based on principles from the biologic, physical, and social sciences which have been integrated into a nursing science.

Why are we evaluating? The purpose of such assessment is to determine the patient's (or the family's) need. We are trying to appraise the situation of the patient to learn what we as professionals can do for him.

Thus, the prime element in the process of evaluation or diagnosis is identification of individual needs. The second element is clear definition of goals for the patient's care. One such goal, in the physical realm, might be to obtain the maximum possible improvement in the patient's condition. Another goal might have to be more modest, such as the maintenance of his present condition without further deterioration. An even more modest but imperative goal must be the prevention of superimposed disabilities(3). A different kind of goal might be to increase the patient's verbal interaction with his roommates. Several categories of goals must be packaged together, since the patient being diagnosed is a person with a variety of responses, facets, and problems. Therefore, goals include desired physical, functional, and behavioral targets.

The nurse making a diagnosis determines which of the identified care needs are amenable to nursing. Once nursing problems have been defined clearly by the diagnosis, a course of nursing activities purposefully directed toward increasing the positive health of the patient can be initiated. The nurse selects the appropriate methods, resources, and personnel to meet the identified needs. Those needs which are beyond the scope of nursing are referred to the appropriate health workers. Thus, the unique function of the professional nurse is

being performed—that of the diagnosis of the patient's need for nursing services and the decision upon a course of action to follow(4).

We have now moved into the realm of nursing therapy. Nursing therapy is defined as knowledgeable intervention in the form of nursing activities, based on the nursing diagnosis, and directed at moving the individual toward positive health(5). Nursing care plans are a step toward nursing therapy. There is absolutely no point in making a nursing diagnosis, unless it leads directly to action in the form of nursing therapy. And, of course, appropriate comprehensive nursing therapy is impossible without a prior diagnosis of need. Nursing therapy is derived specifically from the diagnosis. Direction for the nursing intervention is given by the nursing diagnosis. The three elements of diagnosis—identification of individual need, establishment of goals, and selection of appropriate methods—together provide the knowledge required in order to act appropriately to move the individual toward more positive health.

New knowledge in the health sciences is expanding and pyramiding at a fantastic rate. Predictions about nursing practice of the future, made only five years ago, were considered by a majority of nurses to be science fiction, but today are reality. Nurses are working with patients treated in hyperbaric chambers, with bioelectric monitoring devices, with elec-

tronic cardiac, bladder, and muscle pacemaker and implants. Microminiaturization techniques developed for outer space explorations have opened untold opportunities for the alleviation of man's physical ills.

In view of these technological changes, what happens to the fragility and importance of the individual? One way to meet the challenge is to consciously and clear-sightedly assess the patient's needs as an individual utilizing keen professional observation plus all the mechanical gadgets to obtain highly accurate information about his condition and to utilize skilled professional judgment to interpret and evaluate the information. Then, at all times remembering that all people have a diversity of needs, make a diagnosis and institute a plan of therapy to meet the individual problems of the person in our care.

REFERENCES

1. Abdellah, Faye. *Meeting Patients Needs—An Approach to Teaching.* Paper presented at biennial convention of the National League for Nursing, Cleveland, Ohio, April 10-14, 1961.
2. Manpower in health. *Progressive Health Services* 10:May 1961.
3. Rothberg, June, ed. Foreword, [to the] Symposium on chronic disease and rehabilitation. *Nursing Clinics of North America* 1:352-354, Sept. 1966.
4. Abdellah, *op. cit.*
5. Bonney, Virginia, and Rothberg, June. *Nursing Diagnosis and Therapy; an Instrument for Evaluation and Measurement.* New York, National League for Nursing, 1963.

II

CARE PLANNING

6 Accentuate the positive

A car must have gasoline in its tank if it is to go the full length of the journey. No matter how new or old the car is or what the road or destination is, it needs the energy source. So it is with nurses. As human beings, nurses have basic needs, and among these needs is the inner energy or fuel required to do the job. A nurse can have a good education and a desire to be of help to others. The nursing process helps her organize and plan her care. In order for a nurse to help her clients identify and use their strengths, the nurse herself should have a positive attitude toward herself and her responsibilities. The energy source to move ahead with her nursing stems from the energy she derives from a feeling of positive self-esteem and job satisfaction. When a nurse runs out of her "gas," her care and caring stop; she has run out of fuel. This is called burnout.

The use of the nursing process cannot be viewed as an isolated entity. Its implementation depends on the resources of the individual nurse whose resources begin with her energy level. The nurse who works with the older adult is at special risk for burnout. Contemporary society undervalues its older population. Persons who work for these older adults are discounted too. For example, nursing homes and senior citizen's groups are not seen as exciting working environments. Pay scales are often lower than in other settings, even though the positions require much nursing expertise. Nurses who work with older adults should be particularly aware of the hazards.

A head nurse was talking with the administrator of a long-term-care facility. He was going on and on, saying such things as, "Nurses have done an outstanding job. They are the ones who really focus on patient contentment and care. They can organize a busy floor. They have done a lot, but they cannot rest on their laurels."

The nurse made no response at the time, for the administrator was in the middle of a tirade about other nurses not doing this and nurses not doing that. To this administrator, nurses were just not at all satisfactory. Quite frankly, the head nurse was bored by the entire monologue. After leaving the office, her initial reflection was, "Nurses cannot rest on their laurels? Why not? Why can't nurses be darn proud of the job they have done so well and just take the time to gloat a bit? Oh, to be able to relish success, to enjoy that feeling of victory and of a job superbly done. Why not slap each other on the back and say 'Terrific!' Where is our cheering section?"

THE GOOD OLD DAYS

What about the following type of comment: "In the old days the nursing care was far better?" To this modern nurses respond, "Oh really. By what measure?" There were far fewer critically ill persons in hospitals in the good old days. Today modern technology supports the ill person through the initial phase of recovery. Years ago, if a person had a myocardial infarction, he never made it to the hospital. Burn victims didn't live long enough to receive treatment. If a person was in renal failure, in a couple of days life ended. The older woman who fell and broke her hip wasn't hospitalized. She stayed at home in her own bedroom until she died of hypostatic pneumonia. She couldn't be operated upon; the anesthetic and fluid replacement therapies were not available to sustain her.

Just think of all those old pictures in journals and textbooks of the good old days. There they are: the really good nurses, when nurses were really nurses. What is seen usually are two rows of beds—perhaps 20 beds in all. The head nurse looks starched right up to her stiff collar. Beside the beds, we see perhaps four or five student nurses all looking equally starched and dour. Look

113

at the clients. All of them are in bed. Maybe one or two are sitting up in a wheelchair. The most extensive equipment seen in the picture is a bandage or two and maybe a leg elevated here and there. No wonder they had the time to keep their caps on straight. What is missing in this picture? Where are the IVs, the respirators, the cardiac monitors, the Levine tubes, the Foley catheters, the injections, the x-ray equipment, the lab slips? Today, these technological aspects of care are common scenes while viewing the hospitalized client. Look for the unit with the burned client, the neurosurgical client, the cardiac client; the renal dialysis client—or any emergency care unit or community health care agency. In addition to the traditional comfort care measures and treatments such as dressings and soaks, the nurse of today has the responsibility of monitoring the very sophisticated equipment that keeps the ill client stabilized. Consider, for example, intravenous therapy. Although IVs are often taken for granted, they are essential life-supporting systems. The older adult's fluid and electrolyte balance is a precarious regulation of the cardiovascular volume and the renal filtration ability. With too much IV fluid, the older adult quickly goes into congestive heart failure; but with too low a circulatory volume, his already diminished nephron function is compromised even further. It takes much time, attention, and often patience to meet the physical and emotional needs of the older adult.

The nurse makes decisions every hour that make the difference between illness and recovery, between pain and relief, between success and failure in a course of care by the health team. Often nurses work until they are bone weary, and work hours beyond their endurance. If a nurse does not seem to care, it is often because she has given her all and is frustrated and discouraged down to her gut. It is sad to hear despair and discouragement among nursing colleagues. It is hard to battle against so many odds. What a shame to see good women fall on the wayside for the want of support and congratulations for a job that is truly well done. Any comment denying nursing the right to drink in the bubbly joy of its successes is not right. Nurses are entitled to reap the rewards for their successes. When the nurse who works in the care of older adults feels worthwhile and valued, then she is more likely to have the energy available to encourage the older person to seek a healthy and satisfied life also.

NURSING PRACTICE IN A HISTORICAL CONTEXT

Modern nursing is closely bound to roots in the military and religious orders of the past. These "angels of mercy" and rigid discipline traditions have fostered nursing's feelings of nonworldliness. Nurses are not angels. Some of the heavenly goals nursing sets for itself are just not attainable. Nurses are human and must be measured in human terms. That means nurses make mistakes, plenty of mistakes. However, there is nothing to be ashamed of, to feel guilty about, or to criticize. Nurses are human, so let nursing not use the criteria of the angels for itself. Autonomy comes only through a positive self-image and self-direction. The care of the older adult as a particular specialty has not been considered dramatic and exciting in this era of technology and youth. As a result of these attitudes, nurses in this area of practice run a special risk of discouragement and lowered self-esteem.

VALUE OF POSITIVE SELF-ESTEEM

Compliments and praise are not entirely socially acceptable within the nursing ranks. It is almost more acceptable to say such things as: If nursing is to survive we must do such and such. Or, nursing care today is at its poorest ever—in the old days care was really good. Much hand wringing and moans accompany all these comments. These remarks are pretty common in nursing conversations. A response to the remark about nursing not surviving is nonsense. The care of the ill is an essential service, but there is more to nursing than that. Nursing focuses on support of health and high-level wellness. As long as there are people, they will need nursing, and nursing will be here to serve them.

What is esteem?

Esteem is a measure of a person's worth, value and respect. There are two sources of self-esteem. One is an experience that evokes sufficient self-approval to be esteeming; this is called an intrinsic source of self-esteem. Another is an esteeming experience that depends largely or entirely upon social approval, and this is an extrinsic source of self-esteem. Extrinsic sources can be tangible, such as objects and material rewards, or intangible, such as compliments or praise.

In human development there is a relationship associated with high self-esteem and a person's readiness to explore both his own attributes and job relevant aspects of the environment. High self-esteem frees a person to see his own assets and talents. The self-approval inherent in the use of intrinsic sources of self-esteem is related to other personal attributes such as self-confidence, independence, assertiveness, and an increase in the probability that exploration will be profitable. These are very desirable traits in all nurses and particularly for those nurses who work with older adults.

Self-esteem can be viewed as an antecedent to achievement or as a consequence of it. This is one of those "Which came first, the chicken or the egg?" situations. Maslow's theory states that self-esteem needs must be met before achievement expectations can be met. Conversely, persons with unmet self-esteem needs are not ready to achieve, do not succeed, and do not receive approval. These are the very people, therefore, who have diminished self-esteem. A client's self-esteem needs must be met, and nurses require similar positive esteem self-perceptions to help clients achieve.

Nurses do not always have their self-esteem needs met. People need extrinsic sources of approval; that is, they need praise, recognition, and rewards. Some examples would be a pat on the back, a handshake of congratulations, and the genuine compliment for a job well done. Self-esteem requires a social approval for reinforcement to help nurses gain the self-esteem required to encourage the development of achievement needs. Persons need opportunities for both self and social approval. Nurses should have these opportunities available to themselves every day. Nurses should stand up and cheer for themselves. When nurses do a fine job, they should acknowledge their own success. On the other hand, let nursing discourage every moan and groan, every word of gloom and doom. Nurses should not see the world through rose-colored glasses; nor should they see the world through dark glasses. Nurses should view their world with clear glass so that they may see reality and accept it for what it is. Self-esteem needs must be met before the need to achieve becomes a motivator of behavior. This has most important implications for self-critical cliches in nursing. Peer recognition must occur every day, with love, laughter, and vigor.

Maslow states that a person must feel accepted if self-esteem needs are to be addressed. It is necessary for an individual to experience acceptance (being esteemed by others) before one can esteem oneself. Self-esteem is anchored in and depends upon social approval. The good feelings a person receives from social approval permit the person to go forth and attempt to master the environment. The relationship between self-esteem and achievement and independence is reciprocal: each experience reinforces the next. It is an upward positive spiral (Fig. 6-1). When a person is mature, more and more self-esteem may be derived from self-approval, but the total reservoir of good feelings

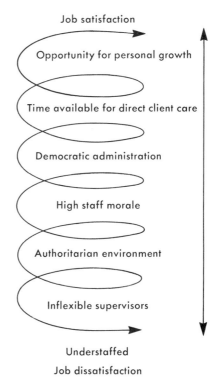

Fig. 6-1. Self-esteem cycle.

about one's self is probably never entirely free from the influence of external approval. Nursing has enormous contributions to make, and nurses work super hard to get things accomplished, only to be defeated or frustrated because of lack of this external or social approval.

As nurses strive toward self-actualization, there are some advantages to this emerging self-esteem and self-actualization. Since nothing or no one is perfect, perfection should not be the measure of success. A positive self-esteem enables nursing to have more accurate perceptions of reality and a more comfortable relationship with it; in addition, acceptance by self and others will be fostered. Nursing should say good-bye to the "they do not like us" attitude and the "nobody appreciates us" posture. The neurotic person is always crippled by unnecessary guilt, shame, and anxiety. What a waste of energy. Those with a positive self-image and a good measure of self-esteem can accept human nature with all of its shortcomings and discrepancies from the ideal image, without feelings of real concern.

All this will decrease nursing's defensiveness. Let nurses take the offensive strategy. Self-esteem promotes a natural spontaneity and creativity, and it lets nursing focus on problem centers. If nurses strive to foster their own self-esteem, the entire profession and the clients will benefit. There will be more energies available to do the real job of nursing. Of what value are exhaustion, frustration, and tears? They are of no value except perhaps to ask, "Where shall I lay the body when the day is over?"

When negative thinking is overcome, the exciting promise of each day can be felt. With positive self-esteem, nursing can give credit to itself for its accomplishments and look upon its shortcomings humanely; when it does examine itself, it will not fall prey to negative ideas that shortchange its estimate of itself.

The put-downs about nurses are wrong. Life can be an adventure; it can be exciting, and it can be purposeful. Uncertainty is merely a fact of life. Confrontations should not be a surprise. Change is inevitable, so why be surprised by it? There is an old saying that goes, "The only man without problems is a dead man." Nursing has problems, but that is a good sign. It means that the organism

is alive. A healthy self-image gives nurses the sense of certainty that is needed to go on. Nurses cannot be loved until nurses love themselves. Self-image will dictate many of the circumstances in which nurses find themselves and will influence how they are handled. An awareness of the good things that happen will bring a feeling of pleasure and contentment. Relish the pleasure. Repetitive thought of something bad builds up frustration and disappointment.

Since self-esteem encourages human interaction, let give and take become natural and rewarding. The positive reinforcement between colleagues encourages positive feelings, which then produce positive action. Permit nursing research to reflect successes, not merely failures. Look at nursing with a sense of humor so that a fall short of an objective is not taken personally. Be gentle with nursing.

When nurses love themselves, their colleagues, and their profession for the fine job they do, they have more personal resources available to offer the client. Older adults in long-term-care facilities, in other agencies, or in the community benefit from nurses who feel good and have energy available as they work. It is important for nurses to take the time to fill up their "gas tank" for themselves and their clients.

BURNOUT

Burnout is a description of the damage done by overworking. It is insidious and tenacious. The result is disillusionment with a career in nursing, casting aside all one's ideals and replacing them with bitterness and disappointment. Burnout is prevalent in the helping professions; nursing, medicine, and social work. These persons become so involved in meeting other people's needs that they do not recognize that their own needs are not being met.

There are physical as well as psychological signs and symptoms of burnout. There are four phases of burnout.

1. Emotional exhaustion
2. Negative and cynical attitudes towards fellow workers and clients
3. Negative feelings about oneself
4. Total disgust

Emotional exhaustion is a part of the syndrome

of not sleeping well, not being able to get out of bed in the morning, and having no feelings of wanting to go to work each day. The physical manifestations are frequent colds, headaches, and various accidents and illnesses. The person feels preoccupied but has difficulty identifying a specific cause.

These vague feelings of discontentment are projected onto the people with whom one works, both colleagues and clients. The person's attitudes, actions, and conversations become cynical, negative, and dehumanized. For example, when the job is discussed with a colleague at lunch, nothing positive is said: the supervisor is described as miserable, the clients are seen as demanding, and the doctors are viewed as overbearing. These kinds of conversations should be a warning sign for a nurse. Reality tells us that nothing is perfect. Every job has good points and bad points. If a situation appears all bad, disequilibrium is occurring, and the nurse should seek insight into her perceptions.

If the disequilibrium is not resolved, the burnout moves into phase three. The negative feelings toward others turn inward on the person herself. The guilt generated is demonstrated by apathy. The nurse merely moves through the paces of each day without being involved. She becomes passive, goes into a shell, and extends herself to no one.

The fourth and final phase is called *terminal burnout.* A feeling of general disgust pervades the individual. Nothing or nobody gives pleasure; the

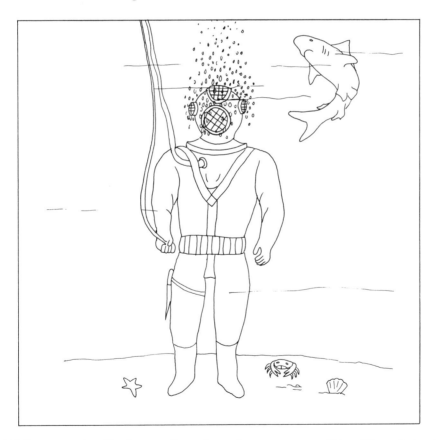

Fig. 6-2. Decompression. The deep sea diver releases the pressure around himself by surfacing slowly. The nurse can surface from the pressure of her professional responsibilities by having social outlets to renew her energy.

individual feels empty and wasted. Fortunately, it is possible to recover from any one of these phases. It is possible to go through burnout more than once. The remedy lies in recognizing the signs and symptoms early and initiating action immediately. It is most important to listen to oneself, to trust one's own feelings, to be fair to oneself. A nurse should ask herself these questions:

1. Does your job seem to take up your entire life?
2. Are you spending more than 8 hours a day doing your job?
3. Do you enjoy the people you work with less now than you used to?
4. Do you have days when you want to avoid your clients?
5. Are you referring to your clients by medical diagnosis or room number rather than by their names?
6. Are you constantly complaining about your job?
7. Are all your friends nurses?
8. Is your time schedule too busy for recreational activity each day? (Look at the word recreational. It is *re-create*. It renews.)

A yes answer to any of the above questions should alert the nurse. Each of these is an early sign of burnout. The more yes answers she has, the more vulnerable she is to burnout.

There is no one answer to stopping burnout. The basic premise is to take care of yourself. If the nurse is not well, then she is not available mentally or physically to care for others. She must recognize the need to vary work with recreation times and have a decompression time after work and before at-home routines begin. Decompression is a process of releasing pressure safely. Just as the deep sea diver must surface slowly and relieve the high underwater pressure on his body (Fig. 6-2), so must the nurse seek a decompression ritual to switch gears from work to private life. Decompression rituals need not take a long time.

- Sit in a nearby park, and look at the sky or trees.
- Walk along the street, and feel the breeze and sunshine on your face.
- Jog for 10 minutes after getting home.
- Sit by yourself in a coffee shop (not in the hospital!) and have a cup of coffee while reading a magazine or romantic love story.
- Enjoy the bus trip home. Sit back, take some deep breaths, close your eyes, and take a nap.
- Don't take the first bus home. Wait for the crowd to pass because you want to be alone. This is your time.

The main rule is to leave work on time and to have at least 15 to 30 minutes to oneself. A supervisor and staff will get used to a nurse leaving on time and putting in only 8 hours, and her family will think she is getting home early. Everyone needs social outlets and support. Without these, a nurse creeps toward burnout without even being aware of it.

JOB SATISFACTION

There are two sides to the job coin. One is burnout, and the other is satisfaction. A nursing position should be a channel for a nurse's personal growth and satisfaction. Seventeen thousand nurses responding to a job satisfaction questionnaire identified a satisfied nurse as one who:

- Has an adequate staff
- Gives direct client care
- Is motivated and stimulated by her work
- Has the authority to make the decisions she must make
- Has good staff morale
- Has a good relationship with her supervisor
- Receives praise and rewards for her work
- Has the support needed from nursing administration
- Has input into policies and decisions
- Has the respect of the hospital administration
- Has a feeling of fulfillment at the end of the day's work

Those nurses who belong to the professional organization, go to continuing education programs, and read professional journals report high levels of personal and intellectual growth. Ninety-two percent of the responding nurses state that direct patient care is a most important aspect of job satisfaction and that it is this area that gives them motivation even in the face of major frustrations.

Increased job satisfaction decreases the risk of burnout; therefore a balance can be struck. Areas of job dissatisfaction, on the other hand, increase stress in the work situation for the nurse and can foster burnout. Nurses in this study identified some areas of major dissatisfaction:

- Apathetic staff

- Little time for patient care
- Indifferent management
- Keeping up with technological advances

Keeping the work stress level within reasonable bounds demands that open lines of communications between nursing staff and nursing administration be maintained. Quality nursing care cannot be rendered when working conditions are intolerable. Active participation by staff nurses in policy-making decisions affecting client care units permits dialogue leading to mutual understanding by staff and administrators.

SUMMARY

The energy source that fuels the nurses' ability to provide care stems from positive self-esteem and job satisfaction. Before others will value the work nurses do, nursing as a group must value itself. The nurse's personal needs for self-esteem must be met before she can render effective care to others. Burnout is a term used to describe the emotional and physical outcome of overwork. The signs and symptoms of burnout are identifiable and can be treated. Closely tied to burnout are the areas of job satisfaction/dissatisfaction. The higher the level of job satisfaction, the lower the risk of burnout.

REFERENCES

Boccuzzi, N. K.: Head nurse growth: a priority for the supervisor, Am. J. Nurs. **79**:1388, August 1979.

Brock, A. M., and Madison, A. S.: The challenge in gerontological nursing, Nurs. Forum **16**(1):95, 1977.

Brooten, L., and Naylor, M.: Leadership for change: a guide for the frustrated nurse, Philadelphia, 1978, J. B. Lippincott Co.

Calhoun, G., and Perrin, M.: Management, motivation and conflict. Topics Clin. Nurs. **1**:3, 1979.

Chamberlin, A. B.: Providing motivation, Am. J. Nurs. **78**(1):80, 1978.

Chenevert, M.: Special techniques in assertiveness training for women in the health professions, St. Louis, 1978, The C. V. Mosby Co.

Cowan, E.: The most rewarding work, Geriatr. Nurs. **1**:30, May-June 1980.

Donnelly, G.: The assertive nurse or. . . . how to say what you mean without shaking or shouting, Nurs. '78:65-69, January 1978.

Dropkin, M.: Complaint behavior and changed body image, Am. J. Nurs. **79**:1249, July 1979.

Godfrey, M. A.: Job satisfaction or should that be dissatisfaction? Nurs. 78:81, June 1978.

Goldman, R.: Geriatric education at the undergraduate level, J. Am. Geriatr. Soc. **25**:485, November 1977.

Maslow, A.: Dominance, self-esteem, self-actualization, ed. 2, New York, 1970, Harper & Row, Publishers.

Mortenson, I.: Why work with the aged? Geriatr. Nurs. **1**:28, May-June 1980.

Moses, E., and Roth, A.: Nursepower: what do statistics reveal about the nation's nurses? Am. J. Nurs. **79**:1945, October 1979.

Norris, C.: Going over the hill, Geriatr. Nurs. **1**:40, May-June, 1980.

Pinel, C.: Geriatrics as a specialty, Nurs. Times **72**:1601, October 1976.

Robb, S. S.: Attitudes and intentions of baccalaureate nursing students toward the elderly, Nurs. Res. **28**:43, January-February 1979.

Robb, S. S., Peterson, M., and Nagy, J. W., Jr.: Advocacy for the aged, Am. J. Nurs. **79**:1736, October 1979.

Roberts, I.: Should geriatric nursing be a specialty? Nurs. Times **73**:1566, October 6, 1977.

Storlie, F. J.: Burnout: the elaboration of a concept, Am. J. Nurs. **79**:2108, December 1979.

Weaver, P.: You, inc.: a detailed escape route to being your own boss, Garden City, N.Y., 1973, Doubleday & Co., Inc.

7 An ethical approach

ETHICS DEFINED

The Greeks used the word *ethics* to describe customs, usual conduct, and character. It refers to one's moral philosophy or beliefs. Ethics or moral beliefs form the basis for rules of conduct, motivation for behavior, and decision making. Socrates insisted that reason must determine ethical decisions rather than having these decisions made by emotion. An ethical decision is not a consensus of a group's beliefs, because they might be wrong. An ethical decision is determined after seeking informed reasoning. Informed reasoning is accomplished by accumulating factual information about the case and keeping a focus on the rightness or wrongness of the outcomes. An ethical decision is not based on what will happen to us as a result of the decision. It does not matter what others think of us, or what our feelings are regarding the case. It is doing what is morally "right." Groups as well as individuals develop standards of conduct. A list of right or moral behaviors is called a code of ethics. Codes of ethics for health care workers serve two purposes:

1. They make health professionals and the lay public aware of ethical issues as policies for health care are being developed.
2. They help organize issues so that related ethical issues can be identified, which in turn makes complex situations more approachable.

A "right" code of ethical practice for a professional group is then operationally defined in terms of the client's *right* to expect this behavior from the professional. Right and duty are correlated in the eyes of the law. The professional person has the duty to provide the client with the best possible care as defined in the code of ethical behaviors of the profession. Before the nursing process can continue into the planning, intervention, and evaluation phases, ethical beliefs must be addressed. With an understanding of the rights of the client and the duties of the nurse, moral guidance is available to the nurse as she addresses her clients' nursing requirements.

There are two general nursing codes of ethical behaviors. One is the International Council of Nurses Code of Ethics written in Geneva in 1973, and the second is the American Nurses' Association Code of Ethics for Nurses.

The International Council of Nurses Code of Ethics describes the rights, duties, and obligations the nurse has toward her client.

International Council of Nurses Code for Nurses*

Ethical concepts applied to nursing

The fundamental responsibility of the nurse is fourfold: to promote health, to prevent illness, to restore health, and to alleviate suffering.

The need for nursing is universal. Inherent in nursing is respect for life, dignity, and rights of man. It is unrestricted by considerations of nationality, race, creed, color, age, sex, politics, or social status.

Nurses render health services to the individual, the family, and the community, and coordinate their services with those of related groups.

Nurses and people

The nurse's primary responsibility is to those people who require nursing care.

The nurse, in providing care, respects the beliefs, values, and customs of the individual.

The nurse holds in confidence personal information and uses judgment in sharing information.

Nurses and practice

The nurse carries personal responsibility for nursing practice and for maintaining competence by continual learning.

The nurse maintains the highest standards of nursing

---

*Reprinted with permission of the International Council of Nurses.

care possible within the reality of the specific situation.

The nurse uses judgement in relation to individual competence when accepting and delegating responsibilities.

The nurse when acting in a professional capacity should at all times maintain standards of personal conduct that would reflect credit upon the profession.

Nurses and society

The nurse shares with other citizens the responsibility for initiating and supporting action to meet the health and social needs of the public.

Nurses and co-workers

The nurse sustains a cooperative relationship with co-workers in nursing and other fields.

The nurse takes appropriate action to safeguard the individual when his care is endangered by a co-worker or any other person.

Nurses and the profession

The nurse plays the major role in determining and implementing desirable standards of nursing practice and nursing education.

The nurse is active in developing a core of professional knowledge.

The nurse, acting through the professional organization, participates in establishing and maintaining equitable social and economic working conditions in nursing.

The code of ethics of the American Nurses' Association is a self-regulating mechanism acknowledging the consumer's trust in the actions of individual nurses in the course of daily care. The code is the minimum ethical basis for practice. Violations of the code subject the nurse to reprimand, censure, suspension, or expulsion by the American Nurses' Association.

American Nurses' Association Code of Ethics for Nurses*

1. The nurse provides services with respect for human dignity and the uniqueness of the client unrestricted by considerations of social or economic status, personal attributes or the nature of health problems.
2. The nurse safeguards the client's right to privacy by judiciously protecting information of a confidential nature.

*From the American Nurses' Association and reprinted with the permission of the ANA. From Code for nurses with interpretive statements, 1976, The Association.

3. The nurse acts to safeguard the client and the public when health care and safety are affected by the incompetent, unethical, or illegal practice of any person.
4. The nurse assumes responsibility and accountability for individual nursing judgments and actions.
5. The nurse maintains competence in nursing.
6. The nurse exercises informed judgment and uses individual competence and qualifications as criteria in seeking consultations, accepting responsibilities, and delegating nursing activities to others.
7. The nurse participates in activities that contribute to the ongoing development of the profession's body of knowledge.
8. The nurse participates in the profession's efforts to implement and improve standards of nursing.
9. The nurse participates in the profession's efforts to establish and maintain conditions of employment conducive to high quality nursing care.
10. The nurse participates in the profession's effort to protect the public from misinformation and misrepresentation and to maintain the integrity of nursing.
11. The nurse collaborates with members of the health professions and other citizens in promoting community and national efforts to meet the health needs of the public.

Formal censure is seldom invoked against an individual nurse for violation of the ethical code. Nevertheless, the quality of nursing care within an agency is a measure of the ethical performance of the nurses practicing there. For example, when a hospital extends dignified, safe, and competent nursing care to clients, it reflects the standard expectations of the nurses who give care there. Because the nurses assume individual responsibility for the care, attending in-service and continuing education courses, reading journals, and other educational activities are a part of the overall nursing expectations in that hospital. The code of ethics can be used by the nurse as she reviews the agency in which she works. If the agency supports her ethical practice, quality client care is encouraged.

The American Hospital Association has formulated a Patient's Bill of Rights. Keep in mind these rights are not "given" to the client, but flow from his intrinsic rights as a human being. Some critics of this document call it timid and paternalistic. It certainly does not address the competency level of the practitioners within the agency. It is a beginning recognition of the client as a consumer.

A Patient's Bill of Rights*

The patient has the right to:
1. Considerate and respectful care.
2. Obtain from his physician complete current information concerning his diagnosis, treatment, and prognosis in terms the patient can be reasonably expected to understand. When it is not medically advisable to give such information to the patient, the information should be made available to an appropriate person in his behalf. He has the right to know by name, the physician responsible for coordinating his care.
3. Receive from his physician information necessary to give informed consent prior to the start of any procedure and/or treatment. Except in emergencies, such information for informed consent, should include but not necessarily be limited to the specific procedure and/or treatment, the medically significant risks involved, and the probable duration of incapacitation. Where medically significant alternatives for care or treatment exist, or when the patient requests information concerning medical alternatives, the patient has the right to such information. The patient also has the right to know the name of the person responsible for the procedure and/or treatment.
4. Refuse treatment to the extent permitted by law, and to be informed of the medical consequences of his action.
5. Every consideration of his privacy concerning his own medical care program. Case discussion, consultation, examination, and treatment are confidential and should be conducted discreetly. Those not directly involved in his care must have the permission of the patient to be present.
6. Expect that all communications and records pertaining to his care should be treated as confidential.
7. Expect that within its capacity, a hospital must make reasonable response to the request of a patient for services. The hospital must provide evaluation, service, and/or referral as indicated by the urgency of the case. When medically permissible, a patient may be transferred to another facility only after he has received complete information and explanation concerning the needs for and alternatives to such a transfer. The institution to which the patient is to be transferred must first have accepted the patient for transfer.
8. Obtain information as to any relationship of his hospital to other health care and educational institutions insofar as his care is concerned. The patient has the right to obtain information as to the existence of any professional relationships among individuals, by name, who are treating him.
9. Be advised if the hospital proposes to engage in or perform human experimentation affecting his care or treatment. The patient has the right to refuse to participate in such research projects.
10. Expect reasonable continuity of care. He has the right to know in advance what appointment times and physicians are available and where. The patient has the right to expect that the hospital will provide a mechanism whereby he is informed by his physician or a delegate of the physician of the patient's continuing health care requirements following discharge.
11. Examine and receive an explanation of his bill regardless of source of payment.
12. Know what hospital rules and regulations apply to his conduct as a patient.

Nurses' rights*

1. The right to find dignity in self-expression and self-enhancement through the use of our special abilities and educational background.
2. The right to recognition for our contribution through the provision of an environment for its practice, and proper, professional economic rewards.
3. The right to a work environment which will minimize physical and emotional stress and health risks.
4. The right to control what is professional practice within the limits of the law.
5. The right to set standards for excellence in nursing.
6. The right to participate in policy making affecting nursing.
7. The right to social and political action in behalf of nursing and health care.

Understanding intent of nursing codes of ethics and Patient's Bill of Rights

The codes for ethical nursing practice and the American Hospital Association's Patient's Bill of Rights are examples of codes of behavioral expectations for persons in the health care system. The federal government and many individual states have addressed the special needs of the older adult in intermediate and skilled long-term-care facilities. A particularly useful guide to client rights in such agencies is included in the Medicare/Medicaid Skilled Nursing Facility Survey Report (form

---

*Reprinted with the permission of the American Hospital Association, copyright 1975.

*Copyrighted by the American Journal of Nursing Co. and reprinted from Fagin, C.: Nurses' rights, Am. J. Nurs. **75**(1):82, 1975.

HCFA-1569 (11-76), U.S. Government Printing Office). The following exercises from the Hillhaven Foundation are designed to have the nurse apply these codes of ethics and bill of rights to actual client situations.

ETHICAL CONSIDERATIONS EXERCISES*

Situation: You are the head nurse of a 30-bed unit in a skilled nursing facility. At the beginning of each day, you check your mail, and the following situations are presented to you. During the nursing report, you will have an opportunity to discuss with the staff the ethical considerations involved.

Discuss your concerns regarding the client's rights, the needs of the staff and other clients, and the many ramifications of the decisions made. Give particular attention to the rights of the client and his family and the ethical implications for the nursing staff.

Exercise No. 1: The move

A note in your mail basket indicates that Mr. Rock, an 88-year-old resident has written to the Director of Nursing "demanding my rights."

Mr. Rock had been brought to the home in an ambulance from the community hospital about 2½ months ago. At that point, there was some question that he had had a stroke. Mr. Rock's records indicated no next of kin and a series of previous residences in apartments and hotels. His social and medical history are both sorely lacking, and staff attempts to gather more information have not been successful.

About 2 weeks ago, Mr. Rock suddenly started disappearing for several hours at a time. When he would reappear, he appeared somewhat unsteady. Four days ago, he was returned in a squad car, after an off-duty policeman had noticed his arm bracelet while in a local saloon and cajoled him into returning.

Following this incident, staff members had discussed Mr. Rock's behavior at a team conference. There were some feelings that he should be moved to another facility; others felt able to provide care for him, at least at the present time.

On hearing of the meeting, Mr. Rock was irate. He indicated to the head nurse that if they were going to discuss him, he should have been present. Since such "gossip" was the policy of this home, he formally requested assistance in retrieving his belongings from central storage and planned to leave in the morning.

Attached to the note indicating that Mr. Rock wanted to know of his rights, was a note from the Director of

Nursing that she had indicated that he could not leave because of the potential interactive effects of alcohol and his drugs.

In preparing to answer Mr. Rock's call, you try to get your thoughts together on the following:

1. What are your legal responsibilities in this matter?
2. What do you want to do?
3. Does the Patient's Bill of Rights offer *you* any guidance in the larger issue of the move? (Which rights?)
4. What about his right to leave for short periods and drink?
5. Have any of his rights been abridged? If so, which ones and how?
   a. What will you respond to Mr. Rock?
   b. What amends need to be made to him?
   c. What topics need to be reviewed with the staff?

Exercise No. 2: The prescription

Dr. Salient, the attending physician, and Mrs. McCarthy, Director of Nursing, have a difference of opinion regarding Mrs. Emory's plan of care. Mrs. Emory has been calling out and showing agitation with other residents and with the staff. This is a recent turn of events, and no one is quite sure of the precipitating circumstances.

Dr. Salient proposes calming her with medications; he indicates that these will stabilize her moods and make her easier to care for. He is concerned that attending to her is taking time from other residents in the home.

Mrs. McCarthy has been working to develop a range of services for the mentally impaired. She has had staff trained in remotivation and in some of the newer techniques of human development. Mrs. McCarthy feels that to utilize pharmacy first may detract from the staff's ability to keep Mrs. Emory awake and alert, and limit their potential to help her develop coping strategies.

Dr. Salient indicates that the pharmacy approach is the one most typically used. Mrs. McCarthy feels that the staff should have the opportunity to work with her for a couple of weeks first. Dr. Salient does not want to take the responsibility for an increase in her agitation that might result from not administering the medications.

1. Does Mrs. Emory have any rights in this situation?
2. How can this situation be resolved, perhaps through convening the appropriate family, staff, and other input? What would you have each of these participants bring or prepare for this type of meeting?
3. How could you determine whether the physician understands the Patient's Bill of Rights?
4. Are there conflicts of interest between the individual items on the Patient's Bill of Rights and the regulations governing a physician's responsibilities?
5. What aspects of the Patient's Bill of Rights might

---

*From the Hillhaven Foundation, Tacoma, Wash. 98411. Reprinted with permission from the conference on The Patient's Rights, April 1977.

apply to this situation and/or be helped in resolving the dilemma?

6. What might several alternative strategies be for reducing the conflict while continuing to respect Mrs. Emory's individual rights?

7. What should be done to respect the rights of other people involved?

8. Is there a difference between short- and long-term commitment to patient's rights? What are the implications of this in this situation?

9. Are the nurses' rights being protected?

Exercise No. 3: Mail routing

In your mail today is a formal letter from Mr. and Mrs. Brown. They "respectfully request" that you collect and forward "all important looking mail" for their mother, Mrs. Rose, and send it, unopened, to them. They indicate that they want their mother to be "free of worries" about her financial matters.

In preparing your response, you consider the following:

1. What are your responsibilities in terms of Mrs. Rose's rights?

2. What additional information do you need? For exam-

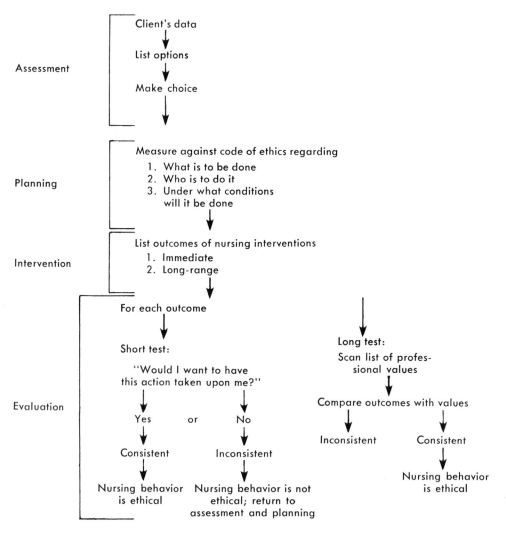

Fig. 7-1. Ethical matrix for nursing behavior.

ple, would your decision or answer be affected by information indicating that:

    a. The Browns are a very caring family?

    b. The Browns are seeking control in a family dispute over control of Mrs. Rose's estate?

    c. The Browns have power of attorney for Mrs. Rose?

    d. Mrs. Rose opposes the opening of her mail?

    e. Mrs. Rose has never been asked about the opening of her mail?

    f. So much mail comes that you don't know how to judge its importance without opening it yourself?

3. How are your current goals for rehabilitation and patient self-care consistent with this issue?

4. What steps might you take to eliminate or reduce the likelihood of this problem in the future?

5. What will you specifically answer to the Browns?

6. What could you do with families or significant others of your current resident population to alleviate recurrence of this problem?

7. Under what circumstances do you have the right to open mail of residents? Who in the facility or family has that right?

Fig. 7-1 refers to a pathway of ethical thinking for the nurse as she makes plans for her nursing intervention. The long form goes through the test against professional values, and the short form asks, "would I want it done to me?"

CARING

Nursing is intimately identified with the act of caring. But what is caring, and how is it related to the ethics of nursing? The act of caring describes a responsibility to watch over somebody with close attention. Caring is an act that gives testimony to a person's respect and regard for another. It is also biological impulse in human nature that is either encouraged or hampered by the circumstances within the setting or environment. Caring is more than a passing feeling of good wishes or liking someone; it is a relationship free of domination, possessiveness, or manipulation. "Being nice to a client" then is not the hallmark of a caring nurse. The commitment a nurse has to the client's well-being measures the extent of her caring and demonstrates an important aspect of her ethical or "right" behavior as a professional health team person.

There are eight important parts to a caring approach to a client:

1. Knowledge
2. Alternating rhythms
3. Patience
4. Honesty
5. Trust
6. Humility
7. Hope
8. Courage

Knowledge is the foundation of the caring relationship. When the nurse knows what to do and why she does it, she is freed from the shackles of mere good intentions. The nursing activities are purposeful; they have organization and direction. For example, Mrs. Lester is a nurse caring for Mrs. Rodney in a clinic of a large manufacturing firm. Mrs. Rodney decided not to retire when eligible several years before and is now 68 years old. She describes to the nurses her interest in her work, but explains how discouraged she is becoming because she is not as "quick" as she was in the past to get her paperwork done at her desk, and her growing fatigue increases at the end of the day. The nurse does a health assessment on Mrs. Rodney and finds all her systems to be within normal limits for an older adult. Because Mrs. Lester is well grounded in the physiology of the older adult, she understands what is happening to Mrs. Rodney as a result of the aging process. This nurse can now share this knowledge with her client and offer the client suggestions for coping with these physical alterations. Without this knowledge base, the nurse is in no position to assist her client and might be left with just the impression of the common social stereotype of the aging process, "Oh, that's too bad, but you are just getting old."

The ability to alternate rhythms is a sign of the nurse's flexibility in working with clients. Some clients require a more relaxed approach, and others need a faster approach to meet their needs. Alternate styles of nursing intervention are often needed even for the same client. It depends on the situation and resources available to the client.

Patience is ethical caring when it is an active perception of the client's time frame rather than a passive watching of what is happening. When the nurse observes the client dressing himself very slowly, she is actively patient if she is noting his success in independence and enjoying his accomplishment. She is passively patient if she appears bored and is daydreaming about what she is going to make for dinner when she gets home.

Honesty is an open, forthright confrontation with the reality of a situation. Other persons' needs are taken seriously and respected without imposing one's values on them or judging their behavior.

Trust implies a recognition and appreciation of the independent existence of the client. The client has a right to go his own way and make his decisions free from reprimand.

Humility enables the nurse to learn about others, and being open to learn more about herself. A humble person knows his own limitations and can acknowledge them openly.

Hope permits the nurse to be forward looking and to plan with her client. It can be a valuable resource when the immediate situation is difficult for the nurse and the client.

Courage affords the nurse the strength to put her value system into action. A new graduate is working evenings in an intermediate-care facility. After a few weeks she knows that she cannot give quality care to her clients with the staffing ratio of one nurse to 35 clients. Even with the two nursing assistants who work on the unit with her, only the minimum physical nursing care can be given the clients on her shift. It takes courage for this young nurse to discuss this with her supervisor.

She might be putting her job on the line if she cannot come to an agreement with administration regarding the level of care given to the clients.

ASSERTIVENESS AS ETHICAL RESPONSIBILITY

Client advocacy is no assignment for the passive, nonassertive uncommitted nurse. Advocacy requires commitment, perseverance, initiative, and leadership to develop strategies to change the older adult health care delivery system. It is an overwhelming task. Where and how do you start? Each nurse starts with herself first. Remember that assertiveness is your new pattern of behavior and your feelings about yourself. Go out and buy one of the "how to be assertive" books listed in the bibliography. Make your feelings known by being direct and beginning your statements with "I." "I am unhappy with the time schedule because I have to work 9 days before my weekend off." "I feel uncomfortable when you correct me in front of clients." "I find referring to the client in that manner very annoying." Make sure that your nonverbal body movements and cues correspond to your verbal tone and positive communication manner to make sure your message carries weight. Begin your new assertiveness behavior by taking small achievable steps. Try keeping an assertiveness log, such as the one in Table 7-1 for a week and then evaluate your behavior. Let your actions for the week be guided by what Melodie Chenevert says

Table 7-1. Assertiveness log

Assertiveness incident	My body language, physical reaction, feelings	My statement—manner of my response	What I really wanted to say	What stopped me from saying it?

in her book, *Special Techniques in Assertiveness Training for Women in the Health Professions.* "To live with yourself and to be able to stay in the health professions a lifetime, there is only one question that you have to answer: 'Is what I am doing or about to do in the best interest of my patient?' " (Chenevert, 1978, p. 4). Exercise the following rights as outlined by Chenevert.*

Ten basic rights for women in the health professions

1. You have the right to be treated with respect.
2. You have the right to a reasonable workload.
3. You have a right to an equitable wage.
4. You have the right to determine your own priorities.
5. You have the right to ask for what you want.
6. You have the right to refuse without making excuses or feeling guilty.
7. You have the right to make mistakes and be responsible for them.
8. You have the right to give and receive information as a professional.
9. You have the right to act in the best interest of the patient.
10. You have the right to be human.

Carry a copy of these rights in your uniform pocket. Take them out during work and read them to remind yourself that you have basic rights. This will help counterbalance your enormous feeling of responsibilities with your few perceived rights. Practice in front of a mirror the assertiveness communication techniques, and during the week use the communication techniques and responses that lend themselves to the situation.

Pat yourself on the back when you do a good job and ask for help when you need it. Commend co-workers who do a good job. You will be surprised at the impact of the self-enhancing behavior of your assertiveness.

Nursing has long been known for its client advocacy role. Nursing was the first health profession to receive national publicity when it took a stand to support legislation for Medicare. Nursing's concern for the right to quality health care for older adults has been commendable. Today, we are rallying to assure equal access to health services through national health insurance for all clients, and reimbursement for nursing services.

*From Chenevert, M.: Special techniques in assertiveness training for women in the health professions, St. Louis, 1978, The C. V. Mosby Co., p. 39.

Our professional nursing organizations, ANA and NLN, have endorsed many resolutions addressing the plight and care of the older adult. Nursing is dealing with politics more and learning to use power to insist on its right to be acknowledged in the political arena. Nursing has strength in numbers, and our actions have been recognized and appreciated by the health consumer. Now, individual nurses are asserting themselves to speak up for their rights along with the client's rights. Many articles and nursing texts are addressing the nurse's right to insist on her "rights." Assertiveness training workshops and courses are popping up all over the health care industry. Nurses are told that they are vulnerable by virtue of their own feminism and the fact that over 80 percent of the caretakers are women. These same women receive orders from males (doctors, administrators) who are on the top rung of the health care industry hierarchy. Assertiveness, according to Webster, is characterized by taking a positive stand; being confident in your statements or position in a persistent way. The nurse works in settings and in situations that necessitate that she speak frankly, candidly, and openly to others. Her distinctive communication technique should be "leveling with others." To be successful in assertive behavior, she needs to like herself, feel comfortable with herself, and have a large measure of self-esteem. Self-esteem is tied into everything. Self-esteem frees you to be happy with yourself.

Nurses were socialized into making statements preceeded by "seems to be" or "appears to be," and cautioned never to diagnose a situation. Even though you saw a client hemorrhaging and recognized blood, it still had to be qualified by "appears to be." No wonder our statements lacked confidence. Assertive behavior is self-enhancing, goal directed, and expressive. Assertiveness is one mode of expressing yourself without hurting, humiliating, or putting another person down or on the defensive. It is also self-enhancing for the other person in the communication. Assertiveness permits you to react to the situation by saying what you mean in a calm, clear manner, defending your behavior without arguing or being reduced to tears. The nurse working with the older adult needs to let others know her position by speaking up and reacting honestly for the good of everyone. This behavioral stance is especially true in order for the nurse to function as an advocate for the older adult.

You are in the best position to look out for "number one." If you don't do it, who will? When each nurse caring for older adults practices advocacy and assertive behavior, we will be able to change the health care delivery system for the older adult. Think about the power we have to make that change.

ASSERTIVENESS COMMUNICATION TECHNIQUES*

Broken record

A systematic assertive communication skill in which you are persistent and keep saying what you want over and over again without getting angry, irritated, or loud.

By practicing to speak like a broken record, you learn to be persistent and to stick to the point of discussion and to continue to say what you want. This technique helps you to ignore all side issues brought up by the other party.

Workable compromise

A technique to utilize with an equally assertive person to work out a compromise. A workable compromise is one in which your self-respect is not in question.

Free information

A listening skill in which you evaluate and then follow up on the free information that people offer about themselves. It accomplishes two things. It makes it easier for you to converse comfortably with people, and it is assertively prompting to others to speak easily and freely to you.

Self-disclosure

Assertively disclosing information about yourself, how you think, feel, and react to the other person's free information, permits social communication to flow both ways. It goes hand-in-hand with Free Information, for in order to elicit more free information, one must be willing to self-disclose.

Fogging

A technique to assertively cope with manipulative criticism in which we *do not deny* any of the criticism, we do not get defensive, and we do not attack with criticism of our own. We send up a fogbank. It is persistent. It cannot be clearly seen through. It offers no resistance to penetration. It does not fight back, and has no hard striking surfaces. Fogging permits you to cope by offering no resistance or hard psychological striking surfaces to critical statements thrown at you.

Negative assertion

A technique in which we cope with criticism or with our own errors and faults by openly acknowledging them. This technique is to be used only in social conflicts, not physical or legal ones. Say, "Yes, I was wrong."

Negative inquiry

An assertive, nondefensive response that is noncritical of the other person and prompts that person to make further critical statements to examine her own structure of right and wrong which she is using in certain situations, for example, "I don't understand. What makes you think nurses are stupid?"

NINE TYPES OF ASSERTIVE RESPONSES*

1. *Assertive talk*. Do not let others take advantage of you. Demand your rights. Insist upon being treated with fairness and justice. Examples: "I was here first." "I'd like more coffee, please." "Excuse me, but I have another appointment." "Please turn down the radio." "You have kept me waiting here for half an hour." "This steak is well done and I ordered it medium-rare."

2. *Feeling talk*. Express your likes and dislikes spontaneously. Be open and frank about your feelings. Do not bottle up emotions. Answer questions honestly. Examples: "What a marvelous shirt!" "I am so sick of that man." "How great you look!" "I hate this cold." "I'm tired as hell." "Since you ask, I much prefer you in another type of outfit."

3. *Greeting talk*. Be outgoing and friendly with people whom you would like to know better. Do not avoid people because of shyness, because you do not know what to say. Smile brightly at people. Look and sound pleased to see them. Examples: "Hi, how are you?" "Hello, I haven't seen you in months." "What are you doing with yourself these days?" "How do you like working at _____?" "Taking any good courses?" "What's been happening with so and so?"

4. *Disagreeing passively and actively*. When you disagree with someone, do not feign agreement for the sake of keeping the peace by smiling, nodding, or paying close attention. Change the topic. Look away. Disagree actively and emotionally when you are sure of your ground.

5. *Asking why*. When you are asked to do something that does not sound reasonable or enjoyable by a person in power or authority, ask why you should do it. You are an adult and should not accept authority alone. Insist

---

*Reprinted from Assertiveness: freeing the nurse to practice, by G. F. Donnelly, Top. Clin. Nurs. **1**:67, April 1979. By permission of Aspen Systems Corp., Germantown, Md. © 1979.

*Reprinted with permission from Journal of Behavior Research and Therapy, **11**:57. Rathus, S. A.: Instigation of assertive behavior through videotape—mediated assertive models and directed practice, copyright 1973, Pergamon Press, Ltd.

upon explanations from teachers, relatives, and other authority figures that are convincing. Have it understood that you will live up to voluntary commitments and be open to reasonable suggestions, but that you are not to be ordered about at anyone's whim.

6. *Talking about oneself.* When you have done something worthwhile or interesting, let others know about it. Let people know how you feel about things. Relate *your* experiences. Do not monopolize conversations, but do not be afraid to bring them around to yourself when it is appropriate.

7. *Agreeing with compliments.* Do not deprecate yourself or become flustered when someone compliments you with sincerity. At the very least, offer an equally sincere "Thank you." Or reward the complimenter by saying, "That's an awfully nice thing to say. I appreciate it." In other words, reward rather than punish others for complimenting you. When appropriate, extend compliments. For example, if someone says, "What a beautiful sweater!" respond, "Isn't it a lovely color? I had a hard time finding it."

8. *Avoiding trying to justify opinions.* Be reasonable in discussions, but when someone goes out of his way to dominate a social interaction by taking issue with any comments you offer, say something like, "Are you always so disagreeable?" or "I have no time to waste arguing with you," or "You seem to have a great deal invested in being right regardless of what you say, don't you."

9. *Looking people in the eye.* Do not avoid the gaze of others. When you argue, express an opinion, or greet a person, look him directly in the eye.

SUMMARY

Ethics are the moral beliefs that form the basis for one's conduct, behavior, and decision making. Professional groups practice under ethical codes that operationally define the expected behavior of the practitioner.

Nursing has two general codes of ethics, the International Council of Nurses' Code of Ethics and the American Nurses' Association Code for Nurses. Inherent in codes of ethics are morally "right" behavioral expectations. Each individual has the right to expect certain behaviors of others. Some of these expectations are spelled out in The Patient's Bill of Rights and Nurses' Rights.

Caring is an ethical responsibility of the nurse. A caring approach to client care is one that has knowledge, alternating rhythms, patience, honesty, trust, humility, hope, and courage.

The nurse has an ethical responsibility to be assertive. As an advocate for the older adult, the assertive nurse can effect change in the health care delivery system to the benefit of both her client and herself.

REFERENCES

Annas, G. J., and Healey, J.: The patient rights advocate; J. Nurs. Admin. **4:**25, May-June 1974.

Annas, G. J.: The rights of hospital patients, an American Civil Liberties Union Handbook, New York, 1975, Avon Books.

Aronson, J.: The right to die, New York, 1974, Decision and Decision Makers.

Aroskar, M.: Anatomy of an ethical dilemma: the theory, the practice, Am. J. Nurs. **80:**658, April 1980.

Baker, D. E.: The elderly: a challenge to nursing—16. Future care for the elderly, Nurs. Times **74:**237, 9 Feb. 1978.

Bandman, E., and Bandman, B.: There is nothing automatic about rights, Am. J. Nurs. **77:**5, 1977.

Berkowitz, S.: Informed consent, research and the elderly, Gerontologist **18:**237, June 1978.

Besch, L. B.: Informed consent: a patient's right, Nurs. Outlook **27:**32, January 1979.

Brody, H.: Introduction to ethical decisions in medicine, 1975, Michigan State University, Ann Arbor.

Burrows, J.: The elderly: a challenge to nursing—2. The elderly in our society, Nurs. Times **73:**1670, 27 October 1977.

Burnside, I. M.: Eulogy for Ms. Hogue, Am. J. Nurs. **78:**624, April 1978.

Butter, R.: Why survive? Being old in America, New York, 1975, Harper & Row, Publishers.

Carnevali, D., and Patrick, M.: Nursing management for the elderly, Philadelphia, 1979, J. B. Lippincott Co.

Cawley, M. A.: Euthanasia: should it be a choice? Am. J. Nurs. **77:**5, 1977.

Chisholm, M. K.: The nurse's responsibilities when caring for the elderly, Nurs. Times **73:**1509, 29 September 1977.

Cohen, E. S.: Law and aging, lawyers and gerontologists (editorial). Gerontologist **18:**229, June 1978.

Deets, C. A.: Methodological concerns in the testing of nursing interventions, A.N.S. 802:1, January 1980.

Elkowitz, E. B.: Death and the elderly patient, J. Am. Geriatr. Soc. **26:**36, January 1978.

Epstein, R. L.: The patients' right to refuse, Hospitals **47:**38, August 16, 1973.

Füsgen, I., and Summa, J. D.: How much sense is there is an attempt to resuscitate an aged person? Gerontology **24**(1):37, 1978.

Galinsky, D., Herschkoren, H., Kaplan, M., and Alyagon, R.: The need for a new approach to neglected elderly patients, Geriatrics **33:**103, January 1978.

GAO and U.S. Commission on Civil Rights assess programs for the elderly. Geriatrics **33:**15, March 1978.

Gelperin, A.: Our elderly, who are they? J. Am. Geriatr. Soc. **26:**318, July 1978.

Horsley, J.: When you can safely refuse an assignment, R.N. **43:**99, February 1980.

Johnson, P.: The gray areas—who decides? Am. J. Nurs. **77:**5, 1977.

Kahana, E.: The humane treatment of old people in institutions, Gerontologist, Part I, 282, Autumn 1973.

Kelley, V. R., and Weston, H. B.: Civil liberties in mental health facilities, Social Work, January 1974, p. 48.

Kelly, C.: 70 plus and going strong: profile of a Panther, Geriatr. Nurs. **1**:81, May-June, 1980.

Kelly, K., and McClelland, E.: Signed consent: protection or contraints? Nurs. Outlook **27**:40, January 1979.

Kramer, K.: The subtle subversion of patients' rights by hospital staff members, Hosp. Comm. Psychiatry **25**:475, July 7, 1974.

Levy, C. S.: On the development of a code of ethics, Social Work, March 1974, p. 207.

Leader, M. A., and Neuwirth, E.: Clinical research and the non-institutional elderly: a model for subject recruitment, J. Am. Geriatr. Soc. **26**:27, January 1978.

Lestz, P.: A committee to decide the quality of life, Am. J. Nurs. **77**:5, 1977.

Levine, M. E.: Nursing ethics and the ethical nurse, Am. J. Nurs. **77**:5, 1977.

Levine, M. E.: The intransigent patient, Am. J. Nurs. **70**:2106, October 1970.

Litigation and Mental Health Services: DHEW Publication No. 76-261 (ADM), 1976, National Institute of Mental Health, U.S. Department of Health, Education, and Welfare.

Lore, A.: Supporting the hospitalized elderly person, Am. J. Nurs. **79**:496, March 1979.

McKinney, J. C., and de Vyver, F. T.: Aging and social policy, New York, 1966, Appleton-Century-Crofts.

Monaghan, J. C.: Whatever happened to the Patients' Bill of Rights? Med. Econ., **52**:109, August 4, 1975.

Norton, D.: The elderly: a challenge to nursing—1. Geriatric nursing—what it is and what it is not. Nurs. Times **73**:1622, 20 October 1977.

The Nursing Home Law Handbook, Los Angeles, 1975, The National Senior Citizens Law Center.

The Nursing Home Law Letter, published by *National Senior Citizens Law Center,* 1709 West 8th Street, Suite 600, Los Angeles, Calif. 90017, first issue, January 5, 1976.

Palmore, E.: Are the aged a minority group? J. Am. Geriatr. Soc. **26**:214, May 1978.

Pankratz, L., and Pankratz, D.: Nursing autonomy and patients' rights: development of a nursing attitude scale, J. Health Soc. Behav. **15**:211, September 1974.

Patients' Nursing Care Rights Stated in Ohio: Am. J. Nurs. **75**:1112, July 1975.

Patients' Bill of Rights: Today's Health **51**:71, November 1973.

Ramanell, P.: Ethics, moral conflicts, and choice, Am. J. Nurs. **77**:5, 1977.

Ramsden, E. L.: Patients' right to know: implications for inter-personal communications process, Phys. Therapy **55**:133, February 1975.

Rawnsley, M. M.: The six A's of assertiveness, J. Contin. Educ. Nurs. **11**:15, January-February 1980.

Regan, T. T.: Intervention through adult protective service programs, Gerontologist **18**:250, June 1978.

Reichel, W.: Final recommendations of the American Geriatrics Society Conference on geriatric education, J. Am. Geriatr. Soc. **25**:510, November 1977.

"Resident's Advocate Program, Inc.", April 15, 1976, 111 South Fairchild Street, Suite 304, Madison, Wisconsin 53703.

Robb, S. S., Peterson, M., and Nagy, J. W., Jr.: Advocacy for the aged, Am. J. Nurs. **79**:1736, October 1979.

Scheideman, J. M.: Problem patients do not exist, Am. J. Nurs. **79**:1082, June 1979.

Schiff, M. A.: Ombudsmen serve as "environmentalists" for nursing home patients, Geriatrics **30**:38, May 1975.

Schwab, M.: Nursing care in nursing homes, Am. J. Nurs. **75**:1812, October 1975.

Schwab, M.: A commentary on ANA's recommendations on long-term care, Hosp. Prog. **56**:55, November 1975.

Snook, I. D.: Patients' rights, Hospitals **48**:177, April 1, 1974.

Taube, K.: Geriatric jurisprudence (a poem), Social Work **21**:17, July 1976.

Tavani, C.: Meeting the needs of the oldest of the old, Aging (291-292):2, January-February 1979.

Train, G. J.: The aged—with tender interest and concern, Psychosomatics, **16**:79, Second Quarter 1975.

Wales, J. B., and Treybig, D. L.: Recent legislative trends toward protection of human subjects: implications for gerontologists, Gerontologist **18**:244, June 1978.

What Are Your Rights As A Patient?: Better Homes Gardens, **52**:6, April 1974.

Wichita, C.: Everyone wins when you push patient power, R.N. **43**:50, February 1980.

Yawney, B. A., and Slover, D. L.: Relocation of the elderly, Social Work, **18**:86, May 1973.

8 Nursing through objectives

CLIENT CARE PLANS

A client care plan is an organized method of indicating the client goals to be accomplished, listing the actions to be taken to reach the goals, and identifying which discipline is responsible for each element of care. Frequently, the client care plan is coordinated from the Kardex file kept by the nurse. On this card the nursing and medical assessment summaries are listed as the nursing and medical diagnoses. Other treatment modalities, such as respiratory therapy, dietary department, or physical therapy, for example, are specified and integrated into the client care regiment and recorded on the Kardex card. After each discipline records its notes on various chart forms, the treatment schedule is recorded on the nurses' client care Kardex card. The client care plan facilitates the individualization of care for the client. Interdisciplinary client care conferences are responsible for the comprehensive client care program. Nursing contributes much information regarding the client's needs and his progress through the nursing portion of the client care plan. The nurse is part of the interdisciplinary team effort, and the written client care plan serves as her communication for sharing nursing information with the rest of the team.

Written care plan by nurse

The concepts of written care plans in nursing have developed over many years. Early textbooks in the 1930s and 1940s mention care plans. They were, however, directed exclusively toward a list of treatments, skill-oriented tasks. For example, if a client was to have a warm soak or medications, the care plan specified when and how the warm soak was to be given. This design of the care plan did not address the client's individual needs—only nursing skills and their techniques. They were nursing care plans, not client care plans. The vast majority of notes on the care plans addressed the needs of the medical model. These needs, although important to the client, mention only medications, treatments, monitoring of vital signs, intake and output sheets, diagnostic studies to be done, IVs, oxygen therapy, the dates for going to the operating room, and operative procedure. The medical model style of Kardex cards is still in use in many institutions.

Care plans were strictly job centered, not client centered. They focused on the things the nurse had to do. What was missing and what detracted from individualized care were the nursing assessments regarding the client's family and the client's psychological, sociological, and physical adaptations to the illness. Contemporary nursing legislation mandates that nurses look at the client's response to health situations and deviations from health and address nursing action toward meeting those needs. This nursing legislation, or the Nursing Practice Acts, proposes that the ultimate goal of nursing is health maintenance. Rehabilitation goals and discharge plans are basic nursing responsibilities inherent to health maintenance when the client is acutely ill in a hospital or in a nursing home. These goals help the nurse identify the client's optimum levels of performance.

In the early 1950s, the concept of nursing through team action or team nursing forced the development of written nursing care plans. It was necessary to have some method of written communications during the shift because a variety of nursing team members were caring for the client. The professional nurse, however, was the person responsible for writing the care plan and making the nursing decisions that were incorporated into it. After 1952, the literature in nursing journals regarding nursing care plans became more prolific. It was emphasized that care plans should be written within a framework of planning for safety for the client, for continuity of care, and for the establishment of cooperation between interdisciplinary team members. The care goal was oriented toward the team effort. Stated were the purpose of team action, who was to do what, and in what ways. Care plans on the Kardex became the basis for making assignments for nursing and auxiliary staff. In the late 1950s care plans evolved to focus on client's needs. The client became the starting point for the goal stated on the care plans and not just the object of the treatments to be given to him. The care plan, as interpreted on the Kardex card, helped the nonprofessional team worker understand the goals for the client and have direction in giving care to the client. The transition from job-centered to client-centered care plans is documented by Kron (1961) when she states that the purpose of care plans is to include not the disease of the client, but the extent to which the disease affects the client's physical and emotional aspects of nursing care.

Wagner (1969) states that care plans were used by nursing educators as instruments for teaching students. The student could see care plans as the reflection of the objectives of care and the steps used to arrive at these objectives. It was stressed that the objectives should be based on scientific principles. This was a major breakthrough in developing the nursing process framework of data collection as a part of assessment. The thinking process of the nurse went from assessment to nursing diagnosis, from nursing diagnosis to plan of care, then to implementation and evaluation. The care plan is a reflection of the logical systematic collection of data and decision-making processes.

Care plans as mandate

Without a doubt, accrediting and surveying agencies have added significant impetus to the development of care plans. For example, the Joint Commission on Hospital Accreditation lists care plans as an essential component of the client's care record. State bureaus of public health for licensing and certification of long-term-care facilities and community health agencies mandate that the plan of care be a written, ongoing record of the individual assessment of each client. In order to get reimbursement on Medicare/Medicaid claims, the health provider must document the

level of care. In nursing, this documentation is the care plan. Evaluation of the client's needs as stated in the care plan will determine whether an agency is providing skilled nursing care or intermediate level care. Rates and payment schedules and number of days allocated of Medicare and Medicaid skilled services are all documented on the client care plan.

Objections to care planning

When faced with writing care plans, many nurses raise objections.

1. It doesn't matter if I do them or not, I'm still professional.
2. We don't have enough staff to have individualized programs of care plans.
3. We have too much paperwork already. It is too much of a burden.
4. Staff will set the goals—that part is easy—and then just goof off.
5. It's trivial work; I like to really be with the patient at the bedside.

Advantages to care planning

There are some decided advantages for using care plans. Some of these advantages directly answer the objections raised about care plans. Written care plans prevent the nurse from being sidetracked into attending to only obvious issues. Because care plans insist that the nurse state goals in a time framework, it directs her attention to the priority of goals and helps her formulate a schedule of care. Care plans are clear and specific. Because they address the specific activities, auxiliary personnel and volunteers can be added to the nursing team. Rather than being complex, care plans are actually quite simple, and when learned, can be instituted easily. The overall implementation of care becomes far easier with the care plan. Because the client has been involved in the treatment development, there is a better chance that he will understand why things are being done. When there is a written care plan, the nurse can use other nurses as a resource regarding nursing treatment rather than asking the client to make nursing decisions.

Mrs. Smith is an 80-year-old woman admitted to an extended care facility for a 3-week period of rehabilitation after a repair of a fractured hip. Several times each day she is addressed by nurses who begin their statements by saying, "What did they do for you, Mrs. Smith? Are you getting out of bed yet? How did they get you out of bed?" Mrs. Smith is being asked to make nursing decisions. Mrs. Smith must restate her care to the nurses each time she is about to begin activities. Little progress is made from that point because it is always repeated. With a written care plan for Mrs. Smith, the nurse would look and see what ROM and transfer activities are to be done, if they have been successful, and what revisions would be made. She then goes to Mrs. Smith and doesn't have to get the information from the client once again. The client has the opportunity to address other subjects rather than just the standard physical treatment of care.

Mr. Clancy is a 67-year-old man who had abdominal surgery 4 days ago. The nurse, without the care plan, comes into his room and says, "Well, Mr. Clancy, how are they changing your dressings? Do you still have a drain in place?" The nurse with the written care plan will know that Mr. Clancy has had his drain removed and that six small gauze pads are necessary under the combine for the dressing. Instead of asking Mr. Clancy how to do the nursing care, the nurse can use the time to teach Mr. Clancy the aseptic principles and some concepts about healing. She is making the nursing decisions and still has time for health teaching.

Documenting quality care

The primary incentive for writing care plans should not be to please the nursing supervisor or Medicare or the JCAH visit surveyor; however, it often is the case. The care plan is basic to the role of a nurse. Quality nursing care must be planned and directed by the nurse, and when it is done, it must be documented in writing. The care plans represent the documentation of the method of organizing the client's care. Mere documentation of care does not guarantee that indeed the stated care was given. It does, however, raise the nurse's level of consciousness regarding the care. If it is not documented, it is viewed as not having been done. Since a nurse would never consider carrying out the medical regimen of care without written doctor's order, why should she consider carrying

out a nursing plan of care without written nursing orders? The argument that it is done verbally and just not written fails because a verbal word or statement cannot be evaluated. Once the nurse is off the unit, the written care plan stands as a resource for other members of the nursing care team who will come to care for that client. Even years after the client has been discharged, the written record stands to validate before everyone the quality of the care. The plan of care begins immediately upon the client's admission and continues day by day, incorporating short- and long-term objectives until the time of discharge. Plans are revised and kept current through notations as necessary.

A well-conceived plan of care individualizes and gives direction and continuity to the client's care. Assignments can be planned on a priority based on information in the nursing plan. When care plans are being used as a basis for staff assignments, remember that professional judgment cannot be delegated. Auxiliary personnel can often do nursing activities, but this is the duty aspect of the care. Judgments and decision making need the knowledge base of the nurse. The nurse continues to monitor the progress of the implementation of care, collects information from both the client and her staff, and adjusts the care plan accordingly.

When the client is transferred from one agency to another (such as from a hospital to an extended care facility), a copy of the care plan should be sent along with the transfer records. It will be a useful resource for the admitting nurse and provide a full understanding of what has transpired in regard to the client's plan of care. If an agency's policy does not permit a copy of the care plan to accompany the client upon transfer, make sure that, within the transfer summary, the important data that specify the client's plan of care are included for the nurses in the new facility to use as a guide.

Management support of care plan policies

Adequate care plan writing does not begin with the individual nurse alone. Agency administration and nursing administration must value written care plans as a vehicle for quality client care and demonstrate that by actions as well as words. Policies set by the agency must incorporate the writing of care plans as a requirement of nursing care. Recognition and reward must be provided for nurses to have the incentive to write nursing care plans. For example, skill in writing care plans must be a part of the evaluation done by the head nurse and staff nurse. If the staff nurse and head nurse see that writing care plans is recognized as a part of professional practice by nursing and administration, then they will have the incentive to take time to write care plans. The agency administration and nursing management may state that nursing care plans are important. However, if they do not include competency in care planning in evaluating the nurses or do not provide in-service education opportunities for the nurse regarding care plans, then care planning is devalued in the eyes of the nurse. When care plan writing is a recognized, noted part of the nurse's professional practice, then the nurse receives a positive message regarding doing care plans. On the other hand, at times the message the nurse receives is that writing client care plans is important because the JCAH or Medicaid visitors are looking for them, but they are to be done only for that. In such cases, the care plans are done for the visitors and not for the clients. What often occurs just before the visitors' accreditation survey is a flurry of activity in the nursing station to get the Kardexes up to date and have goals written.

Time must be made available for the nurse to carry out this written phase of the nursing care process. She must collect data and make a nursing diagnosis, both components of the written care plan. The nurse-client ratio must be examined to permit the nurse the opportunity in the 8-hour shift to perform these written works. With skill, writing care plans does not require a lot of time. It is a skill, like other skills, that can be learned, and there are rules that can be followed. Before we discuss how to write client goals and objectives, the broader topic of what goals and objectives are will be presented.

OF GOALS AND OBJECTIVES

If you are going to take a car ride, how do you know what road to take if you do not know where you are going? Goals and plans are the nurses' road map to quality client care. This road map can be read by other nurses caring for the client, auxiliary personnel, and the client himself. When it comes time to evaluate the care given to the client, the goals for the client become the focal point of the question, "Did the client get to the point of optimum health?" In other words, were the goals reached, did he get to where he was supposed to go?

A goal is the place at which a trip or race ends, the place at which one strives to arrive. A plan is the scheme or program for making that trip to the goal. The difference between a goal and a plan is the difference between an object and the objectives. The object is the place or goal one wants to reach, and the objectives are the plans made to reach that object. The goal or object describes the outcome to be reached, and the objectives or plans describe the steps needed to make the trip. The goal/object is the product of the work and the objectives/plans are the process of the work. The objectives/plans describe what must be done.

Process and product of client care

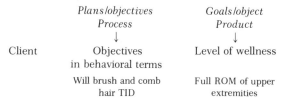

Roadmap to Philadelphia destination via a particular road

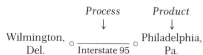

Care plan to reach client wellness destination via a special client objective

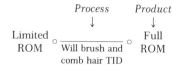

Objectives stated in terms of the client's behavior facilitate active participation of the client in the process of keeping well and recovering full function. When the plans are made in concert with the client, he understands what is expected of him and can offer suggestions to ensure the success of the activity. In the preceding example, the client's goal was full ROM of the upper extremities. This could have been achieved by wall climbing exercises, rope turning exercises, or ball throwing exercises. The client stated that she finds repetitive exercises boring. Some alternatives were offered, one of which was hair combing and brushing activity as a part of daily grooming. Objectives give information upon which to direct activities. Not only does this objective encourage attainment of the goal, but also; it is integrated into the client's usual lifestyle. The active participation of the individual in the process of care demonstrates the philosophical difference between a client and a patient. This client has active participation in the planning and outcome of her care. She is not passive.

The setting of client goals and the evaluation of the success in the achievement of the goal are closely related. Evaluation or measurement of the outcome of nursing care is impossible without having goals to measure. Knowing that full ROM of upper extremities is the desired outcome, the nurse can observe whether or not the client has reached full ROM of the upper extremities. Day-by-day progress can be noted on the chart and can be discussed with the client. All nursing personnel involved with the client's care are aware that, because of morning stiffness, the client's mobility in arms and shoulders is limited but that full ROM is being encouraged. If the client is not able to reach the goal, this can also be discussed and other options made available to meet the goal can be offered.

A goal is reviewed several times. These periods of review are called formative and summative evaluations. When a goal is set, a tentative date of achievement is proposed. For example, the goal is full ROM of upper extremities by October 20. The nurse does not wait until October 20 to assess whether or not the goal has been achieved, but notes the progress the client is making toward that goal before that date. She does a formative evaluation of the client's progress, which gives her the opportunity to adjust the client's activities or to supply additional information or materials so that the client will be in the best possible position to reach the goal. For example, the nurse should observe the client during the hair combing and brushing activity at least once. A formative evaluation of the client's progress might indicate that the nurse should provide the client with a larger comb or with a brush with a longer handle. Or perhaps the nurse might suggest to the client a certain number of strokes or length of time the activity should last to get full muscle and joint involvement. At this time also the nurse should let the client know how successful the activity has been and what else might be done to ensure attainment of the goal. The nurse might say, "You are doing a very good job with the range of motion for your arms. Take care to include the back of your head also because that action demands full shoulder joint activity and will help you loosen up that painful joint."

On October 20 the nurse makes a summative evaluation of the goal attainment. The purpose of the summative evaluation is to appraise the overall effectiveness of a particular plan of care. The data from the summative evaluation is not for modifying the activity but for assessing if it was appropriate for the client and if the goal was reached. More information relating to evaluating plans of care is included in Chapter 11.

Client objectives in behavioral terms

After the nurse makes the nursing diagnosis, she has before her a list of the client's nursing needs. The next step is to set client goals and to describe the behavior of the client that will enable him to reach the goals. This case study demonstrates objectives written in terms of client behaviors.

Mr. Thomason is an 88-year-old man with extensive varicose veins in both legs. His physician suggests that he be seen by the visiting nurse once a week until his acute course of numbness and tingling and mottled skin improves. When the nurse visits Mr. Thomason, she notes the complaints of leg ache and muscle fatigue as well as extremity coldness, slightly mottled skin, and a small amount of swelling in the right leg. The nurse understands that the incompetent veins in Mr. Thomason's legs are causing blood to pool in his extremities with sluggish return of blood to the central circulation. His health history indicates that he wears calf garters on his socks, and his daily profile indicates that he works for 5 or 6 hours each afternoon making music boxes in his basement.

Medical diagnosis

Varicosities of great saphenous veins

Nursing diagnosis

Impaired venous peripheral circulation

Client goals	Client objectives
1. Improved venous return from the legs	Mr. Thomason will: Apply elastic stockings upon arising each morning. Elevate legs on stool for 20 minutes after each meal. Ambulate for 10 minutes of each 2 hours while working on music boxes. Elevate foot of mattress on 6-inch blocks. Wear socks without calf garters. Do range of motion exercises for legs each evening while preparing for bed.
2. Protection of legs from potential physical injury.	Inspect the skin on legs each evening for color, temperature, and signs of redness, cuts, bruises, or areas of pain or tenderness. This inspection will be done in the bathroom with the two lights on. Wear closed toe shoes and slippers.
3. Knowledge regarding peripheral vascular system physiology.	State the function of the veins in the legs. Describe a varicose vein. Explain how change in activities will help relieve discomforts associated with varicose veins.

Date of planning session: October 11
Target date for goal achievement: October 25

Nursing orders

Measure client for knee-high elastic stockings and order from surgical supply house.
Explain the correct technique for elevating legs.
Measure ankle circumferences bilaterally.
Teach re: Correct ankle and leg position when sitting, standing, and recumbent.
Demonstrate ROM of legs.
Teach re: Proper footwear and legwear and application of elastic stockings.
Teach re: Anatomy and physiology of venous system and the signs and symptoms of skin breakdown on legs and feet.
Give client written instruction sheet of all information reviewed.
Give client business card with agency phone number in case any questions arise.

This nurse has evaluated Mr. Thomason's individual needs and addressed them comprehensively through her nursing diagnosis, client goals and objectives, and nursing orders. Her client care plan reflects her philosophy (1) that the client should assume responsibility in the caregiving regimen, (2) that health teaching is an integral part of her role as nurse, and (3) that potential health threats are anticipated as a part of planning. The nursing activities are clearly documented and are easily reviewed. The nursing orders constituted the nurses' notes for this particular visit. This agency's stationery is designed to include a flowsheet approach to care planning. It took this nurse only a few minutes to complete the client care plan. On her next visit on October 18, she will use her nursing orders to do a formative evaluation of Mr. Thomason's progress. If Mr. Thomason has any difficulties or questions, he knows how to reach his nurse. By keeping communications open with a telephone call between visits, the nurse uses a cost-effective method to do a client goal achievement check before the target date. If adjustments in the client care plan have to be made, it is possible that she could make suggestions during the telephone call.

The nurse describes in specific detail client action that will demonstrate how he will be behaving when the goal is reached. When the target date is set in advance, assessment of the behavior that can be observed and measured is easy. Target dates can be moved if necessary, either forward or back, depending on the client's response and progress; but the target date does give the client and the nurse something to look forward to and a framework in which to set evaluation measures. Because the client behavior is spelled out in specific detail, other persons who care for the client can read the plan and know exactly what is to be done and what the client is doing.

To ensure clear, precise, and concise objectives, the nurse should check the objectives for the following points:

Points	Examples
1. List only one behavior in each objective.	Ambulate length of hall two times a day.
	Eat a midmorning snack of juice or a piece of fruit.
2. Begin each objective with an *action* verb describing the behavior expected.	Some examples of action verbs:

Attend	Drink	Participate
Administer	Eat	Perform
Ambulate	Elevate	Read
Apply	Exercise	Recognize
Ask	Explain	Restate
Bathe	Express	Select
Brush	Give	Show
Button	Irrigate	Stand
Choose	Inspect	State
Clean	Listen	Strain
Cover	Make	Suction
Decide	Match	Talk
Demonstrate	Measure	Take
Distribute	Moisten	Tell
Describe	Monitor	Test
Do	Observe	Walk
Discuss	Order	Wear
Draw	Paint	Write
Dress		

Points	Examples
3. State any special conditions under which the behavior should be performed	Test urine for sugar and acetone ½ hour before each meal.
	Take a shower once a week using a shower chair.
	Apply lotion to feet at night before retiring.
4. Limit objective to as few words as possible.	Perform breast self-examination on the first of each month.
	Demonstrate ROM exercises.
5. List each objective on a separate line. It facilitates reading objectives and identifying target dates.	

General guidelines in goal planning

As the nurse approaches goal planning, there are some overall guidelines that will help her formulate her client care plan.

1. Include the client and the family in the planning process from the beginning.

2. Focus on the client's assets.
3. Set realistic goals.
4. State the client goals in specific terms.
5. Write the nursing orders necessary to reach each goal.

The client's particular desires, his likes and dislikes, should be a part of each goal. These desires and preferences of the client are part of the assessment phase of the nursing process. To as great an extent as possible, the client participates in setting the goals. In addition to the client, the family or significant others are also included. The goals are always explained to the client and the family and questions answered regarding them. A lucid description of the regimen of care, both medical and nursing, facilitates client and family interaction. By including the family and the client very early in the caregiving process, the nurse actually saves herself time in the long run. When the client and the family understand exactly what is going on, they are less likely to have negative feelings about the nursing care, offer fewer complaints, or question the motives and outcome of the care being given. This nurse is, in effect, treating the client and family the way she herself might like to be treated.

The nurse focuses on the client's assets rather than on his limitations. The nurse reviews the data collected in the first step of the nursing process, and notes the client's assets. Included are those things the client can do, things that he likes, and in what ways and to what extent he is independent. A list is made of possible client goal areas, keeping in mind that the potential goal areas should be stated in positive terms because positive terms accentuate his assets. When the client's needs are identified and goals stated in negative terms or phrases, it emphasizes his limitations. For example, compare the possible phrasing of these nursing statements:

Negative statement	Positive statement
Feels that she is useless.	*Wants to feel that she is useful.*
Focus is on limitations:	Focus is on assets:
79 years old	Former schoolteacher
Arthritis	Likes music
Osteoporosis	Devout Baptist
Has no visitors	Enjoys reading

Negative statement—cont'd

Both statements address the topic of feelings of self-worth. A negative statement connotes a dead-end situation. The emphasis is on the client's physical limitations. This predisposes both the client and the nurse to measure what the client cannot do because of her age, arthritis, osteoporosis, and limited social contacts, rather than visualize the scope of the client's assets.

Positive statement—cont'd

When client goals are phrased in a positive statement, options for remedy are more readily identified. The nurse and the client review the data collected and these assets become the options that translate into client goals. Because these are the self-stated characteristics of the client, they are indeed individualized goals. The goals are what the client can do, and what she likes to do, and they incorporate the behavior of her life-style.

Nursing diagnosis

Altered self-concept

Client goal	Target dates	Client objectives
To feel useful	10/11	Mrs. Lee will: Select three songs for residents' Wednesday recreation hour.
	10/15	Distribute the song sheets
	10/15	Lead the group in sing-along.
	10/26	Attend community Baptist prayer services.
	11/4	Write a story for the residents' monthly newsletter, *Table Talk*.

Nursing orders

1. Have recreational therapist provide song books to choose songs.
2. Bring cartons of song books to day room. Arrange nursing care and medications so she will be free by 6:30 PM.
3. Have recreational therapist introduce her to group.
4. Provide her with writing materials and the telephone number of the secretary who types *Table Talk*. Give her back copies to review.
5. Have recreational therapist make arrangements for her to attend Community Baptist Church prayer services.

Setting realistic goals is as important as any of the other guidelines for client care planning. The nurse must set goals that are attainable for the individual client. The nurse considers the client's level of functioning, particular medical and nursing diagnoses, and his available assets at the particular time. The nurse, as part of a health care team, must be involved in setting reasonable goals and must have a good understanding of what can logically be expected to be accomplished while the client is under the team's care. For example, Mrs. Lombard is admitted to a long-term-care facility after having had a CVA. During her hospitalization at a nearby general hospital, full rehabilitative measures were instituted, but she still has extensive neurological impairment on her left side. An unreasonable goal for Mrs. Lombard would be that she will walk independently again, for the neurological damage is permanent and irreversible. However, a goal that she will walk again with braces or will have mobility in a wheelchair is certainly within a reasonable expectation for goal planning.

Client goals are written in specific rather than general terms. Goals such as (1) to ensure optimum well-being or (2) to restore to independence are too global. These are overall goals that apply to all clients. Specific goals address the unique areas of the client's individual concerns. Such specific goals as (1) to include four vegetable/fruit servings in each day's food intake or (2) to button one's shirt are specific and discrete for the particular client's needs.

To encourage specifically stated client goals, it is useful if the agency's Kardex form has the overall objective printed as a part of the Kardex stationery. Having these statements before her encourages the nurse to zero in on specific goals to reach these overall goals.

The last general guideline in goal planning is the writing of nursing orders. Nursing orders can be described as specific nursing actions leading to the successful reaching of the goals. When a nursing order is written, it stands as the documentation of the planned nursing intervention. Because it is a written and not a verbal description of care to be given, nursing activity is not left to memory, and misunderstandings are avoided.

Nursing orders are best written in a precise and concise format. Included in each nursing order should be a statement of what the nursing activity is to be for the particular client. Use specific terms in short sentences. Long, rambling sentences distract from the central point of the nursing order. If a nursing activity is to be repeated or carried out for a particular length of time, this should be stated quantitatively. For example, when a nurse wants to encourage a client to drink fluids, she might write the following nursing orders:

Encourage PO fluids—2800 ml/day including fluids with
   meals and snacks.
  Distribute throughout day as follows:
     1500 days
     1100 evenings
      200 nights
  Encourage OJ, H_2O, tea, and broth between meals.
  Teach re: Doing self I & O sheet.

All nursing personnel are aware of what the nursing actions should be, and so nursing intervention can be individualized on each shift.

Areas of decision-making responsibility

When nurses write care plans designed to include the client as a part of the decision-making process, the question sometimes arises, "What is a nursing decision, and what is a client decision?" The nurse must decide what nursing measures are needed, and the client participates in the area of how the nursing measure is to be implemented. After collecting as much information as possible about the client, the nurse makes the nursing diagnosis. The client does not make the nursing diagnosis, but certainly does contribute information leading to it. The nurse makes her diagnosis and her plans based on her wide and in-depth knowledge of nursing, social sciences, and biological sciences. She has the right and the responsibility to make these decisions because she has the education to do it; and actually, that is exactly what she is being paid to do by the client. Client decision-making enters when options for implementing activities to reach the goals are being discussed. The following example demonstrates client participation in his care planning.

The nurse notices that Mr. Alexander, a resident in Oakdale Nursing Home, seems sad after hearing that his daughter will be moving to another state and will not be able to visit as often as she has been in the past. His appetite and fluid intake have decreased. The nurse understands the potential emotional and physical implications of the situation. She monitors Mr. Alexander closely and decides that the nursing diagnoses should be:

Inadequate emotional support related to anticipated loss
Potential fluid imbalance related to decreased appetite
   and fluid intake.

The nurse discusses her decisions with Mr. Alexander. He agrees that he is saddened by his daughter's move and that his grief is taking its toll on his emotional and physical health. They mutually arrive at the client goals of preventing further emotional injury and maintaining his adequate nutritional status.

A brief discussion between Mr. Alexander and his nurse during morning care sets care objectives in specific terms. Mr. Alexander would like the nurse to talk to his daughter about the move because it makes him uncomfortable to bring up the subject. Since the nurse understands that she should not usurp his relationship with his daughter, she agrees to discuss the matter with his daughter with the understanding that he will discuss it with her also. He agrees that his lack of participation in recreational activities fosters more loneliness and isolation but states that he doesn't have the energy for daily participation. He agrees to participate every other day. Since mealtime has not been used as a source of socialization, he agrees to take his meals with Mr. Fox.

Client care plan

Client goals	Date	Client objectives
To prevent emotional injury	10/24	Mr. Alexander will: Verbalize reasons for daughter's move. Discuss alternative communication/contact plans with daughter. Participate in agency social activities four times a week.

Client care plan—cont'd

Client goals	Date	Client objectives
To maintain adequate nutritional status	10/24	Record his fluid intake on I & O Sheet. Eat his meals with friend, Mr. Fox in adjacent room. Discuss food preferences with dietician.

Planning Date: 10/21
Nursing orders
  1. Speak with daughter
     Inform her of his concerns.
     Ask her to clearly state to him the reasons for the move.
     Discuss the communication options that will be available after her move, such as telephone calls, letters, and anticipated frequency of visits.
     Discuss the feasibility of having Mr. Alexander transferred to a facility near her new home.
  2. Nursing aide will play cards with him each afternoon for 20 minutes.
  3. Recreation therapist notified of need to be included in more activities.
  4. Teach re: Self-recording of fluid balance sheet.
  5. Notify dietician re:
     Need for special food preference to increase desire to eat.
     Arrangement to have tray delivered with Mr. Fox's tray.
  6. Dietary aide notified to deliver Mr. Alexander's and Mr. Fox's trays together in Mr. Fox's room.

CLIENT CARE CONFERENCES

Client care conferences come in all shapes and sizes. A conference may be simply structured to include a few health care personnel or elaborately structured to include an interdisciplinary health care team and department representation. Why are conferences needed, and who benefits from them? Conferences are another tool used as a source for gathering information in the first component of the nursing process. The conference may be used to clarify client assets and goals. It lends itself to input from other personnel and disciplines to clarify clients' needs and approaches to meet these needs. It can identify nursing diagnosis, nursing orders, and nursing intervention. The conference is an arena for the interdisciplinary team to develop a collaborative framework that uses the expertise of each team member to en-

sure quality care. It facilitates communication between the interdisciplinary team and departments within the agency or facility. It clarifies the specifics of the client care plan, including the goals and outcome behavior, and identifies the responsibility of each team member for executing his section of the plan. Conferences are excellent evaluation tools. The team may decide that they need more information from the assessment or diagnostic stage, that the therapeutic modalities need adjustment, that the goals are too general, that nursing orders need to be changed, or that the care plan and goals are being met and the client's response is positive. Formative evaluations are done at each conference, and needed modifications are made.

Organizing client care conferences

The same excuses for not writing care plans apply to not doing client conferences. The best approach is to just schedule the conferences and do them. Winning is beginning, and to win the conference battle you have to begin having conferences. One time frame is to have a nursing client conference after the initial assessment by each health team member is completed. Some agencies and facilities recommend a conference within a minimum of 6 days and a maximum of 14 days after admission. Most assessments are completed and the diagnostic results recorded within a week. It is easy to get to all new admissions and schedule a conference, but what about the other clients? Along with the new admissions, determine how many long-standing clients you want to include in the conference. Schedule a weekly day and time for the conference.

Nursing can take the initiative by conducting client conferences on the unit. These conferences would include the nursing staff involved with the client and at least one nurse from another shift.

Setting

The charge nurse arranges for a room for the conference, preferably one on the unit or in close proximity to the unit. It should be comfortable, well lighted, and ventilated, with a table with a sufficient number of chairs for participants. When the same room is used each week, it becomes known as "our conference room."

Format for client conference

1. Charge nurse schedules a conference room.
2. Charge nurse designates another nurse as nurse recorder.
3. Charge nurse states name of client under discussion.
4. Nurse assigned to client briefly presents assessment data.
5. Group discussion to collect more data.
6. Nursing diagnosis formulated.
7. Client brought in and introduced to group.
8. Client's preferences related to possible goals are elicited.
9. Client can either stay or leave while nursing orders are being written.
10. The date and time for evaluation are scheduled as target dates are reached.
11. A client is identified for the next weekly conference, so the nurse responsible for the client can prepare her information.

Duties of participants

The charge nurse serves as the group leader and resource person for the group's activities. It is important that she sees that the conference is held each week. As the routine for the conference is being established, it is imperative that the conference begin at the specified time. Personnel will soon be programmed to expect a conference as part of that day's routine.

The charge nurse presents a brief nursing assessment and health status of the client. The charge nurse leads the discussion addressing one or two areas of client needs. The recorder of the conference is a nurse, because she is best able to translate the discussion and decisions into the client goals, nursing diagnosis, and orders. A time limit should be set for conference per client. In order to be realistic and avoid the pitfall of having the conference become a burden, ½ hour per client is usually sufficient. If two clients are to be presented each conference day, then only 1 hour need be allocated for client conferences. Note that the term, *time taken out,* for conferences was not used. Just as physicians and business people make decisions using the conference method, so too can nursing decisions be made during conferences as a part of nursing practice. Nurses, however, need the support of administration to recognize that

part of the hands-on dimension of nursing duties includes client care conferences.

As conferences are established, clients also become familiar with the conferencing process. It has been the experience of nurses who conduct conferences that, at first, the clients are timid about participating in a conference, but then come to enjoy it when they see that they are getting individualized attention. Often, being the conference's focus gives the client added status with peers. The charge nurse prepares the client a day or two before by explaining the purpose of the conference. She introduces him to the conference members as his participation in the conference begins. The charge nurse makes sure that the client is included in the discussion, that is, that the people are not talking around him, but including him in the conversation. She translates the discussion into lay terms, if needed, for the client and leads the group back to including the client in the discussion.

The charge nurse is also responsible for keeping the group members on the topic and helping the group keep to the time frame of the meeting. When the conference is ending, the charge nurse summarizes the group's finding and helps the nurse recorder complete the client conference minutes, as shown in the boxed material on p. 142, and then places the minutes in the client's chart. A copy of the minutes is usually forwarded to the nursing supervisor or the Director of Nursing. The client's Kardex is then brought up to date by either the charge nurse or the nurse who is primarily responsible for his care.

The conference recorder documents the conference decisions by summarizing the identified nursing assessment, nursing diagnosis, client goals, target date, and nursing orders on the client conference minutes sheet. Recorded duties can be assigned to one nurse permanently or can be rotated. One advantage to rotating the recorder duties is that each nurse has the opportunity to learn to write brief nursing summaries. It is a challenge.

Conference members are responsible for arranging their care schedules to be available and on time for client care conferences. When a client of theirs is to be presented, the conference member should prepare by reviewing the client's record

---

Client conference minutes

Client's name _____

Unit _____ Shift _____ Date _____

Charge nurse conducting conference _____

Members of conference:

RNs   **LPNs**   **Nursing assistants**

1. Brief nursing assessment presented by _____
    a. _____
    b. _____
    c. _____
    d. _____
2. Nursing diagnosis
    a. _____
    b. _____
    c. _____
    d. _____
3. Client goals   **Target date**
    a. _____   _____
    b. _____   _____
    c. _____
4. Nursing orders   **Target date**
    a. _____   _____
    b. _____   _____
    c. _____   _____
    d. _____   _____

---

and be ready to present relevant information regarding the client to the conference group. Group members are expected to listen to the presentation thoughtfully and to share their ideas with the group.

Expanding from a nursing care conference to an interdisciplinary care conference

Interdisciplinary team members

Physician	Occupational therapist
Nurse	Activities director
Social worker	Psychologist
Chaplain	Speech therapist
Physical therapist	Dietician
	Other significant individuals

Minutes of the interdisciplinary team conference are taken, just as they are in client care conferences conducted by nursing (see boxed material on p. 143). Each discipline presents its individual assessment and brief evaluation summary with goals to the group. The conference team makes specific recommendations regarding client care and sets an interim date for review. A summary is placed on the client's chart. The nursing Kardex is used to record the discipline's suggested modalities of the client's care schedule and coordinate the interdisciplinary goals.

The expertise and experience that nursing has gained in conducting their own conferences can be applied to the interdisciplinary team conference as nursing participates as a member. The

Interdisciplinary conference client care plan

Client _____ Date of conference _____ Interim conference date _____

Diagnosis _____ Admission date _____ Attending physician _____

Client/interdisciplinary team goals _____

_____

_____

_____

Medical regime care objectives	Nursing care objectives	Social worker objectives
Physician MD	Nurse RN	Social worker MSW

Occupational therapist objectives	Physical therapist objectives	Speech therapist objectives
OT/Activity director OT	Physical therapist PT	Speech therapist

Nutritional objectives	Religious objectives	Client's preferences
Dietician	Chaplain	

Client conference recommendations   **Interim conference date**

1. _____ _____

2. _____ _____

3. _____ _____

concept of federally mandated interdisciplinary team conferences is on the horizon. The format for an interdisciplinary team conference is that of a client care conference.

RATIONALE FOR DISCHARGE PLANNING

For the older adult, a discharge may occur from the hospital into a long-term-care facility, or from the facility to a hospital, or from either facility back into the client's home. If the client's death is inevitable, then his discharge plan relates to sustaining him. Discharge planning begins with the client's admission. Discharge planning is an integral part of utilization review in hospitals and long-term-care facilities. The need for continuous stay must be documented by the client's requirement for the specified level of nursing care. Nursing cannot wait to develop a plan for the continuation of nursing care until the day of discharge or the day that the utilization review committee denies the client continuous stay status under Medicare. The client has the right to have a plan for discharge as part of his client care plan. Social service is often called on to assist in the development of a plan. The federal government (U.S. Department of Health and Human Services, formerly HEW) mandates a discharge plan for Medicare clients documented on the client care plan before they leave the facility for home or another agency.

A hospitalized older adult needs continuity of health care to assure his ease of return to the community. The older adult may have several options for medical and nursing care. Continuity of care may be provided temporarily or permanently by a long-term-care facility, a community health nurse, the family, and the use of community resources. The client should have some input in deciding the option that addresses the scope of his health care needs.

Nursing contributes to the assessment of the health status of the individual and the selection of appropriate actions, which enable the older adult to maintain a balance between dependent and independent functioning within his discharge environment. Nursing can plan and implement nursing behaviors based on a comprehensive understanding of the theories of aging and the mutual simultaneous interaction between the older adult and his environment.

The human system of the older adult is continuously adapting to stressors or conditions that impair adequate functioning. In order to maintain equilibrium, the human system must initiate some degree of adaptation to the three levels of health: preventive, maintenance, and sustaining.

Nursing must address itself to signs and symptoms of changes in the older adult's system by maintenance of the client's integrity through consistency of care, predictability of events, and reduction of the factors that might affect the client's physical and emotional condition.

The discharge plan for the older adult must address:

1. A plan for discharge to another environment (home or institution), that is, *preventive* and *maintenance* aspects of health care.
2. A plan for death and dying, that is, *sustaining* the client.

Discharge to another environment

In the long-term-care facility, a plan for discharge may be developed by the charge nurse, the director of nursing, a discharge nurse coordinator, or social service. Many hospitals have discharge planning departments that are responsible for developing and implementing a plan. The hospital client's nurse initiates the discharge plan on the care plan. The nurse coordinator or discharge planning department is responsible for initiating, implementing, and coordinating any discharge activities. They may incorporate the help and expertise of other health team members, community agencies, and social service. The nurse coordinator is responsible for identifying a safe environment satisfactory to the client and his family and conducive to health.

Functions of the discharge coordinator

The coordinator assesses the potential need for discharge planning within 7 days of the client's admission into a long-term-care facility and upon admission into the hospital. She periodically re-evaluates the revises each client's discharge and makes the discharge plan available to the utilization review committee. Plans can be made to discharge the client to any of the following:

Hospital from a long-term care facility
Rehabilitation center
State institution

Long-term-care facility from a hospital

Residential center

Private home or apartment (alone or with family members)

The discharge environment is selected with attention to the client's assets, health teaching needs, preference, financial resources, nursing care needs, and family relationships. The nurse gathers all available data from the chart, nursing history, client care plan, and clinical conferences, and then reassesses plans according to new information.

Often a referral is made to a public health or community agency. If the nurse is unable to make a visit to the discharge environment, she may elicit a request for a home evaluation from the community health nurse or social worker.

The evaluation of the environment and family will add new information, thus expanding the data base.

Major areas of concern at discharge

A number of standard areas of concern are included in discharge planning. The nurse assesses the health teaching needs for the client and his family, including:

Medications

Special procedures/demonstrations

Equipment and its use

Diet instruction

Other special needs, such as transportation and assistance in the home

Financial abilities of the client and family are also explored. The social worker secures communication with other agencies and financial sources that are available within the community. She secures needed equipment and makes arrangements for payment by means of insurance or Medicare. Often additional resources must be sought, such as:

Registered nurse

Licensed practical nurse

Companion

Home health aide

Housekeeper

Homemaker services

Meals on wheels

Family service

Laboratory work

The older adult may require community sources of help for working out initial problems of adjustment. The community health nurse may be called upon for guidance, support, or referrals to a mental health counselor.

When the client needs additional medical care, nursing, or physical therapy treatments, transportation arrangements must be made as part of discharge planning. An appointment for therapy may be available, but of little use if the client cannot get to it. Many communities have volunteer drivers who are available to the client if arrangements are made in advance.

Discharge plan form

For effective organization of the client's discharge plan, it is very helpful to use a discharge plan form. Included on the form are the client's medical and rehabilitation potential and a summary of the nursing assessment and plans. Discharge goals are outlined and periodically reevaluated. The discharge data are collected sequentially during the client's stay. Such areas as the client's activities of daily living, and medication, dietary, and treatment regimens are all reviewed. Inherent in discharge planning are client and family conferences to assure their input and understanding of the discharge process. Interdisciplinary conferences facilitate the ease of transfer from the facility to another environment by anticipating client needs and coordinating supportive health activities. The client's initial adjustment to the new environment actually begins before transfer, and he has the opportunity to work out questions and feelings with his nurse while she is still close at hand. The client discharge plan is completed when the transfer sheet is sent to the new agency. When the follow-up plans are executed by the discharge coordinator, the client's discharge plan form becomes part of the permanent medical record of the client (see pp. 146-148).

The discharge environment evaluation should be done as an on-site visit. The nurse discharge coordinator, visiting nurse, or social worker are appropriate health professionals to make such an assessment.

The environmental evaluation should include basic client data (see pp. 149-150). The psychosocial climate prevailing in the proposed environment for the client is assessed. In addition, the

Text continued on p. 150.

Convalescent center client discharge plan

Name _____ Room No. _____

Admission date _____ Anticipated discharge date _____

Admitting diagnosis _____

Assessment of potential need for discharge planning to another environment by nurse coordinator: _____
_____
_____

Medical goals and rehabilitation potential: _____
_____

Nursing history: _____
_____

Nursing assessment and diagnosis: _____
_____

Nursing orders: _____
_____
_____
_____
_____

Reevaluation of discharge goals: _____
_____

Dates: _____ _____ _____ _____
Anticipated discharge environment: _____
_____
_____

Level of independence: ☐ Totally independent ☐ Moderately dependent ☐ Totally dependent. Explain
level of activity: _____
_____
_____

Client instructions: _____
_____
_____
_____
_____

Medication and dosage, schedule and mode of self-administration, and precautions and reactions that client
should observe: _____
_____
_____

If client is unable to administer medication himself, instructions were given to: _____

Does person so instructed demonstrate an understanding of the above information? ☐ Yes ☐ No
Explain: _____
_____
_____

Convalescent center client discharge plan—cont'd

Instructed in special treatments and/or procedures, equipment and its use: _____

Client: _____

Family: _____

Person instructed (_____) demonstrates an understanding of the above information: ☐ Yes ☐ No

Explain: _____

Diet instructions: _____

Special diet: _____

Client instructed by: _____

Family member (if instructed): _____ Relationship: _____

Do persons instructed demonstrate an understanding of the diet, its preparation and restrictions? ☐ Yes ☐ No

Explain: _____

Additional instructions given to the client or family: _____

Needed equipment: _____

Plans for securing equipment: _____

Additional resources that must be sought for discharge planning

☐ RN   ☐ Housekeeper   ☐ Meals on Wheels
☐ LPN   ☐ Home health aide   ☐ Social service
☐ Companion   ☐ Family service   ☐ Homemaker service

Others: _____

Plans for securing needed resources: _____

Financial abilities of client and family: _____

Physician/coordinator conference: ☐ Yes ☐ No

Recommendations: _____

Referrals with physician approval:
☐ Social worker   ☐ Occupational therapist
☐ Public health nurse   ☐ Medical care
☐ Community health nurse   ☐ Dentist
☐ Speech therapist   ☐ Podiatrist
☐ Physical therapist   ☐ Family service
☐ Others: _____

Continued.

Convalescent center client discharge plan—cont'd

Mode of transportation to referrals if needed: _____

Anticipated initial problems of adjustment and sources of help: _____

Plans for follow-up care: _____

Recommendations for client/coordinator conference: _____

Recommend family/client/coordinator conference: ☐ Yes ☐ No
Recommendations: _____

Discharge plan approved by: _____
Attending physician: _____
Utilization review committee dates: _____ . _____ _____ _____
Date of discharge: _____ Time: _____ AM _____ PM _____
Mode of discharge: ☐ Wheelchair ☐ Ambulatory ☐ Stretcher
Accompanied by: _____
Discharge environment: ☐ Home ☐ Other Explain: _____

Condition of client on discharge (check progress note) _____

Level of independence: ☐ Totally independent ☐ Moderately dependent ☐ Totally dependent. Explain
level of activity: _____

Form of health at time of discharge if appropriate: _____

☐ Preventive ☐ Maintenance ☐ Sustaining
Final diagnosis: _____

Transfer sheet sent to other agency? ☐ Yes ☐ No

Plan for follow-up by coordinator: _____

_____
Signature

Convalescent center request for home and/or environment evaluation

To: _____
     (Name of agency or individual)

Date: _____

From: _____
      Discharge nurse coordinator's name

Re: _____
     (Name, address, telephone number of client environment to be evaluated)

The above client is presently at our facility. To help us plan for his/her future discharge, we would greatly appreciate your assessment of his/her future environment.

Facility's data

Date of admission: _____

Person or relative to contact: _____
_____

Insurance plan: _____

Diagnosis and/or problems: _____
_____
_____

Nursing history: _____
_____
_____

Nursing assessment and nursing diagnosis: _____
_____
_____

Nursing orders: _____
_____
_____

Data to assess, collect and evaluate if appropriate:

1. What is the family's attitude toward the client's return home or transfer to other environment? _____
_____

2. Does the family accept the limitations and/or aging process and developmental tasks of the client? ____
_____

3. What concerns does the family have about the client? _____
_____
_____

4. Who is assuming responsibility for the client and his/her care? _____

5. Does the climate of the environment seem conducive for the client's form of health—preventive, maintenance, or sustaining—as well as for the physical and emotional well-being of the client? _____
_____

6. Is the environment adaptable to meet the client's needs within his/her limitations? _____
_____

Continued.

Convalescent center request for home and/or environment evaluation—cont'd

7. Is the environment conducive for respecting and maintaining the rights and values of the client? _____

8. Resources: Do you feel that the client needs any of the following services?

       ☐ RN   ☐ Homemaker service   ☐ Transportation

       ☐ LPN   ☐ Physical therapy   ☐ Meals on Wheels

       ☐ Companion   ☐ Occupational therapy   ☐ Family service

       ☐ Home health aide   ☐ Social worker   ☐ Equipment

   Other: _____

9. Additional comments: _____

_____

_____

                                  _____

                                  Signature of interviewer

Please return to:
Nurse coordinator
Sunshine Convalescent Center
Holladay Road
Robin, Pennsylvania

---

evaluator assesses whether or not the health-related aspects of the environment are in accord with the client's anticipated health status. Recommendations are made regarding what added health personnel and/or services and community resources will be needed by the client. When the environment evaluation is done at least one full week in advance, there is ample time available to carry out the evaluator's recommendations.

Plan for death and dying

Nurses as health care providers are in a unique position to begin the *sustaining* measures required when the client will be discharged because of death. Nursing coordinates and synchronizes medical and other related professional and technical services, as required for *sustaining* the client. Nursing sustains the client by involving the individual, family, and appropriate religious groups. She also helps other nurses and personnel understand their feelings about death and their behavior in contacts with the dying client through staff development programs. The nurse assists the client and provides added strength to help the client feel safe and secure to face dying with courage and dignity.

The physician will outline the medical regimen on the chart. The nurse is responsible for executing the medical regimen of care. Also, the nurse assesses the nursing needs of the client and develops a nursing care plan, keeping in mind the client's perceptions, attitude, and response to dying. Client-oriented clinical conferences involve the staff in the dying process, and help them recognize and interpret the behavioral reactions of the client to dying, and the adjustive responses of the client, family, staff, and community. With the client himself, the nurse assists with sustaining and promoting the individual's psychological adjustment to himself and his perception of death. She must consider the biomedical, psychosocial, and cultural variables that determine how well he can understand nursing activities as death approaches. As the discharge planning continues, the nurse observes, describes, and explains the interrelationship between the nurse, client, staff, and others. She does nursing care, explaining it to the client, and understands the mutuality of her experience with dying clients.

Discharge planning for the dying client helps the nurse coordinate and synchronize medical and other related professional and technical services, in order to sustain the dying client by intradisciplinary and interdisciplinary collaboration. When the death occurs, the nurse secures medical assistance and pronouncement of death. The nurse recognizes body changes that follow death and the need for caring for the body in order to preserve a natural, comfortable-appearing client in preparation for family viewing and transfer to the mortician.

Steps in discharge-planning process

In the discharge-planning process, the health team reviews the attainment of the stated goals for the client. They determine if the client is ready for discharge and what additional arrangements must be made to facilitate an easy transition (Fig. 8-1).

The following 11 steps constitute a common discharge planning protocol for implementation by a nurse in a hospital or long-term-care facility. These steps resemble a retrospective audit (see Chapter 12) because, in effect, the discharge planners are reviewing the client's progress during his stay and his readiness for discharge. Examine the medical record to collect data in order to:

1. Evaluate the plan that was used for the client to ascertain if the purposes of the plan were met.
   ☐ Yes   ☐ No   ☐ To a degree
   Explain: _____

Model for discharge using nursing process

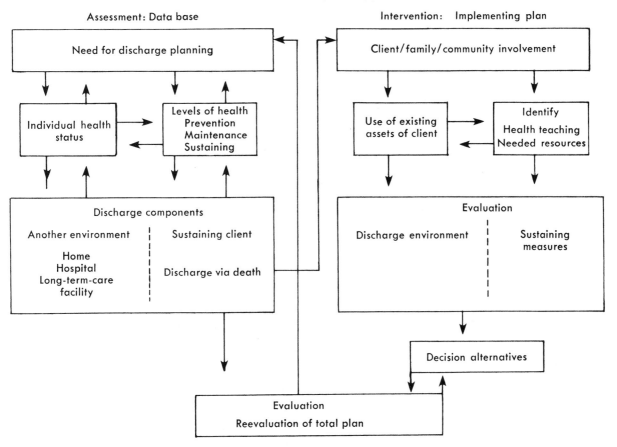

Fig. 8-1. Guides to nursing objectives.

2. Evaluate the client's goals and their attainment.
3. Evaluate the client's plan of care and clinical conference.
4. Arrange for an interdisciplinary conference of all health team members involved in the care of the client to evaluate the collaboration in the delivery of comprehensive health services needed to maintain the client's transfer to another environment, or services needed for the sustaining of the client's approaching death.
5. Evaluate the effectiveness of staff development programs and classes for the staff to help sustain the client or prepare the client for discharge to another environment.
6. Evaluate the adequacy of reference material and audiovisual and library sources available.
7. Conduct a nursing audit if needed.
8. Evaluate follow-up reports from staff, as well as from:
   Referral agencies and individuals
   Families
   Clients
   Physicians
   Hospitals
   Nursing homes
   Rehabilitation center
   Residential center
   Clergy
   Social worker
   Community health nurse
   Speech therapist
   Physical therapist
   Occupational therapist
   Dentist
   Podiatrist
   Other
9. Determine if there was a follow-up on-site visit of the discharge environment by the nurse coordinator or other individual.
   ☐ Yes   ☐ No
   Results of the visit: _____
10. Evaluate clients discharged to another environment immediately and again within six months.
11. Make recommendations.

The chart below lists tools that may be used to gather data for making a discharge plan.

Data collection tools for discharge planning

Tools that have been used to collect data	Check data collected	Date for conferences
1. Medical record		
2. Client care plan		
3. Clinical conferences		
4. Physician conferences		
5. Client conferences		
6. Family conferences		
7. Client/family conferences		
8. Questionnaires		
9. On-site visits of environment		
10. Referrals		
11. Environment evaluation form		
12. Follow-up reports and evaluation		
13. Data from other health team members; interdisciplinary and intradisciplinary conferences as needed		
14. Community agencies		
15. Social service consultant		
16. Audiovisual aids		
17. Staff development programs		
18. Reference material		

SUMMARY

Nursing through objectives enables the nurse to design and organize plans for client care. When these plans are written, they serve as both a guide and a source for documenting and evaluating nursing intervention. Care plans are no longer a matter of choice, but are mandated as a part of government and third-party reimbursement policies.

The prospect of having to write out client care plans is frequently a difficult thing for some nurses to address. However, with an understanding of the importance of documenting quality care and the support of management, written client care plans can become a reality.

Objectives and plans describe what must be done for the client. They describe the process component of the care. The product of the care is the goal or level of wellness that the client has achieved as a result of the nursing intervention. When client objectives are stated in behavioral terms, they can be measured in an evaluative process.

Goal planning should include the client and his family and focus on the client's assets, yet be realistic. After writing specific client goals, the nurse spells out the nursing orders needed to reach those goals. She realizes that, although the client has input into the discussions regarding nursing actions, the nurse herself is ultimately responsible for the nursing decisions.

Client care conferences can be limited to the nursing staff alone or can include the entire interdisciplinary team. On either level, the purpose of the client care conference is to design a comprehensive and organized plan of care for the individual client.

The ultimate outcome of all client care planning is to take the client to the point of discharge from the agency. Whether the discharge is because of death or to another environment, discharge planning reduces the stress factors for the client and significant others.

REFERENCES

Brock, A. M., and Madison, A. S.: The challenge in gerontological nursing, Nurs. Forum **16**(1):95, 1977.

Cantor, M. M.: Achieving nursing care standards internal and external, Wakefield, Mass., 1978, Nursing Resources, Inc.

Ebersole, P., and Hess, E.: Care of the aged: nursing roles and functions, St. Louis, 1981, The C. V. Mosby Co.

Elkowitz, E. B.: Death and the elderly patient. J. Am. Geriatr. Soc. **26**:36, January 1978.

Eulogy for Ms. Hogue Burnside. Am. J. Nurs. **78**:624, April 1978.

Greiner, D., and Mason, D.: Secrets in administrative systems, Topics Clin. Nurs. **1**:3, 1979.

Kron, T.: Nursing team leadership, Philadelphia, 1961, W. B. Saunders Co.

Lazarus, I. W.: A program for the elderly at a private psychiatric hospital, Gerontologist **16**:125, April 1976.

Marriner, A.: Applying the research process to quality assurance, Am. J. Nurs. **79**:2158, December 1979.

Norton, D.: The elderly: a challenge to nursing—1. Geriatric nursing—what it is and what it is not, Nurs. Times **73**:1622, 20 October 1977.

Pattee, J. J.: Training objectives of a well-developed geriatrics program, J. Am. Geriatr. Soc. **26**:167, April 1978.

Polliack, M. R., and Shavitt, N.: Utilization of hospital in-patient services by the elderly, J. Am. Geriatr. Soc. **25**:364, August 1977.

Sacher, G. A.: 1976 Robert W. Kleemeier Award lecture: longevity, aging, and death: an evolutionary perspective, Gerontologist **18**:112, April 1978.

Seelbach, W. C., and Sauer, W. J.: Filial responsibility expectations and morale among aged parents, Gerontologist **17**:492, December 1977.

Segerberger, O.: The immortality factor, New York, 1974, E. P. Dutton and Co., Inc.

Smith, J. A., Buckalew, J., and Rosales, S. M.: Making the right moves in discharge planning: coordinating a workable system, Am. J. Nurs. **79**:1439, August 1979.

Vitale, B. A., Latterner, N. S., and Nugent, P. M.: A problem solving approach to nursing care plans, ed. 2, St. Louis, 1978, The C. V. Mosby Co.

Wagner, B. M.: Care plans—right, reasonable, and reachable, Am. J. Nurs. May 1969, p. 986.

Wolanin, M. O., and Phillips, L. R. F.: Confusion: prevention and care, St. Louis, 1981, The C. V. Mosby Co.

III

INTERVENTION

9 Communication: establishing a relationship

Each day, more than half our waking hours are spent in communication. To help make that communication more effective, this ninth chapter does three things. First, it enables nurses to clarify some principles of communication so that a basis for data collection can be established. Second, the ideas presented may be used in various health delivery environments, wherever older adults are found. Third, a global use of the word *communication* is developed for older adults. Included are communications from the basic level of interpersonal communication, within the individual as a being having an internal environment and an external environment, to the complex communication of the group to the media and the world in general. Having this perception of communication, the nurse may form a knowledge base from which to view the nature of communication throughout the nursing process. Nurses might use these suggestions as a vantage point from which to create a framework for dialogue among older adults and other nurses. These perceptions can also be used in articulating reasonable alternatives in health delivery to older adults.

COMMUNICATION
Values and use of communication

Communication's importance and uses are demonstrated on several planes. It can be the use of self to establish rapport. As social beings, individuals have social interactive needs. Older adults can use communication to express a full gambit of feelings and ideas, to test reality, and to negotiate their place in the system. Nurses focus on the client's assets of readiness for communication. They use all available technology and methods, telephones, radios, TV, intercom systems, as well as game playing, planned activities, and such activities of daily living norms as socializing at the mailbox. Nurses also need to reach out to meet older adults who function successfully in society, to interview them in action, at home, taking trips, in the library, and in the work force.

It is important for the nurse to participate in exercises to break stereotypes for older adults. Consider the life-style of an older couple who have moved and now make their home in the sunshine of Arizona or Florida. Their communication skills are fully functioning for them as they reach out to meet new friends, sightsee, and encounter totally new experiences. The nurse who takes courses in schools and colleges can observe older adults using communication skills to share their beliefs and expectations with the younger students. Their contributions in class mark the group as heterogeneous in the broadest possible application of the term.

Reciprocity is extended to the younger college student in programs such as one designed by the History Department at Temple University in Philadelphia. Students are sent out into the community to interview older adults who have lived through World War I, World War II, the Depression, and other massive events, to learn about history firsthand from people who have actually experienced the events. These interactions enrich the students' knowledge of history and enable older persons to share their wealth of knowledge and experiences. Such interactions serve as time-binders and facilitate intergenerational awareness.

Definition of communication

The essential components of communication described in most communication texts are the communicator, the message, and the receiver (Fig. 9-1). Through the components of communication,

157

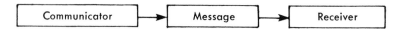

Fig. 9-1. Components of a communication.

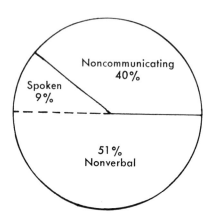

Fig. 9-2. Communication and noncommunication portions of a day.

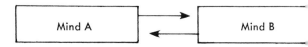

Fig. 9-3. Communication as a process.

knowledge can be imparted, information revealed, and a sharing occurs. As the message passes from one place to another, there is a partaking, a level of intercourse.

It is estimated that 60 percent of the day is spent in communication (Fig. 9-2). Of this 60 percent, only 9 percent is contributed by the spoken word. That leaves 51 percent of daily communication time available for the really important kinds of communications: nonverbal. Of all of the nonverbal time, much of it is devoted to perceptual awareness. This includes the continuous awareness of the voice tone, the style in which something is said. There are mental, physical, and emotional messages being sent simultaneously with each communication.

The remaining nonverbal time is spent in listening. Listening includes seeing with the eyes. All of these are ways of perceiving or receiving information. Specifically, the receiver chooses all or part of the message selectively based on his own effective beliefs. Attitudes, values, and judgments flavor every message; and as we listen to verbal and nonverbal cues in a communication, attention to this effective level will help clarify all the com-

ponents operating. Simon and colleagues (1972) view values as a set of personal beliefs and attitudes about the truth, beauty, and worth of any thought, object, or behavior. They are action-oriented and give direction and meaning to one's life.

Used in the broadest sense, the word communication includes all methods by which one mind is affected by another in all human behavior. Included are oral and written modes, all of the fine arts, work, and political interaction.

In Fig. 9-3 person A and person B are attempting meaningful communication in order that each may grow in knowledge as a result of the information he sends and receives. It is a relationship similar to the teacher-student dyad. Roles are not fixed; each is at one time a student, at another time, a teacher. Each has information that may be valuable to the other in the formation of thoughts, ideas, feelings, and values in the transformation of that complex phenomenon that he calls *myself.*

Communication and our mortality

Webster defines the phenomenon of *age* as: "1. The time that a person or a thing has existed since birth or beginning; 2. The life time; 3. A stage of life; 4. The condition of being old; old age (worn with age)." Communication with the older adult lends itself to interpersonal relationships that arouse the nurse's independent feelings about old age in general, her own old age, and her own mortality in particular. The biggest obstacle to overcome in communicating with the older adult is focusing on the so-called "age" of the client and the nurse's age. Even though most nursing personnel prefer to work with age groups other than the older adult, eventually nurses will encounter the older adults in their practices because of the longer life span and rapid increase in the 20 million persons in the older population.

Research has cited that the caregiver's age and psychological response to her own acceptance of aging and life crisis situations may have a negative anxiety-provoking effect on her therapeutic communication with the older adult. The middle-aged nurse may find it just as difficult to communicate with the older adult as it is for the parent to communicate with the teenager. Naturally, the nurse is not to assume the parenting role or attitude when dealing with the older adult. However, the nurse's discomfort and anxiety may be due to the fact that confrontation with other human beings who are going through a perceived negative life experience is both painful and threatening. Our contemporary society has held aging as a strong taboo as it reminds us of our own mortality. This taboo is called *agism.*

Maggie Kuhn, founder of the Gray Panthers, says that "Agism permeates our Western culture and institutions. It infects us and the aging and the aged, when we reject ourselves and despise our powerlessness, wrinkled skin, and physical limitations. It's revealed when we succumb to apathy and complacent acceptance of things that society does to diminish us. Thus, a symptom of our sickness is that we feel complimented when others tell us we do not look or act our age" (1971).

Older adults communicate well with adolescents, children, and other older adults. However, they do not always communicate well with middle-aged persons. This is often described as alternate-generational compatibility versus adjacent-generational dissonance.

The middle-aged nurse must consider the variables of the agism taboo, as well as possible defense mechanisms on her part, such as denial or projection, as she explores her own values when communicating with older adults. Dissonance is aroused in this nurse as she is threatened by the ambiguity presented in the older adult. She may see herself, her own aging process, and her own destiny projected by the client. This will cast a huge, nonverbal dimension into her communication style and content with older adults.

Overt agism, discrimination based on age, is pervasive in our society. Stereotyping has older adults in a double bind. Often they are seen as too old to engage in certain activities, such as sex, driving a car, disco dancing, and skin diving. The older adult who chooses to do the activity is laughed at because he looks funny. When he chooses not to participate, he is still put down as worn out. Either way, he doesn't come across as a positive image.

Derogatory names such as, "dirty old man," "old goat," "old maid," "old crab" are labels placed on older adults going about their business. If they were younger, they would be making reasonable requests. Agism distorts the legitimacy of their requests.

For example, several people (two women, one gentleman, one teenager, and one older adult) are at a deli counter waiting for service. Two clerks suddenly appear to wait on the people and proceed to ignore the older woman, Miss Bell, who was there first. She speaks up and asks for help and is told, "I'll be with you in a minute." The other people at the counter actually push ahead of the older woman and get served first. She wants to speak up, but does not because she knows she only has a small order and needs help reading the small numbers on the price signs.

Mr. and Mrs. Finn, an older adult couple living next door to a family with four teenagers, have to constantly remind the adolescents and their friends not to play baseball near the tomato plants. The baseball always manages to end up in the tomato patch. The youngsters get angry at being yelled at, and the couple become the "old crabs."

Preoccupation and infatuation with the young is often seen, especially in advertising. Youth is good, old is bad. The young are shown as having all the answers. The older generation is told that they messed up and now youth has to solve all the problems. Few ads show people over the age of 40. The message being sent is that older adults do not eat, sleep, or drink. Seldom are children shown with older adults. They are regarded as a class or a group, not as individuals.

It is a fact that there are more in-group differences in an aggregate of older adults than in other age groupings. This dramatic heterogenous make-up of a group of older adults is characterized by wide differences in individuals within the group.

These differences develop as a result of various life experiences.

When they are included in advertisements, it is usually in a posture of weakness, such as using denture cleansers, remedies for diarrhea, vitamins, and iron supplements for "iron-poor, tired blood." These images of older adults are transferred to us, reinforcing our myths and shaping our attitudes.

The nursing process permits individualization. Through our nursing diagnosis and the goals we set for older adults, we communicate to the person our interest in him as an individual with a unique past, specific needs for the present, and personalized goal setting for the future. Without the nursing process, the individual remains lumped in the large mass known as the aged, a useless scrap heap of worn out leftovers.

The vocabulary of our language reinforces agism. We are told to think young, wear Forever Young dresses, and live in leisure villages. Consider the euphemism of "senior citizen, golden years" to describe the older adult years. Euphemism means to substitute a delicate or pleasing expression in place of that which is offensive or indelicate. The offensive word in this case is *old.* When a middle-aged adult is told, "You're running out of time," a chill of horror goes up his spine. The society is communicating to him that his day is over and he will soon be replaced. This changes the whole frame of reference for the person in the middle adult years (Fig. 9-4).

An example regarding retirement is Mr. Antico, a 54-year-old assistant vice president who has climbed up the corporate ladder in a large banking organization. When the executive vice president position becomes available, he expects to take another step up to the next higher position. This time, however, he is stopped. When told that a 35-year-old man will take the position, his dreams of becoming bank president are shattered. He is seen as "too old" for the job.

Verbal communication: too much and too little

Much is said about verbal communication, and a great deal can be done to enhance verbal communication, particularly with older adults. Verbal communication is not an isolated phenomenon; it occurs in a full setting of all communication maps and territories. Our knowledge of the world and where we are in it is derived from words.

S. I. Hayakawa described the phenomena of the verbal world around us as the "Niagara of words" in our culture (1965). Are all of the torrents of words from our noisy era a form of cultural shock for the older adults who are from a more quiet era before radio and TV?

In earlier days, communication was within the narrow scope of their personal lives, their families, and immediate community. Today, the mass media brings the entire world action into the home.

Data collection is needed regarding the client's perception of the value of verbal communication and preferred styles and modes, interpersonal and intrapersonal (fantasy) communications.

On the other hand, with no touching, no sounds, no loving, there is muscle wasting, mind deterioration, and death. The older adult needs verbal interaction, interpersonal contact, and regular interaction with the environment. Food, shelter, and communication are each essential for living. Consider the environment as being both internal and external to the individual; that is, the internal physical world of the individual is bound with the physical external world into one unit. In this context, internal and external feelings of high-level wellness, self-esteem, and body image are tested and accepted. Every sound, every verbal word in the

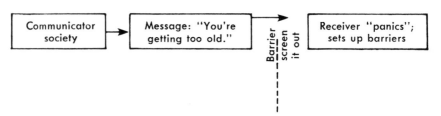

Fig. 9-4. Society's communication.

environment has a feeling tone and sends a message for the older adult.

The purpose of verbal communication is to give information back and forth between two or more persons to foster a sense of comprehension and mutual cooperation toward a goal. The nurse can do this by practicing active verbal communication skills of speaking, of going into the phase of listener, and then observing the verbal and nonverbal responses of the client.

The nearest individual in the room or in the next apartment or in the park is a communicator for the older adult. Verbal stimulation must be available to each person, whether it be direct verbal-to-verbal, face-to-face interaction or the product of technology. One telephone call or letter can be extremely meaningful. The nurse as an intervenor can give the person tasks by which to reach out verbally to others as a part of the planned nursing care. In data collection, it is important to assess how much verbal interaction is required for a particular client. How many times a day does the person have to have verbal interaction to prevent feeling lonely? Is a response expected by the person? What are the responsibilities of the older adult to reach out for verbal interaction?

Therapeutic communication

There are two different levels of verbal communications. These are called *therapeutic* style and *nontherapeutic* or *social* style. Both have advantages, and the therapeutic style has a distinct advantage of having a specific goal in mind. Because the nurse has anticipated some kinds of barriers that might arise, she stays with the particular topic without wandering, and gives a sense of valuing the verbal interaction by her attention to it. The therapeutic style of communication can help the nurse collect data, carry out a plan, and help the client participate in the care being given. It develops, trains, and inspires as well as informs. The more casual or nontherapeutic style of communication is the form of socialization frequently seen by nurses as they care for clients. The nurse should recognize, however, that it is not goal oriented and it is not supportive to "wellness" in a particular systematic way. When the nurse goes into a client's home or room and just passes the time of day lightly, telling jokes and stories, dis-

playing authority, or gossiping, this is merely social interaction and is not designed to meet the client's particular needs. What the nurse is doing is meeting her own needs for socialization and personal ego building.

The social and biological benefits of therapeutic communication are many. Everyone develops an individualized style that complements his beliefs and personality. The nurse should enter a situation expecting a good level of communication. Fear of the situation frequently leads the nurse to lower expectations and goals regarding the success of verbal nursing. Consider the following example of a nursing student's verbal fear.

A nursing student, Miss Pedone, tells her instructor, "Mr. Clark doesn't want to talk to me." Upon discussing the situation, Miss Pedone recognizes that it is she who is hesitating to open communication lines with Mr. Clark because she is afraid that he will speak of his wife's recent death in an auto accident.

Set the scene first with a brief social period and then engage in goal-directed therapeutic communications. Let your own personality style be known. Let the client know that you can change your style and be flexible if needed. The goals should be jointly developed and pursued by you and your client. The client then grows in the expectations of the nurse as a teacher and counselor through the use of verbal skills.

Therapeutic communication can help us make our verbal interactions effective and efficient. There are four steps generally held as important when setting up a communication. The nurse should:

1. Establish the appropriate climate.
2. Facilitate accuracy of the communication.
3. Validate the information being received.
4. Evaluate the results.

When a climate is established, it is understood that the proper timing of the conversation, focusing on the particular goal in mind, is essential. The nurse is collecting data regarding the client's ability to listen to a person at a particular time. The nurse chooses the correct vocabulary and level of phrasing that will help the listener understand the communication. When using the right words, the nurse can explain, give information and direction, and focus on the emphasis of the important parts of the communication with ease and clarity. Facilitating accuracy involves identifying areas of lack of information and misinterpretation. In addition, the recognition of personality differences and status differences between the nurse and the client will help remove barriers to communications. Voice tones and particular inflections in the sentence both have an emotional content that the nurse is sharing with the client. Anything but positive attitudes tends to make the verbal communication a negative one. Questions or phrasing comments in the most positive manner is one positive approach that helps in the client's reception of the information.

In order to validate a communication, the nurse checks on the understanding level of the client regarding the information that she has given. She asks the client if there are any suggestions he might like to offer regarding the level of understanding or content of the verbal communication. She should observe the answers to the questions she asks the client to see if they are appropriate, and by all means encourage active verbal participation on the part of the client.

Whatever the setting, there is a possibility of integrating both social or nontherapeutic styles of communication. It is very useful to make the first few minutes of any visit with the client a social interaction. This is the first of the two phases of verbal communications with clients. The social interaction enables the nurse to set up the orientation for the older adult and then loosen up the interactions to make both persons very comfortable before getting down to business. If the social phase is kept to no more than just a few minutes, the client becomes used to changing gears and getting into the therapeutic level of communications directed toward the particular goals for the interactions.

A history of loneliness and decreased use of verbal communication skills might require practice on the part of the client to improve skills. A sense of trust must be established. The nurse should plan for verbal communication care just as carefully as she organizes for physical care. As with physical care, data are collected, plans made, and then as the implementation phase begins, the goal can be reached. It is essential to set up an accepting atmosphere in which all expressions of emotion are permitted, especially the emotional expressions of laughter and joyful memories, but not to brush off unhappy memories either.

The client can describe the culture and influences to help you assess his former life-style. Since this was an environment of choice in the past, perhaps it can be modified for satisfactory living today. How were communication needs met in the recent and distant past? For example, was there much conversation at meals? Does the client mix with all-male or all-female groups? What is the status of verbal communication within the family? When with a group of clients, storytelling or singing is a good way to begin verbal interactive skills. When the modality of choice is known, it is a cue for the nursing diagnosis and plan.

The client should fully understand that communication is an important component of the plan of care and work with the nurse to have experience available for himself. The client and the nurse should plan to use what is available in the person's environment, as basic as it may be. For example, a radio can be the means of keeping in touch with what is going on in the world. Shows include a wide variety of music, news, discussion, self-help, and consumer shows. Church groups and school volunteer services open up dialogues between older adults themselves or other age groups. Consider the verbal interactions within a senior citizens group or a group such as the Gray Panthers that have developed a high-level stylization of political communications. They speak out for the use of power in legislation. The nurse should see verbal communications as a vehicle in self-esteem and self-actualization. Not only should nurses encourage the experiential framework, allowing the client to share his or her experiences with nurses, both as a therapeutic form of interaction as well as data collection; but nurses should also give permission, a "yes you can do it" attitude with no limits set on the growth that clients can plan for themselves.

How nice it is in any setting to have a group of persons together and use a social style, yet within the therapeutic frame. How can this be done? Read horoscopes from the newspaper, read "Dear Abby's" column, read those charming comic strips or a favorite columnist. Many older adults enjoy cartoon strips such as Hagar the Horrible, or

Broomhilda, or Beetle Bailey. It is verbal communication of a social nature, but it is also therapeutic when the nurse is striving for a higher frequency of verbal interaction or group interaction. It is enjoyable for both the nurse and the client to have a laughing and sharing period. Many nurses implement verbal, social, and therapeutic communication in their practices.

The community health nurse sees Mrs. Coffee three times a week. They have established a good rapport, and one part of their social interaction time includes reading the horoscope in the daily paper. After this brief social interlude, they get down to the serious business of changing Mrs. Coffee's burn dressings.

Reminiscence as a therapeutic tool. In 1961 Dr. Robert N. Butler identified reminiscence as a part of life review that the older adult experiences during his final years in preparation for death. Review of one's life occurs as a natural process of unraveling events, including specific details within various time frames of the individual's life. These recalled events may be reviewed with satisfaction, sorrow, grief, nostalgia, or approval. Life review offers the older adult a procedure for assessing his life and working through resolutions to personal conflicts. Reminiscence is now accepted as a valuable therapeutic tool for the giver as well as the recipient. Reminiscence provides for the older adult a way of reliving, reexperiencing, or savoring events of the past that are personally significant. Nurses no longer think of reminiscence as "crazy talk" or "living in the past" but as a therapeutic communication outlet for the older adult. It helps them maintain self-esteem and reinforces a sense of identity. They may recall many happy hours with family, friends, job activities, achievements, and life goals. Also, the negative aspects of the past may be verbalized and put in perspective. Reviewing one's life and the past provides an outlet for coping with the current stresses that must be dealt with today. Reminiscence provides the information that the nurse needs to help the client relate to the aging process by constructively identifying his stresses within the framework of his past experiences. The information provides the link between the past and the present. The nurse is better able to understand the client's present behavior from the knowledge gained. Reminiscence communication with the client gives the nurse a historical perspective on the client and adds to her data collection for development of nursing diagnoses, planning care, and resources for others.

How does the nurse begin reminiscent therapy? She simply sits down and talks to the client. Information pertaining to the client's occupation, country of birth, previous life-style, roles, or residence, as well as events such as a wedding, birth of a child, the Depression, World War I or II may be used as primers to get the client to open up and divulge his history. It is important that the nurse not appear that she is pressed for time or just nosy. A real concern and interest in the client's past experiences must be transmitted. A nurse might share plans for her wedding with a woman or man client and encourage the client to relate experiences surrounding his or her own wedding. A nurse with teenagers or one who has traveled or likes needlework may compare experiences or memorable events associated with a craft or child rearing. What might evolve is a story of how the nuns taught the client the skill in a convent school years ago.

Reminiscence differs from social communications in that it is goal directed and directly affects the amount of data collected by the nurse. It puts an end to the rote, 20-questions style of data collection. It is very useful as a rapport-establishing strategy. It has an ego-strengthening advantage for the client and eliminates the dehumanizing factor for the nurse. Her client becomes a unique individual, no longer just a name. The client has shared some funny, sad, and pointed stories with the nurse that set him apart from the group. Reminiscence broadens the nurse's knowledge base and is a scientific part of data collection of general information on the older adult.

Nonverbal communication

As valuable as verbal communications are, it is the nonverbal dimension of the interaction that packs the wallop. Affect (from the Greek root *affekt*) addresses the emotion or feeling tone attached to an idea or statement. It is often the stimulus in arousing the emotional mood or feeling within a communication.

A message has two components: a thinking or

cognitive domain and a feeling or affective domain. If you consider that most of the verbal message is the idea or cognitive component, the total remainder of the message is the affective component, most of which is nonverbal.

Because all therapeutic nursing action is goal oriented, the communication should be based on a conceptual framework. Having a frame of reference has the advantages of minimizing undirected communications on the part of the nurse as well as giving a context in which to evaluate the effectiveness of her communications.

Considering nonverbal communication as a part of the affective domain facilitates a way of measuring. There are five levels defined as part of the affective domain. Although not yet all-inclusive or a perfect system, the affective domain has proved to be very useful when writing nursing objectives in behavioral terms. Since the nonverbal component constitutes the major proportion of behaviors in a communication, it is well to have some way to measure it.

Affective domain. The terms used to address the categories of the affective domain follow:

1. Receiving
2. Responding
3. Valuing
4. Organization
5. Value complex

Receiving is that process of gaining the older adult's attention, and can range from a basic awareness that there is an interaction in progress to a full keying in to a message. This identifies the receiver as receiving a message. Receiving represents the lowest level of response to a communication in the affective domain.

The next level is called *responding,* and identifies the receiver as an active participant in the communication. He or she is not only receiving or attending to the communication, but is reacting to it in some manner.

Valuing is a measure of the worth or value a person attaches to a particular communication. It is this level of the affective domain categories that spells out the existence of internalization of sets of specific values. Cues to these values are expressed in overt nonverbal behavior. You cannot hide your message. You might be verbalizing one thing, but your voice tone, facial expressions, hand

and body positions, and eye movement speak out on the values you have within yourself as a communicator or receiver of a message. As defined by Krathwohl (1964), "Internalization is the change or inner growth that occurs in an individual as he becomes aware of and adopts certain attitudes and principles which are inherent in forming selected value judgments and behaving according to his values." Things that we call "attitudes" or things that we say we "appreciate" come into this category of valuing. If there is one thing that is true about this level in the affective domain, it is that once the beliefs or attitudes are in place, they are seen with consistency and stability. Each time they appear in our communication, they reinforce the internalized value. Consider the following example.

Mr. Cook, admitted to the CCU, is addressed by his nurse as Grandpa. While giving evening care, the nurse says, "I am going to change your gown now, Grandpa." Feeling hurt and insulted, Mr. Cook responds to the nurse, "Sweetie, I am not your grandfather." The nurse is surprised and embarrassed and realizes that Mr. Cook is correct in his observation. The nurse likes to be called by her name, Mrs. Pendagast, and she should extend Mr. Cook the same courtesy.

The next level of the affective domain is that of *organization.* This category becomes operational only after the nurse as a communicator has explored her beliefs in some depth. It arises out of a philosophical position taken consciously by the nurse as she works with older adults. Organization is concerned with bringing together different values, resolving conflicts between them, and beginning the building of an internally consistent value system. Organization is demonstrated in the nurse's communication when there is uniformity in the spoken and nonverbal message.

The fifth and most advanced of the major categories in the affective domain is called *value complex.* This is a step above the organizational level in that conflicts have been resolved and the nurse has in fact developed a nonjudgmental style in her communications that is pervasive and predictable. She no longer must go through the trial-and-error exercises of the organizational level. Her communication behaviors are automatic.

For example, a visiting nurse is interviewing an

older couple, Joseph Davis and Carol Symes, in their apartment. They state they are not married but living together as an economic consequence of the Social Security laws. This living situation is at odds with the nurse's value system. She has, however, examined her communication behavior and understands and accepts that there are beliefs other than her own set of values. Because she has come to terms with these opposing value systems, she is able to be nonjudgmental as she helps them set their health goals.

Kinesics. Kinesics is the study of bodily movements and facial expressions, the nonverbal communication that accompanies speech. A common term used for kinesics is body language. Body language is socially learned much the same way a person learns verbal communication. Data support the theory that cultural ethnic background, socioeconomic class, role socialization, region of the country one resides in, and experiences all influence the individual's use of the body in communicating. For example, Northern European cultures dictate direct eye contact during communications to connote honesty and forthrightness. In Hispanic cultures, downcast eyes when being spoken to by a superior are a mark of respect to the person. Arm position with arms folded over the chest conveys a lack of openness on the part of the speaker or receiver. The arms act as a physical barrier. In much the same way, people remove their glasses when they want to emphasize a point.

Many times there are inconsistent meanings between the verbal elements and the body elements transmitted in communication. The communicator may be unaware that there is an inconsistency between his spoken word and kinesic language. Studies estimate that this inconsistency may happen as much as two thirds of the time. It has been found that women can translate kinesic communication better than men. Several studies have indicated that people with absolutely no background in kinesics can accurately interpret a sender's message at least 60 percent of the time.

Both positive and negative feelings are transmitted by body language. In addition, eye contact, gestures, posture, facial expressions, touch, and the use of the environment also demonstrate nonverbal communications. Even in a crowd, the individual who chooses to disengage from interactions is communicating his desire for privacy. The client may communicate many messages to the nurse through kinesics. The data collected during the assessment phase of the nursing process can be used as a knowledge base for interpreting the client's messages accurately. For example, in a nurse communication with an older adult woman native of India, the nurse nods yes, which means no in India, and is very distracting to the client.

The nurse, when approaching an important communication with the client, should strive for appropriate eye interaction, keep arms in an open position, and be sitting or standing at the same level as the receiver with her body turned in the direction of the receiver of the message. This communicates nonverbally to her client that she is ready for full communications with him and does not seek to dictate to but interact with him.

As a profession represented largely by women, nursing can take advantage of its communication assets. The nurse should cue in on the verbal language the client is throwing out to her and respond to the nonverbal cues just as much as she would to the verbal cues.

The nurse should put the Kardex or other equipment at least to the side of her body if she intends to discuss anything with the client. With this material in her arms, the client is more likely to look at the equipment or Kardex and wonder if it is about him instead of focusing on the words the nurse is saying to him.

When the client is relating some particular details about himself, the nurse should move her body forward just a little, keeping facial and neck muscles relaxed so that it doesn't appear that she wants to speak. Appropriate nods of approval will move the conversation along. This communicates to the receiver yes, I want to listen to what you have to say. With a relaxed body stance, and feet in a nonmoving position, you do not appear pressed for time; even though you may have only 30 seconds available, at least the time you are spending with the person is his time, and you are saying it with your body.

Touching. Touching is a basic human need, and almost everyone can identify with being held and touched by his mother. Remember when mother would kiss the injured part and make it all better? Individuals grow up on touching as a form of nourishment for the human organism. Tactile communication has kept us oriented to the world around us: the temperature, objects, texture—soft, hard, rough, silky, hairy, and smooth. Touching as a form of healing can be traced to biblical writings and hieroglyphics. Nursing has been identified as an art, and the artful use of the hands in nursing intervention has been readily accepted by clients. A common example of this is the soothing back rub. However, touch is not always appropriate or appreciated. People who are experiencing anxiety, dependency, or acute forms of loneliness may need careful and prolonged support on a verbal level before physical contact will be effective or welcome.

There is a current movement abreast acclaiming the therapeutic power of touch through the transmission of healing energy through the laying on of hands. Nurses are investigating this phenomenon, and some are incorporating it into their nursing practice. It is believed that older adults have a great need for human touch. This need exists partly because aging—and the accompanying wrinkles, graying hair, and changing shape—causes a change in a person's body image; hence, aging may intensify the need for communication of acceptance. Also, skin and circulatory changes decrease sensitivity to touch, so it is possible that the older adult might need more tactile stimulation. Psychologist Dr. Sidney M. Jourard (1971) believes that people become sick when their spirit and sense of self-worth are low. He goes on to further explain that this may be canceled out and replaced by "wellness" when one's individuality is respected and acknowledged, that being handled and touched by a person who cares seems to reinforce identity, mobilize spirit, and promote self-healing. A primary means of promoting wellness in the older adult is for nurses to maintain the client's self-esteem and dignity through the use of communication. The message the nurse must communicate to maintain wellness is that of respect and appreciation for the client's heritage, values, feelings, and wisdom.

Proxemics. Proxemics is the study of the special needs of humans and the behaviors derived from these needs. Central to the study of proxemics is the concept of territoriality.

Territoriality. Territoriality is a concept referring to the observable behaviors of animals in which they hold firmly to their own territory geographically and fight off would-be intruders. Humans, including the older adult, have a need to identify their territory and defend it. They value and cherish their own space or place. Therefore, the communicator is wise to secure permission to enter the territory of the older adult before attempting to establish rapport.

As a concept, territoriality addresses people's need for (1) identity, (2) security, and (3) stimulation. Although all persons require these three needs, they are the same needs that society tries to take away from the older adult.

IDENTITY. The body image, usually established by the age of 4 years, does not remain constant, but changes with aging throughout the life span. The client's sense of his identity and self-esteem may have decreased because of the loss of mobility, roles, spouse, and friends and changes in health status and finances. The space the body occupies within the environment gradually decreases because of increasing changes in the skeletal system and weight loss. The body space is usually considered to be from 18 inches to 4 feet about the body of the person. Cultural and socioeconomic orientations will make a difference in these measurements. The Japanese, for instance, operate within closer proximity to each other. What could be called a "proxemics dance" can be observed when American and Northern European businessmen have a discussion. The Dutch man advances towards the American, and the American backs away, seeking a wider distancing. Body space may be viewed as portable territory and possessions as concrete or nonportable territory. The imaginary bubble of body space moves about with the person. Concrete possessions are separate from the person's body itself. The space is outlined by an imaginary bubble that is respected by other persons. Invasion of this bubble for close bodily contact must be sought and welcomed by the client.

Included in identity are the client's material belongings. Possessions collected over a lifetime make a statement about the person's interests, economic worth, and life-style. These possessions are the link between the person's identity and the social milieu to which he subscribes.

SECURITY. A sense of security is fostered when

a client perceives that he is in charge of his particular territory and free from anxiety. To have mastery over familiar surroundings lends the client a sense of control. These feelings of mastery and control put him at ease. Combined with the sense of emotional security must be a sense of physical security. The environmental safety includes things and persons within the immediate territory. Freedom from physical danger is a prerequisite for a sense of personal security.

STIMULATION. Stimulation provides a reason for living. Stimulation may be provided by interaction of person to person, person to animals, person to insects, and person to inanimate objects. The care of his territorial property and possessions gives the client freedom from boredom. The personal time and energy expanded in territorial portection give the client a sense of mission and personal accomplishment. The client's own territoriality is an environment that renders personal internal and external stimulation to the client. Studies have shown that removing older adults from their territory has affected their identity, security, and stimulation. Research is being done in the area of relocation trauma for older adults.

Institutional proxemics. Consider the use of side rails in the hospital. It is automatic for everyone over 65 years of age to have them in place. From our perspective, we are providing safety, which is certainly a reasonable objective. However, what have we done from the client's perspective? We have assaulted his territoriality. When he responds with a loud, "I don't want these here, I don't need them, I am not going to fall out of bed," he is taking great risk of being labeled difficult. The institution is saying that it has the right of proxemics. The institution relieves the person of his territoriality. His mastery over his surroundings is diminished, and he is denied the right to define his own boundaries. When the nurse puts up the side rails, she is nonverbally reinforcing the institution's dominance over the individual. When the man comes across loud and clear with the message that he does not like his territory limited, he is exercising his full right as an adult. The nurse and the client must negotiate the terms necessary to accommodate the proxemics and safety needs of the client. At the time of admission when the nurse is introducing the client to agency routine and policies, the nurse includes the topic of side rails. The policy is stated that side rails must be up for all clients over age 65. The rationale for the policy is explained. Some persons become confused when sleeping in a new bed, and the rails are applied as a safety measure. If the client expresses displeasure, the nurse can negotiate and say that they will only be up at night, or she can move the bed to a wall so only one rail needs to be up. The nurse must investigate the specific reason for displeasure. If, for example, the client has nocturia, then he will have to be up during the night to go to the bathroom. The nurse understands that she can protect the territorial rights by keeping the urinal close at hand and lights bright enough for the client to see it. Falls occur because a client with a distended bladder cannot reach a urinal or get to the bathroom. Eventually, he voids in bed simply because he cannot retain the urine any longer in the distended bladder. The bed becomes wet and cold and to escape the immediate uncomfortable territory, he climbs over the side rail and falls.

The following is an example of territoriality's identity, security, and stimulation. Mrs. Hollis, a recent widow, has been living in a house all her life. Circumstances force her to move into smaller and less expensive accommodations. She must now adapt to the loss of many of her cherished household furnishings, as well as to the greatly reduced territory of a one-room apartment versus an eight-room, two-bath house. She tells her friends that she misses her possessions and feels as if she's living in a cell and the four walls are closing in on her. This woman who has made her household care a major focus in her life now finds she has little work to do within the studio apartment. Many hours of the day are spent with no purposeful activity.

Coping with the environment

What does it mean to the person who has a cerebral vascular accident or other medical condition that suddenly renders him unable to speak to others, and communicate his feelings, needs, plans, happiness, or sadness? Life is going on all around him, in the hospital room, the long-term care facility, and at home. How can we include him in our world and touch his new speechless world? First, every opportunity must be taken to include him in our world. Do not talk about him in his presence or as if he were an inanimate object such as a chair. Talking about a client in his presence without including him in the conversation identifies him as being socially, if not physically, invisible.

Our operational stance is that the cognitive faculties are functioning. Explore other means of communication, such as having him blink eyes, move a finger, anything that symbolizes yes, no, agreement, or disagreement with phrases, sentences, and the conversation.

The nurse enters the client's room to give morning care. He has recently had a stroke and is aphasic. She perceives herself as actively communicating with him; she is talking about the things she is doing for him. As she shaves him, she notices that he is grunting and gesturing, but she does not understand what he is trying to communicate to her and continues with her care. After the bath is finished and linen changed, the nurse feels very proud that she has done a fine job, and he looks refreshed and comfortable. When the family comes in to visit, there is a loud commotion and the nurse comes to the bedside to investigate. The wife explains to the nurse that she has never seen her husband without a mustache in the 30 years she has known him. The nurse turns to the client and says "That's what you were trying to tell me while I was shaving you." Because the beard was overgrown, the mustache was not obvious.

Short sentences are best when a physical yes or no response is to be demonstrated. The burden is put on the sender to open up other communication channels for the receiver. Exploring and experimenting with listening, touching, smelling, and tasting may be found to be a dynamic creative way to relate to each other. The level of aphasia today is not necessarily the level of aphasia in that person tomorrow. Because the aphasic can improve, ongoing evaluation is required.

Including the client with aphasia in functions at the long-term-care facility such as parties and other activities can be rewarding both to the client and staff. One nurse recalls how a client would delight in selecting a pretty dress, combing her hair, and applying lipstick to go to the weekly cocktail party. They would circulate the wheelchair around the lounge, giving everyone attending an opportunity to comment on how pretty the client looked, to touch and talk to her. The expression in the eyes and on the aphasic client's face related her return message of greetings.

Establish a sense of communication rapport based on respect and trust. A good way of looking at communication is through the transactional analysis formula of parent-adult-child tapes. Tapes are the memories of communications stored in the brain cells. Every experience, sensation, and event is on the permanent, inexhaustible recording tape of the mind. Since no two persons' life experiences are the same, everyone's tapes are different. Parent, adult, and child tape designations are broad categories for communication.

Parent tapes cover all the no's, don't do that's, should not's, ought not's, and I told you so's. Although a good part of these recordings related to the lifesaving information (for instance, look both ways before you cross the street), they are the words of domination of one person over the other. Child tapes deal mainly with the feeling level of communications. These feelings relate most often to being less than adequate. These tapes record feelings of being helpless, stupid, or clumsy. When an adult has these feelings, he is resurrecting child tapes. The feelings of inadequacy are being relived. Adult tapes begin recording before the end of the first year. The major function is to collect data from the world for the individual to make realistic decisions. The adult tape recognizes that neither the world nor himself is perfect. So, his expectations of both are reason-

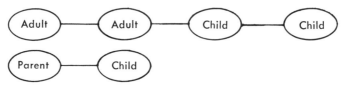

Fig. 9-5. Transactional analysis formula of parent-adult-child tapes.

able. Nothing or nobody is perfect. The adult tape plays feelings of satisfaction and self-worth to the individual.

If the parent tape plays, the individual's communication is filled with "you ought to and you should." It is a parent-child communication. If two adult tapes are playing, there is a mutual exchange of information and independent decision making.

Miss Adamson walks cheerfully into Mr. Horoshack's room and announces, "We're going to have our shower now." Mr. Horoshack refuses to take a shower and says, "No, no, no, I'm not taking a shower." He is saying no because this is the only area in which he sees that he has control and can make a decision. And he has decided not to take a shower.

Using the frame given in transactional analysis, the nurse should look at her communication style and examine it for adult-adult tapes (Fig. 9-5).

The stereotype of the older adult describes a dependent, passive, non-decision-making, "second childhood" type person. Cued in on such a stereotype, the nurse might turn on adult-child tapes. In doing this, the nurse is forfeiting the individual's prerogative for information, for decision making, for options, for input regarding his own destiny. In addition, weighing heavily in this adult-child tape is the attitudinal message of condescension, even disrespect. Such messages lead to the inevitable self-fulfilling prophecy. Another possible alternative is anger on the part of the older adult. But anger is not a feeling permitted to older adults. Even justifiable anger meets with hostile response from others.

REALITY ORIENTATION AS AN INTERVENTION MODALITY

Reality orientation is the term given to a simple communication intervention for making the client aware of time, place, and person. It is a procedure we all do throughout the day during our nursing practice. Every time you say, "Good morning, Mrs. Jones. It is 10:00 A.M. Today is Tuesday," or "Good evening, it is cold out," you are engaging in reality orientation. It sounds simple, and it is simple. It is also an inexpensive technique for nursing to use to keep the well older adult in touch with

cognitive reality. And, of course, it is essential to bring the older adult who is not well to reality rather than leave him in states of confusion, disorientation, or apathy.

James C. Folsom, MD, formerly the Director of the Veterans' Administration Hospital at Tuscaloosa, Alabama, was the first to identify reality orientation as a modality. This is not to be confused with the medical abbreviation of R/O (rule out) to state the process of ruling out an arm-long list of medical pathological conditions that could be afflicting the client. Taking a wellness-oriented nursing focus, we will use the abbreviation RO for reality orientation as a goal for all of our clients. Dr. Folsom defines RO as "an early phase of rehabilitation of older adult or brain-damaged patients with a moderate to severe degree of confusion, disorientation, and memory loss" (1973).

Rehabilitation

Let us examine the word *rehabilitation* in Folsom's definition from a nursing perspective. Because he works from an illness framework, he sees rehabilitation starting immediately at the time of illness. This is a nice point of view, but when using the nursing perspective we must go back before the illness, on the wellness-illness continuum, to a point before the illness became manifest and see rehabilitation as a health maintenance tool.

The National League for Nursing describes reality orientation as an extension from infancy when the initial communication between mother and child has a bonding function. The inside self differentiates itself from fantasy or a make-believe world, and establishes in the mind of the individual a reality world based on fact. This accomplishment is the task of reality testing. It is the responsibility of the caregiver to alter the environment to communicate to the person sufficient stimuli to permit reality testing. In the infant, the drive for need satisfaction and a love-bonding are both critical for survival. Without a love-bond, marasmus, a failure to thrive, ensues, with death as the outcome.

Confusion/disorientation

When the environment provides insufficient information or messages, or when stress reduces

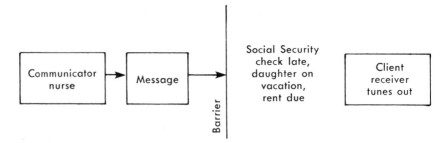

Fig. 9-6. Disruptions in a message.

message tolerance, disorientation occurs. The individual appears confused, and indeed is. Confusion can happen to anybody, not just the older adult. The messages sent by the environment are not being received appropriately by the individual. The nurse should recognize the environment as a mode of communication, anticipate disruption in the message by the receiver, and intervene appropriately (Fig. 9-6).

The previous discussion identified confusion as a major threat to the health of the older adult as he is going into a new environment or under a situation of physical or emotional stress. To maintain health, the nurse should automatically implement RO. Why wait for disintegration of the self-esteem or all the correlates that go with it?

Nurses anticipate confusion and disorientation in the older adult when addressed by stress or change in the environment. Older adults as a group anticipate it also. Many older adults voice their concerns about becoming disoriented and confused. If they forget to mail a letter, or if they forget to phone a friend, or if they forget something that they were told the day before, they will laugh and say, "I guess I'm becoming senile," as a joke and pass it off. But in the back of their minds, they are concerned.

Consider the inference communicated by the word *senile*. It connotes the end of their cognitive life, and an end of their physical life, when in reality, people over 65 have roughly a 10 percent prevalence of cognitive loss and over the age of 80, it rises to 30 percent. These data are a negative view rather than a positive view of the facts. A nursing model demands that nurses communicate to older adult clients the fact that 90 percent of all people over 65 have full cognitive faculties and 70

percent of all people over 80 are also fully alert. Through nursing intervention, nurses communicate to clients and their families the data base needed to dispel the myth of cognitive deterioration and provide them with the incentive to maintain their own level of "wellness." In addition, the next level of intervention sets the nurse up as the mediator between the client and the environment in times of stress. The nurse translates the garbled message from the environment to the client, communication occurs, stress is reduced, and coping mechanisms engage.

The following is an example of relocation adjustment and territoriality.

The nurse understands that Mrs. Pedone is having a difficult time adjusting to the nursing home. Everything is new and strange. She has lived in only two other places in her life, the home she lived in with her parents and her own house after marriage. She misses her old surroundings and personal belongings.

While talking with Mrs. Pedone's son, the nurse makes arrangements for him to bring in her old easy chair, which he kept after her house was sold. The comfortable and functional piece of Mrs. Pedone's past now serves her well as she makes her adjustment.

Goals of reality orientation program

The reality orientation program may be implemented in any environment, and the major goals of the program follow.

1. Minimize confusion, disorientation, and physical regression.
2. Maintain the individual's level of awareness.
3. Restore the individual's sense of reality.
4. Improve socialization.

5. Restore the individual to the maximum level of independent functioning.

Principles of reality orientation

A therapeutic plan of communication can be outlined, initiated, and implemented by the nursing staff. The recipe for stimulating the client, giving him a sense of identity, and adding to his security and serenity incorporates the following 10 basic essential ingredients:

1. Establish a calm environment; avoid excessive stimuli.
2. Maintain a set routine.
3. State clear, simple responses to client's questions, and ask clients clear and simple questions.
4. Speak directly to clients, avoiding loud and childlike conversations.
5. Direct clients by giving clear instructions, or guide them to and from their destination.
6. Remind clients of the date, time, and place.
7. Avoid permitting clients to remain confused by allowing them to ramble in speech or actions. Direct them back to reality.
8. Be firm but gentle.
9. Be sincere.
10. Be consistent.

The 10 guidelines can be carried out in any environment—the client's home, long-term-care facility, or hospital. The essential objective is to start the modality at the first sign of confusion or threat to personal integrity. The significant increase in the number of hospitalized older adult clients makes it very important for the nursing personnel to be psychologically prepared and emotionally armed with a positive attitude toward older adults. Any change from the older adult's usual environment can lead to slight disorientation, which is compounded by sleeping pills, sedation, the stress of a hospital admission, operation, anesthesia, and the hundreds of things to which we subject the hospitalized individual.

Nurse Practice Act and reality orientation

In many states, professional nursing is defined as "the diagnosing and treating of human responses to actual or potential physical and emotional health problems through such services as case finding, health teaching, health counseling, and provision of care supportive to or restorative of life and well-being." *

Given this definition of professional nursing, then it is less than good practice if nurses do not predict that there will be confusion and incorporate reality orientation as a part of the therapeutic approach to communications automatically when dealing with the older adult. It is also less than good practice if nurses do not initiate RO immediately upon diagnosing communication disruption. RO is the treatment of choice and within the scope of the Nurse Practice Act when the nursing diagnosis describes broken communication patterns. Some of these might be withdrawal, altered relationships with others, and reduction in self-awareness and concern for environment, impaired thought process, deprivation, confusion, disorientation, or memory loss. It should not be left to the legal profession to define what is nursing malpractice. Just because a nurse has not been sued yet in a court of law for not anticipating new sensory impacts and their consequences on the older adult, it does not mean that it cannot happen in the future in this type of situation.

Nurses have defined their role as diagnosing and treating potential health threats. Since some health threats are quite predictable, nurses and their peers should hold themselves accountable.

Gunter and Miller (1977) feel that nurses need to do research into the advantages of reality therapy with the older adult and that the data collected would be of great value to nursing and the scientific community at large.

Reality orientation and hospitalized client

When in the hospital, the client is confined, the environment is structured, and there is no ready access to newspapers, communication with friends, and the usual daily schedule. Add to this medication and treatments, and the total of the new messages being sent to him is enormous. The client may say, "Oh, I thought it was Tuesday." when it may actually be Wednesday. The nursing personnel become very upset, and at report that af-

---

*Nurse Practice Act, New Jersey State Board of Nurse Examiners, 1975.

ternoon, the client is labeled confused or disoriented. Have you, the well-oriented, "normal" adult, ever asked, "what day is this anyway?" Without a calendar and clock in the room for the clients to orient themselves to date and time, they often try to orient themselves by watching the routine of the hospital. They learn to know that the bed bath is given in the morning; there is a breakfast, lunch, and dinner tray at certain intervals, and eventually they become familiar with who works which shift. What happens to the messages that the client is receiving when we send in the float nurse, who does not give her name, the context or period of time she is staying with the client, or indeed what she will be doing for the client? Are we overloading the client's ability to handle messages? Consider the example of trying to get a long-distance telephone call through on Christmas Day. There is a communicator, you, the caller, and a message you want to transmit, but it goes nowhere because the lines are overloaded, and the message cannot be transmitted. The recording comes on, "Sorry, because of heavy traffic, there are no lines available. Try again later."

Think about how we use medical jargon in our communication. As the nursing history was taken, data were collected regarding socioeconomic level, culture, education, past experience, and current knowledge base about the health situation. As the nurse approaches her intervention phase, she uses this personal knowledge of the client to choose the vocabulary that will be most useful. She is initiating the evaluation phase as she speaks to the client to assess to what extent the client understands. She validates the level of the client's comprehension. When the client can restate in his own terms the information the nurse communicated, it validates that the message was received. If the message was not received, this is more information with which the nurse has to operate. She begins then to look at the data, chooses other options, and initiates intervention again.

One foreign environment in which we place the older adult is called the *intensive care unit*. With its "outer space equipment," lack of windows, and constant lights, it is enough to scare clients into speechlessness or confusion. This is fertile territory for implementing an RO program. In addition

to the ICU, any hospital unit can be considered a foreign environment for the client. Reality orientation does not have to be limited to one setting.

Reality orientation and the client in the community

Consider another woman now, labeled confused, but in a home environment. It is winter and an urban setting. The woman is 70 years old, independent in her own apartment, and accustomed to going to church, stopping for her groceries in the morning, and seeing her neighbors. She then picks up the newspaper, comes home, has lunch, and watches the soap operas on TV. Let us imagine the middle of winter, and there is a snow storm with much slippery ice. She's afraid to go out because of the risk of slipping on the ice, so she stays at home for 3 days, 4 days, 5 days. Now she has not bought her newspapers or seen her friends. She begins to feel a little bit listless and has vague feelings of anxiety. She says something is wrong, and she does not feel well. She does not feel well because she has not been exposed to her normal stimuli, conversations, and settings—to those things that are appropriate to her life-style. She is well, but her environment is creating stress, and a low level of confusion sets in. She now has some nonspecific complaints of not feeling well, and it is said to be her age. But it is not her age; it is her environment. She is just not getting the stimulation that she needs. Granted, the situation does not have to be extreme or critical. However, when a nurse is planning with the client and family, the nurse should initiate the subject of orientation and see what plans the client and family will make. If they have no idea of what can be done in a situation like this, the nurse should share with them information regarding sensory deprivation and make suitable plans. It might be valuable for community health agencies, visiting nurses' associations, or the nurse in private practice who works with a family with an older adult cannot initiate reality orientation as part of health teaching and health maintenance.

Props

Certain physical equipment is necessary as a part of the RO package. These are called props.

Although designed specifically for long-term-care facilities, any or all of these can be equally effective for home, hospital, or community settings.

Props required to carry out the RO techniques include a calendar and RO board. The RO board is a 24-inch × 24-inch square board to display the following information:

1. Name of agency
2. Location of agency
3. Year
4. Date
5. Day of week
6. Weather
7. Next meal
8. Next holiday

The board can be easily made or purchased from school or photographic supply houses. Bold black letters at least 2 inches high on a white background for legibility are best for communicating the information. One should be hung in each area where clients gather, such as dining rooms, nursing stations, and dayrooms. Portable types are useful for bedridden clients' rooms. The board will visually communicate with clients to stimulate and orient them to reality. The nurse adds verbal communication of the information at every opportunity during conversation with the client. This reinforces reality. The RO process is in effect during the client's waking hours. During every nurse-client encounter, basic current and personal information is presented over and over to the client, beginning with his name, where he is, and the date. People who are at risk for confusion are RO candidates. Each contact the nursing staff has with an at risk client is used to improve awareness of person, time, and place.

All clients should have a calendar in their room. The calendar should be large enough for them to read the numbers and dates of the month. They should be encouraged to cross off each date so that they know what day and date it is.

A client should be told where he is going, the purpose, and what is expected of him. For example, "It is time to go to physical therapy now, Mrs. Jones. You will receive hot pack treatments to your back." "It is lunch time, and you are going to the dining room." At every opportunity, the client should be rewarded for a correct response and

success in finding his way around by praise or other appropriate rewards. Consistency in communication approach is the key to the rehabilitation of the confused client, and each member of the nursing staff has the responsibility to maintain this consistency.

Administration

An important area to look at in reality orientation is administration. In many long-term-care settings, reality orientation programs come under the direction of the therapeutic activities department. The administration of RO is a matter of philosophy. However, it is logical to have RO under the auspices of the nursing department. Nightingale herself established that regulation of the environment of the client is a nursing priority.

Since the administrator assumes the major responsibility for the direction of the RO program, the administrator must believe in RO and support it. The degree of commitment and the inspiration that the administrator projects to the staff can either make or break the RO program. The director of nursing and the licensed professional nursing staff are also key people who create the feeling of dedication, commitment, and responsibility needed for a successful RO program. The attitude of the nursing staff will, for the most part, affect the success or failure of the program. A commitment that extends beyond the daily physical care of the client is vital. The director of nursing must provide the leadership that instills the essential sense of responsibility within the nursing staff for achieving the RO goals. Her enthusiasm and support of the program will be noticed by the personnel and help motivate them. She might take the time to visit the classroom and praise the instructor and commend the nursing staff using the technique. Staff cohesiveness and commitment to the program will foster its success.

Staff development

The director of staff development, or in-service education, is the logical person to coordinate the RO program, orient the staff, select and train instructors. The first requirement is for the director of staff development to successfully complete a certified course in the theory of reality orientation therapy. Then, a comprehensive orientation plan to include employees from all departments and residents' families can be developed and implemented. Lectures, demonstrations, group discussions, role playing, films rented or purchased, and slides help make the orientation workshops interesting and educational. It takes about 2 to 3 months' time to include all departments in the orientation program, but it is well worth the time and effort to orient all employees and secure their cooperation in making the program successful. All departments within the long-term-care facility must know and be familiar with the RO basic 10 principles before launching the program. For instance, housekeeping, dietary, and maintenance workers will all at one time or another interact with a client who is in a long-term-care facility. While the housekeeper is cleaning the room and performing her daily functions, she can also be saying, "Good morning, Mrs. Jones. Today is Tuesday." She reinforces the basic communication idea of the RO program. Likewise, the dietary personnel as they serve the client's meals in the dining room can say, "Today is a sunny Tuesday, and the menu is roast beef, mashed potatoes, and string beans." This brings the client back to reality, and reinforces the type of food he is eating.

A special orientation program for client's families can be developed to encourage their cooperation and support. The medical director can be asked to present a program to orient the medical staff to gain their endorsement and cooperation.

Instructors

The RO instructors are trained individuals who have successfully completed a subscribed course of theory and supervised classroom instruction under the direction of the staff development director. An instructor may be from the ranks of nursing service as charge nurse, staff nurse, or even a professional nursing student. Success of the program is fostered by the instructor's dedication to the RO program and the use of this commitment to foster improvement within the clients.

The instructors' responsibilities include maintaining consistency in holding regular scheduled classes, maintaining records and clients' evaluation forms, and selecting new clients who can benefit from admission into the classes. Daily charting of clients' behavior is useful in showing improvement or weak areas that require a needs assessment. A team approach can be implemented to ensure the clients' sense of security, self-esteem, dignity, comfort, and belonging.

Improvement in the client's orientation and socialization is usually slow in coming and requires patience. Sometimes weekly instructor seminars help lend positive reinforcement to their work. However, the instructor rewards are well worth the effort. Being an instructor gives status to the personnel. This status and esteem are passed on to the RO clients. Self-esteem and job satisfaction derived from helping the older adult break through a state of confusion cannot be measured. The philosophy should be that nursing is successful as long as clients are not regressing.

Classes

To enhance the RO program, clients may be asked to attend a daily half-hour classroom session that is limited to four participants. Midmorning is usually an excellent time to hold class. Clients are usually able to participate at this time of day. Classes are held 5 days a week, Monday through Friday. The classroom climate is one of cheerfulness, quiet privacy, and adequate ventilation, temperature, and size. The trip to the classroom offers stimulation of the senses and a change in environment. The class usually starts and ends with the instructor showing a clock and stating the time.

The instructor then interacts with the group with communication and props. A beginning exercise is introducing the clients to each other and asking them to state their names and shake hands with the person sitting next to them. This may be successful the first day or weeks later. We are culturally grounded since birth in our rituals of hand contact and name identification. This simple introduction–hand shake procedure is remembered by the client and forces him out of his isolation back into the environment. It also provides an opportunity for touch and stimulation of the other senses. The RO board is read by the instructor. The client in turn reads the board and receives immediate positive feedback through touching, eye contact, smiles, and praise. Every opportunity is made to have the client volunteer information about things he can answer. Simple activities are selected, such as identifying common objects or the day of the month on a calendar. The instructor generates communication from correct responses. The nurse's interaction can be guided by the cues the client transmits and be a mutually beneficial experience. If the client does not answer correctly, the instructor tells him the answer and has him repeat it. Since the attention span is short, classes should not exceed 30 minutes. The seasons of the year and holidays are excellent tools to open up communication. You will be surprised how much the client recalls about his holiday experiences, summer vacations, and childhood days.

Families need to participate with the client, nursing staff, and instructor in setting realistic, attainable goals. They need to understand the philosophy and purpose of the RO program and may require more orientation. Families should be encouraged to observe RO classes and participate in them. Be patient with the family, and reinforce the positive aspects of the therapy to gain their cooperation. Teach them the 10 basic rules for RO. This will enable them to be consistent in their manner and approach with their parent or loved one. The family will then understand that they should not encourage rambling speech or rambling activity. They will now know how to reinforce reality. Always teach the family to participate in touching and using familiar names. Tell the client what is going on at home even though he is not there so that he will not be separated and isolated from the home setting. The ultimate goal is, after all, to return the client to self-care and his home.

When the client becomes aware of time, place, and person and successfully completes the exercises in the classroom, he is promoted to the advanced RO class, remotivation group, special interest group, and facility activities. Depending on his physical condition, he may be a candidate for discharge to the home or transfer to a lower level of care area within the facility.

Mrs. Franklin was identified as an RO candidate by the charge nurse; however, her daughter would not give consent for the client's class participation because she thought it was a kindergarten-like activity. The head nurse suggested that she go with her mother to an RO class. After seeing class in session, she consented to having her mother participate. Several weeks later, Mrs. Franklin's daughter remarked how pleased she was to see her mother's progress and attributed it to the RO classes.

Reality orientation client activities

It is the nursing staff's responsibility to assess the level of orientation and recommend the RO program as indicated by findings. Many times the family and staff feel that the confused are happy and let them be. But, again, we must remember that if this behavior is condoned and accepted by the staff, then the client will act the script. Dependency is fostered and self-esteem lowered. Communication and stimulation are needed within the environment to bring the client out of his withdrawal pattern and back to reality. One means of promoting reality orientation is to stimulate the confused by the normal social interaction of mealtime. How many of us like to eat alone, isolated from communication with other people? A group dining area for the confused will permit them to partake of the social interaction and stimulation of having someone sitting beside them. The RO instructor or other nursing personnel can supervise the meal, stimulate communication, and use the techniques of RO. Often, the RO instructors plan activities around a client's birthday, holidays, or special event. The clients participate in the planning and preparation of favors for parties.

Reality orientation is indeed a therapeutic nursing tool that may be implemented in any agency. The rewards to the client and job satisfaction for the nurse are worth the effort involved.

SUMMARY

Communication reaches out to all aspects of our lives. The messenger, the message, and the receiver should always be considered. When we can see a broad view of communication, then we have opened up the world as potential goals are set for the older client. When we can offer them the world as a community and we can see them as active participants, then they can share and give. When we as professionals have a narrow view of communication as verbal person-to-person interaction only, we are seeing the narrowest of all uses of communication. The depth and breadth of a communication interaction is limited only to the extent of the person's resources. When their resources are regarded and treated as rich and full, so will their communications be. The more senses that are used, the clearer the message will be to the older adult. All senses should be focused on. Add to speech, visual stimuli, touch, and even olfactory stimuli as appropriate.

REFERENCES

Achenbaum, W. A., and Stearns, P. N.: Essay: old age and modernization, Gerontologist **18:**307, June 1978.

Alfano, G. J.: There are no routine patients, Am. J. Nurs. **75:** 1804, 1822, October 1975.

Almore, M. G.: Dyadic communication. Am. J. Nurs. **79:**1076, June 1979.

American Hospital Association: This way to reality. A guide for developing a reality orientation program, The Association, 840 North Lake Shore Drive, Chicago, Ill. 60611, 1973.

Ardrey, R.: The social contract, New York, 1970, Atheneum.

Arie, T.: Confusion in old age, Age Ageing Suppl:72, 1978.

Barnett, K.: A theoretical construct concepts of touch, Nurs. Res. **21:**102, March-April 1972.

Barnes, J. A.: Effects of R.O. classroom on memory loss, confusion and disorientation in geriatrics, Gerontologist, April 1974.

Beck, A. T.: The diagnosis and management of depression, Philadelphia, 1973, University of Pennsylvania Press.

Besdine, M. D.: Consultant, National Institute on Aging paper, Reversible causes of cognitive impairment of the elderly—detection, evaluation and treatment. Presented at First Annual Gero-Psychiatry Conference on Depression and Confusion in the Elderly, Marlboro Psychiatric Hospital, Marlboro, N.J. April 1979.

Blazer, D.: Techniques for communicating with your elderly patient, Geriatrics **33:**79, November 1978.

Blazer, D.: Working with the elderly patient's family, Geriatrics **33:**117, February 1978.

Boguslawski, M.: The use of therapeutic touch in nursing, J. Cont. Ed. Nurs. **10:**4, 1979.

Boore, J.: The elderly: a challenge to nurses—4. old people and sensory deprivation, Nurs. Times **73:**1754, 10 November 1977.

Borzilleri, T. C.: The need for a separate consumer price index for older persons. A review and new evidence. Gerontologist **18:**230, June 1978.

Butler, R. N., and Lewis, M. I.: Aging and mental health, ed. 2, St. Louis, 1977, The C. V. Mosby Co.

Carroll, P. J.: The social hour for geropsychiatric patients, J. Am. Geriatr. Soc. **26:**32, January 1978.

Citrin, R. S., and Dixon, D. N.: Reality orientation. A milieu therapy used in an institution for the aged, Gerontologist **17:**39, February 1977.

Connor, M.: Common concern: words and wheelchairs, Geriatr. Nurs. **1:**61, May-June 1980.

D'Addio, D. L.: Reach out and touch, Am. J. Nurs. **79:**1081, June 1979.

DaVito, J.: The interpersonal communication book, New York, 1976, Harper and Row, Publishers.

Ebersole, P.: Reminiscing, Am. J. Nurs. **76:**1304, 1976.

Fallot, Roger D.: The impact on mood of verbal reminiscing in later adulthood, Intl. J. Aging Hum. Dev. **10:**385-400, 1979-80.

Folsom, J. C.: Major problems in the treatment of "senility." Speech presented at the Eighteenth Annual Conference, VA Studies in Mental Health and Behavioral Sciences, March 28-30, 1973.

Forsyth,, G. L.: Analysis of the concept of empathy: illustration of one approach, A.N.S. **80**(2):33, Jan. 1980.

Gasek, G.: How to handle the crotchety, elderly patient, Nursing 80 **10:**70, March 1980.

Gebbie, K., and Lavin, M. A.: Classification of nursing diagnoses, St. Louis, 1975, The C. V. Mosby Co.

Goldman, R.: Geriatric education at the undergraduate level, J. Am. Geriatr. Soc. **25:**485, November 1977.

Gruber, H. W.: Geriatrics—physician attitudes and medical school training, J. Am. Geriatr. Soc. **25:**494, November 1977.

Gunter, L. M., and Miller, J. C.: Toward a nursing gerontology, Nurs. Res. **26:**3, May-June 1977.

Hall, E. T.: The hidden dimension, New York, 1966, Doubleday & Co., Inc.

Hanson, R. G.: Considering social nutrition in assessing geriatric nutrition, Geriatrics **33:**49, March 1978.

Harris, C. S., and Ivory, P. B.: An outcome evaluation of reality orientation therapy with geriatric patients in a state mental hospital, Gerontologist **16:**496, December 1976.

Hayakawa, S. I.: Language in thought and action, ed. 2, New York, 1965, Harcourt Brace Jovanovich, Inc.

Herbert, M.: Studies of sleep in the elderly, Age Ageing Suppl:41, 1978.

Holtzman, J. M., Beck, J. D., Hodgetts, P. G., and others: Geriatrics program for medical students and family practice residents. I. Establishing attitudes toward the aged, J. Am. Geriatr. Soc. **25:**521, November 1976.

Holtzman, J. M., Beck, J. D., and Hodgetts, P. G.: Geriatrics program for medical students. II. Impact of two educational experiences on student attitudes, J. Am. Geriatr. Soc. **26:**355, August 1978.

Hoyter, J.: Positive aspects of aging, J. Gerontol. Nurs. January-February 1976, p. 19.

Hulicka, I. M.: Understanding our client, the geriatric patient, J. Am. Geriatr. Soc. September 1972.

John, A., and Steel, K.: Interest in geriatrics at a university department of medicine. J. Am. Geriatr. Soc. **26:**149, April 1978.

Johnson, F.: Response of territorial intrusion by nursing home residents, stress and adaptation, 1979, Aspen Systems Corp.

Jourard, S. M.: The transparent self, New York, 1971, Van Nostrand Co.

Jungman, L. B.: When your feelings get in the way. Am. J. Nurs. **79:**1074, June 1979.

Kastenbaum, R.: Essay: gerontology's search for understanding, Gerontologist **18:**59, February 1978.

Kazmierczak, F., and others: Communication problems encountered when caring for the elderly individual, J. Gerontol. Nurs. March-April 1975, p. 21.

Kelly, J. T., Hanson, R. G., Garetz, F. K., and others: What the family physician should know about treating elderly patients, Part 2, Geriatrics **32:**79, October 1977.

Krathwohl, D. R., and others: Taxonomy on educational objectives, handbook II: affective domain, New York, 1964, David McKay Co.

Krieger, D., Reper, E., and Ancoli, S.: Therapeutic touch, Am. J. Nurs. **79**:660, April 1979.

Kuhn, M. E.: New life for the elderly—liberation from agism, Enquiry, September, November 1971, revised 1974, Gray Panthers, 3700 Chestnut St., Philadelphia, Pa. 19104.

Lancaster, J.: Macro-system interaction: communication within the health care delivery system, Top. Clin. Nurs. **1**:3, 71, 1979.

Lehr, U., and Rudinger, G.: Consistency and change in social participation in the aged, Hum. Dev. **12**:255, 1969.

Letcher, P. B., Peterson, L. P., and Scarbrough, D.: Reality orientation: an historical study of patient progress. Hosp. Community Psychiatry **25**:801, December 1974.

Loomis, M. E.: Group process for nurses, St. Louis, 1979, The C. V. Mosby Co.

Mead, B. T.: How to relate to the elderly patient, Geriatrics **32**:73, October 1977.

Midler, P., Sr.: Rx for the aging person: attitudes, J. Gerontol. Nurs. March-April 1976.

Murphy, J. C.: Communicating with the dying patient. Am. J. Nurs. **79**:1084, June 1979.

New Jersey State Board of Nursing: Nursing Practice Act, 1975.

Nightingale, F.: Notes on nursing, Philadelphia, 1946, J. B. Lippincott Co.

Nonverbal communication in nursing, Costa Mesa, Calif., 1975, Concept Media.

O'Brien, M. J.: Communications and relationships in nursing, St. Louis, 1974, The C. V. Mosby Co.

O'Brien, M. J.: Communications and relationships in nursing, ed. 2, St. Louis, 1978, The C. V. Mosby Co.

Parsons, V., Sanford, N.: Interpersonal interaction in nursing: basic concepts in nurse-patient communication, Reading, Mass., 1979, Addison-Wesley Publishing Co., Inc.

Penel, C.: Geriatrics as a speciality. Nurs. Times **72**:1601, 14 October 1976.

Pfeiffer, E.: Handling the distressed older patient. Geriatrics **34**:24, February 1979.

Preston, T.: Caring for the aged: when words fail, Am. J. Nurs. **73**:2064, December 1973.

Ramaekers, M. J., Sr.: Communication blocks revisited. Am. J. Nurs. **79**:1079, June 1979.

Rawnsley, M.: The concept of privacy. A.N.S. **80**:25, January 1980.

Retirement: when, why, how? Geriatrics **33**:15, July 1978.

Rule, W. L.: Political alienation and voting attitudes among the elderly. Gerontologist **17**(5 Pt. 1):400, October 1977.

Scarbrough, D.: Reality orientation: a new approach to an old problem, Nursing **4**:12, November 1974.

Secker, B.: Win by cultivating new effective habits for leadership. Paper presented at NLN 14th Biennial Convention, Atlanta, 1979.

Seefeldt, C., Jantz, R. K., Galper, A., and Serock, K.: Using pictures to explore children's attitude toward the elderly. Gerontologist **17**:506, December 1977.

Shannon, C. E., and Weaver, W.: The mathematical theory of communication, Urbana, Ill., 1949, University of Illinois Press.

Sierra-Franco, M. H.: Therapeutic communication in nursing, New York, 1978, McGraw-Hill Book Co.

Simms, L. M., and Lindberg, J. B.: The nurse person developing perspectives for contemporary nursing, New York, 1978, Harper & Row Publishers.

Simon, S., and others: Values clarification: a handbook of practical strategies for teachers and students, New York, 1972, Hart Publishing Company.

Skowronski, S. M.: Proxemics and nursing care. Hosp. Prog. **53**:72, August 1972.

Smith, V. M., and Bass, T. A.: Communication for health professionals, Philadelphia, 1979, J. B. Lippincott Co.

Tharp, T. S., Baker, B. J., and Brower, T. F.: Nursing staff attitudes toward the geriatric nurse practitioner student, Nurs. Res. **28**:299, September-October 1979.

Vosburgh, P.: Treating the psychologically disturbed geriatric patient, Conference Report, Hosp. Comm. Psychiatry, November 1969.

Walsh, J. A., and Kiracofe, N. M.: Change in significant other relationships and life satisfaction in the aged, Intl. J. Aging Hum. Dev. **10**:273-281, 1979-80.

Williams, L. M.: A concept of loneliness in the elderly, J. Am. Geriatr. Soc. **26**:183, April 1978.

10 Modifying nursing approaches for the older adult: physiological needs

This book has established that persons over 65 have general declines in almost all the body systems. The 65-year-old has at least another 12 years of life to anticipate. At 80, many still have 10 years of life before them. The purpose of this chapter and the next is to focus on those nursing interventions that will help the older adult to be comfortable and enjoy his personal environment, family environment, and community environment. These three systems are addressed because they comprise the older adult's complete environment.

This chapter emphasizes the hands-on care for clients at home and in long-term-care facilities. Fundamental nursing skills are modified to meet the particular needs of both the well older adult and the older adult who has a stabilized chronic condition. The purpose of nursing is to support optimum levels of wellness and function of the client. The nursing actions outlined represent the implementation phase of the nursing process. Because nursing diagnosis prescribes what the nursing actions will be, nursing diagnosis is linked with nursing implications in case examples. Nursing intervention is directed to all phases of the life-style, from basic personal hygiene to environmental safety. Anticipation of each of the needs of the body systems of the client and the client's adjustment to environmental situations are included. Because nursing always focuses on actual and potential health problems, anticipatory guidance is offered for prevention of further complications and teaching strategies to broaden the client's knowledge are included. Frequently, community resources are presented to offer the client additional physiological and psychological support systems.

Within the concepts of self-care by the client, the professional nurse integrates basic rehabilitation principles. In nursing, self-care is always the goal. Although it may take longer for the older adult to do a particular task, the ultimate outcome is independence and self-care. Personal care and hygiene tie in with feelings of self-esteem and reinforce the value and advantages of adulthood. Maslow's hierarchy of needs from Chapter I will be threaded throughout the chapter. The physiological needs, such as food, sleep, and clothing, have traditionally been addressed by the family and institutions. These needs must be met before the client can achieve the higher levels of the hierarchy. These physiological needs are discussed in this chapter. The remaining needs—environmental safety, love and belonging, self-esteem and self-actualization—can be satisfied when the client is in a therapeutic setting, either in his own home or in an agency that subscribes to the therapeutic model. These needs are discussed in Chapter 11. The reader is referred to Chapter 3, which compares therapeutic, custodial, Nightingale, and bureaucratic models. Nursing actions are described within the framework of the therapeutic model, which encourages human worth and self-dignity. Each of the body's systems is discussed in correlation with the physiology and altered physiology of aging as presented in Chapter 1.

Nursing actions include the basic concepts of the nurse as the health teacher and health counselor. Many suggestions are offered regarding health teaching, teaching principles and teaching strategies. The nurse is one member of the interdisciplinary health team, and interactions of other health team members are offered as supplements to nursing care where indicated.

PHYSIOLOGICAL NEEDS

The first level of Maslow's hierarchy of needs deals with basic physiological needs for proper body functions (Fig. 10-1). Personal hygiene is presented first, followed by clothing, sleep and rest, exercise, housing, nutrition needs, and sexuality. These first-level needs are the basic building blocks of client wellness. Unless these needs are met, the client cannot progress through the levels to self-actualization. Nursing intervention modified for the special characteristics of the older adult helps the client meet these physiological needs. Health teaching and anticipatory guidance are functions of the nurse that offer the client the knowledge base necessary to make decisions and maintain his independence.

PERSONAL HYGIENE

Most older adults are capable of taking care of their own personal hygiene needs. Data collected by the nurse during assessment will identify any

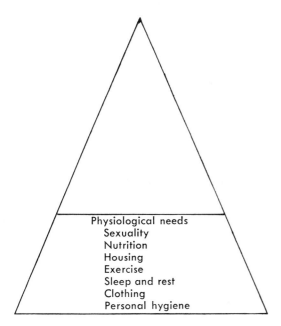

Fig. 10-1. Physiological needs—first level of Maslow's hierarchy of needs.

professional assistance that may be needed by the older adult. The information collected about the client's method of bathing will be helpful in planning care. To maintain independence in personal hygiene, home care bathing activities may need to be simulated, whether it be bathing in a tub, shower, at a sink, or soaking or washing feet in a bucket before cutting toenails.

The assessment is done in depth regarding the personal hygiene habits of the older adult. It is imperative that the older adult have a sense of involvement in the care at the agency. From the time of his admission, he must receive the message that he is expected to participate in the planning of care, and that his preferences will be respected as much as possible. Nursing intervention is carried out based on the plan of care reflecting the client's normal pattern of living. The client should be able to pick the time of day for his personal hygiene. For example, many people have become accustomed to taking a shower or tub bath before retiring in the evening as a means of helping to promote and induce sleep. Other people are used to taking a bath in the morning before or after eating breakfast. Providing an opportunity for an option to the older adult helps maintain his own dignity and self-actualization. Permitting the client to decide the time of the bath may seem like going into very minute detail; however, it is important for the client who has been doing it for over 50 years. It gives the client an opportunity to exercise will and control over institutional style living, whether it be in the hospital or nursing home setting.

If the community health nurse is planning the older adult's move into the home of a son or daughter, a review of the hygiene routines of the older adult should be part of the anticipatory guidance she gives to the family. It eases the assimilation of the older adult into the usual schedule of family activities.

Skin care

Bathing is a major activity in skin care. The older adult's skin and mucous membranes are thin and sensitive to high temperatures and mechanical irritation. Even the well-nourished adult requires modifications in nursing interventions. The older adult's impaired circulation to peripheral cells predisposes him to injury because of the inade-

Areas of hygiene assessment

The following questions relate to areas of preference in your personal hygiene. We will be pleased to accommodate your preference in our daily nursing activities. Please indicate your preference.

Bathing

1. What is your usual pattern of bathing?
   a. Tub
   b. Shower
   c. Sink
2. Do you prefer bathing?
   a. Daily
   b. Every other day
   c. Twice a week
   d. Once a week
3. Time of day preferred for bathing.
   a. Morning
   b. Afternoon
   c. Evening
4. Do you receive assistance with bathing?
   a. No
   b. Yes. If yes, who renders assistance and in what way?
5. Which brand of soap and lotion is preferred?
   a. Ivory
   b. Dial
   c. Dove
   d. Lux
   e. Alpha Keri
   f. Intensive Care
   g. Other

Mouth care

6. Do you wear dentures?
   a. No
   b. Yes. If yes,
      (1) Complete upper, lower
      (2) Partial upper, lower
      (3) Bridge
7. Are your dentures marked with your name?
   a. No
   b. Yes
8. Do you have your own denture cup?
   a. No
   b. Yes
9. Do you cleanse your dentures daily?
   a. No
   b. Yes. If yes,
      (1) In the morning
      (2) At bedtime
      (3) After each meal

10. Do you brush your teeth daily?
    a. No
    b. Yes. If yes,
       (1) In the morning
       (2) At bedtime
       (3) After each meal
11. Do you floss your teeth?
    a. No
    b. Yes
12. Do you need assistance brushing your teeth or dentures?
    a. No
    b. Yes

Nail care

13. Do you cut your own fingernails?
    a. No
    b. Yes
14. Do you do your own manicure?
    a. Yes
    b. No
15. Do you wear nail polish?
    a. Yes
    b. No
16. Does a podiatrist do your foot care?
    a. Yes
    b. No. If no, would you like one to visit you?
       (1) Yes
       (2) No

Hair care

17. A beautician/barber is available by appointment; would you like this service? (Fee schedule available at nurse's desk.)
    a. No
    b. Yes. If yes,
       (1) Wash
       (2) Set
       (3) Cut
       (4) Coloring
       (5) Permanent
18. Do you wash and set your own hair?
    a. No
    b. Yes
19. How often do you do your hair?
20. How often do you shave?
21. Do you use a hair depilatory?
    a. No
    b. Yes

quate circulation. Emaciated and dehydrated clients have skin that is more susceptible to bacterial, mechanical, and chemical injury than the younger adult. Bathing equipment, tubs, and shower stalls should be cleaned thoroughly between clients, particularly so for the older adult. Older women are susceptible to monilia infections (*Candida albicans*). Cross-contamination of vaginal discharge causes vaginitis in these older women, whose normal bacteria flora is altered after menopause.

Water temperatures for the over-60 person should be lowered from 110° F to 100° to 105° F. Most states have a regulation that a safety valve maintains the hot water at no higher than 105° F in long-term-care facilities. The client at home should also have an appropriate mix of hot and cold water in the faucets in the sinks and bath tub or shower stall.

Mechanical injury or irritation can be alleviated by preventing friction and excessive pressure while caring for the skin. Washcloths should be made of a very soft terry cloth or cotton material. Disposable wash cloths should be tested for abrasiveness. Percale linen rather than muslin should be used on beds. Although it is necessary to commercially wash linens in most agencies and use detergents and bleaches, bed linens for the older adult should not be starched. Instead of starch, laundries supplying long-term-care facilities should add oil to the rinse water. Also, antistatic rinses and fabric softeners can be added in the last rinse cycle or in the dryer. The same linen preparations can be done at home as well. With some special attention to the linen used on the older adult's bed, the integrity of the superficial skin is protected. In addition, these measures eliminate the common causes of itching. As with all persons, the bed linens should be free of wrinkles, crumbs, used tissues, or other materials that can damage the skin. The keratotic layer of the older adult's skin lacks the sebaceous secretions of other age groups. The limited resiliency of the skin increases cell loss with friction of movement on coarse, starched linen. Diminished adipose layers predispose the client to the stresses of shearing force against bed linens.

Mechanical injury is a risk during back rubs. Effleurage, the long stroking motion, is the pref-

erable motion for the older adult. It should be the beginning and the end stroke of the massage. The petrissage and tapote, or pinching and tapping strokes, must be used with far less vigorous motion than with a younger person. Thinner muscle masses and spinal column changes make the older adult's back less able to tolerate excessive manipulation or pressure. Although these two steps of massage should not be eliminated, only light to moderate pressure should be used. The back rub is a comfort measure and should not be painful or tiring for the client. The nurse should be aware of her physical size and the strength of her hands as compared with the fragile body of the older adult.

A lubricant must be used on the hands to prevent friction and mechanical injury to the skin. The lubricant of choice for the older adult is an oil base or emollient lotion. It is not uncommon to reapply the lotion several times during the backrub, as the dry skin quickly absorbs the moisturizing lotion. In addition to being comforting, the lotion promotes a skin suppleness, reducing the risk of breakdown. Soaps used for bathing should have a neutral reaction with a pH similar to the skin. Alkaline soaps destroy the protective acidity of the skin secretions. Oil-base soaps are recommended for older adults with dry, sensitive skin. Hexachlorophene soaps are not recommended, because of the increased risk of contact dermatitis.

Alcohol and dusting powders are not appropriate for this age group. These products dry the skin. However, if the client finds the scent of the powder pleasant, it can be applied to axillae, groin, breasts, and buttocks. These areas can become moistened with perspiration, and should be assessed for caking or skin irritation as a result of powdering.

The older adult group is the population who most frequently uses footboards and bed cradles. Both items present considerable mechanical risks to the client's skin. Although most nursing fundamental textbooks emphasize the need to pad these devices, it is extremely important that this protection be provided for the older adults. In the presence of peripheral vascular disease, the skin cannot tolerate any physical injury from these metal, plastic, or wooden bed assessories. Tissue repair is retarded, and so injury must be prevented.

Types of bathtubs

There are many varieties of bathtubs manufactured. Several are particularly suited for the older adult client. A low-sided tub built into the floor permits easy entry and exit while providing enough depth of water for bathing. The walk-in tub features a door built into one side. The client or nurse opens the door for the client's entry into the tub and then closes the door. A watertight seal between the door and tub prevents leakage. The water must be drained completely before the client opens the door to exit from the tub.

The Century tub bath has a hydraulic chair lift and Jacuzzi whirl pool component. The procedure for a Century tub bath will be presented later. One other style of tub is useful for the older adult who is bedridden. This is a freestanding tub of stretcher height. The client can be transferred onto this tub and be completely bathed with safety and minimal exertion.

Tub and shower equipment

Safety is a priority during tub baths and showers. Safety rails or grab bars should be installed in client bath tubs (Fig. 10-2) and shower stalls. They are sold in a variety of sizes and types to fit most requirements. They should be made from metal or plastic material that is resistent to rust, corrosion, wear, and impact damage. When home installation is needed, the client, his family, or the nurse can order these safety handles from a surgical supply house. Many models can be snapped into place without the need for special tools. Other types do require special fixtures to attach them to walls and tubs. Price ranges for this equipment vary.

Tub and shower chairs are a needed safety and comfort accessory for the older adult's tub bath or shower. The model of choice for the older adult is a chair, rather than a stool. The chair should provide back and arm support, as well as have leg bottoms with suction tips for stability. Many manufacturers have chair models with nonlocking wheels on legs instead of suction cups. The mobility of these chairs places the older adult at risk of falling. Assistance must be available continuously while the client is in this type of wheeled shower chair. This reduces the client's independence and privacy.

It is not uncommon to have to choose a backless stool model for the client's home bath tub or shower. The full chair model is larger than many home tubs or showers can accommodate. When a choice has to be made, the most important safety feature is a stool with suction tips on the leg bottoms. Stability is of primary importance in the safety of older adults. Medicaid and Medicare will reimburse the client for at least part of the cost when such safety devices are ordered by the physician.

Scheduling clients' baths

With the belief that clients have a right to continue hygiene practices similar to their lifetime habits, planning nursing intervention for hygiene measures can be done through a rotating bath schedule. Some compromise is useful. For example, most agencies cannot provide a full bath every day. The client can choose the time of the day he

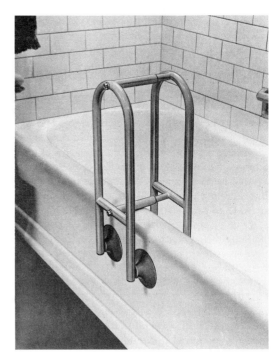

Fig. 10-2. This bathtub safety rail helps the client into and out of the tub. This model has a double handhold for extra support. There are no protrusions to cause injury. (Courtesy Lumex Inc., Bay Shore, N.Y.)

prefers for his bath or shower, and usually can choose two or more days of the week on which to have full hygiene care. For those clients whose hygiene practices have been less than optimum, the requirement of making a choice helps them achieve better hygiene care goals.

With the hygiene practice preference data of her clients, the head nurse develops a hygiene schedule for her unit. Taken into consideration are client preferences, staff availability, and physical facilities. A typical plan for a 32-bed unit is found in Table 10-1.

The client hygiene schedule is divided into the categories of the hygiene facilities available at the agency. The agency has two Century tubs available to this unit, one regular tub and three showers. The nurse lists the client's name in the column designating the type of tub or shower desired, and the time of day preferred. Because staffing policies permit the staff to have every other weekend off, most baths and showers are scheduled for during the week. Those clients wishing baths and showers more frequently than twice a week are accommodated (Clients II, M, and N). The client with decubiti needing frequent dressing changes is scheduled for the Century tub once a day. This rotating schedule accomplishes a staffing goal. It relieves the staff of giving all the complete baths to everyone during the day shift. The primary work load is distributed through the week, Monday to Friday, over two shifts, leaving the weekend with a significantly lighter work load.

Therapeutic bathing

The bath or shower is a source of cleansing the skin, exercising the muscles, and improving circulation for all age groups. For the older adult, it is a particularly important source of exercise and stimulation. It is during the bath that the older adult can put his muscle groups and joints through purposeful range-of-motion activities. It is a refreshing and relaxing modality that provides the nurse and client a one-to-one opportunity for therapeutic communication. Considerable nursing time during the bath is given to assessments of such areas as skin conditions, psychosocial status, muscular skeletal function, and level of self-care.

Century tub bath

In addition to being cleansing and relaxing, baths can be therapeutic. The Century tub bath is particularly well suited for the older adult. This elevated, pastel-colored tub is fitted with a Jacuzzi whirlpool system and a hydraulic chair lift (Fig. 10-3). The tub is filled to one-half capacity with 105° F water and a bath oil is added. The client is seated in the hydraulic lift chair and draped with a bath blanket to prevent chilling and provide privacy. The chair is slowly lowered, and the client is positioned in the tub. The Jacuzzi whirlpool is

Table 10-1. Client hygiene schedule

	Mon/Thurs		Wed		Tues/Fri		Sat/Sun	
	AM	PM	AM	PM	AM	PM	AM	PM
Century tub	A* B C CC	D E F G	CC		AA BB DD EE	FF GG CC		CC
Regular tub	H I J	K II			KK LL MM	HH II JJ		II
Shower	L	M N		M N	OO PP QQ	RR SS M N		M N

*Letters indicate individual clients.

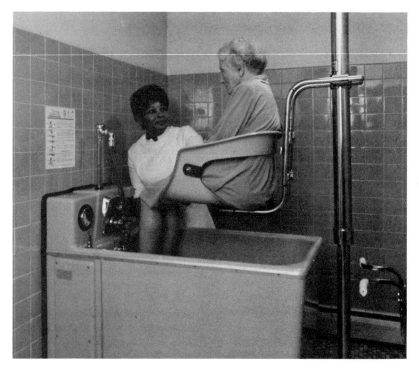

Fig. 10-3. The Century tub bath provides a therapeutic whirlpool water action that cleans the skin while stimulating circulation. (Photo copyright Lawrence S. Williams, Inc.)

started, sending warm swells of water around the client's body to cleanse, stimulate, and refresh. As the client is being removed from the tub in the chair lift, there is a potential safety hazard because of the water dripping on the floor. Sheeting or absorbent mats should be placed on the floor to absorb the water, and the client draped.

It is not uncommon that an older person will refuse a Century tub bath because of fear of the equipment. The nurse can accompany the client to the tub room when it is not in use and explain the use of the Century tub. It is useful for the nurse to demonstrate the chair mechanism and even to have the client sit in the chair before the first actual bath is scheduled. After becoming accustomed to the Century tub, most clients enjoy the warmth and massaging action of the whirlpool stream. For clients at risk for decubitus ulcers, the agitating water action of the bath serves as a form of hydrotherapy, increasing circulation to the skin.

Emollient baths

Starch bath. For the client with dry skin who prefers tub baths, emollient or soothing baths can be ordered. These are particularly suited for the older adult, because they might be familiar to him as an old-fashioned, yet effective, remedy. The substances used can be found in any household, are inexpensive, are not drugs, and do not cause excessive slipperiness in the tub, which would be a hazard. Cornstarch or oatmeal are the most common substances used in emollient baths. To prepare a cornstarch bath, bring 2 quarts of water to a boil. Take 2 cups of corn starch and add enough cold water to make a smooth liquid. Add the liquid starch to the boiling water. Fill the bathtub two thirds full with warm water and add the 2 quarts of liquid starch mixture. After any emollient bath, have the client pat the skin dry with a soft towel.

Aveeno bath. A convenient oatmeal preparation is made by the Musker Foundation, Inc. under the trade name Aveeno. It is a colloid fraction of oatmeal cereal particularly designed for baths. It requires no boiling or straining and dissolves easily in the bath water. One cup is usually added to a tub two thirds full of warm water. If Aveeno is not available, ordinary oatmeal can be used. Boil the oatmeal for 20 minutes in a cheese cloth pack. After cooling, add the strained oatmeal to the running bath water by squeezing the oatmeal through the cheese cloth bag. This straining process eliminates lumps that do not disperse in the water and might clog the plumbing.

For the safest and most soothing action, the temperature of the bath water should be in the neutral or warm range of 92° F to 98° F (33.5° C to 36.5° C). Warmer tub bath temperatures are inappropriate for the older adult. The systemic temperature may rise within minutes after being immersed in hot 104° F (40° C) water. The pulse rate increases 10 beats per degree of increased body temperature, cardiac output falls, and there can be a drop in blood pressure. Although these changes can be tolerated by a younger person, an older adult can feel faint. Warm baths relax and soothe far better than do hot baths.

Towel or lotion bath. The bath of choice for the fragile older adult is the towel bath. This is an in-bed bath using a lotion or a quick-drying solution such as Septi-Soft. A cotton terry towel large enough to cover the client's entire body is saturated in a plastic bag containing the cleansing agent or lotion warmed to a temperature of 96° to 98° F (35.5° to 36.5° C). After the towel is wrung out, it is unrolled up the client's body from the feet to the neck. As the towel is unrolled, the sheet on the client is removed. Beginning with the feet, the nurse uses a gentle rubbing and massaging action. When the lower half of the body has been cleansed, the towel is folded up and a clean sheet is placed over the legs. The neck, ears, and face are completed, then the client is turned and the bath is completed using the clean outside portion of the folded towel. After the back and buttock have been cleansed, the client is dressed and the bottom bed linens are changed. Usually little additional towel drying of the client's skin is needed, as the cleansing solution air dries in seconds. When the cleansing towel has been wrung out almost dry, it serves as both the cleansing and drying towel.

This towel bath is done with less fatigue to the client and is particularly well suited for in-bed clients with dry and itching skin. Older adults in the old-old age group enjoy the gentle, comforting strokes of this type of bath. The towel bath also is useful for the client with arthritis; the warmth of the towel is soothing to stiff, aching joints.

Oil bath or shower. Oil baths can be performed as a bedside basin bath, tub bath, or shower. Alpha Keri is an oil-base commercial product popular with older adults with dry skin. Baby oil is also useful for oil baths and showers. It has a pleasant fragrance and is relatively inexpensive. It can be used in place of soap during the bed bath by adding a capful or two to the basin water. For use in the bathtub, add three to four capfuls to running water. For the client who prefers to shower, two to three capfuls can be added to the face cloth. Extreme caution must be used to prevent slipping. A rubber mat or towel should be placed at the bottom of the bathtub or shower stall. The nurse should recommend that the client not stand in the shower, but use a shower chair or sit on a bath towel placed on the shower floor. After the shower, the client should not stand to leave the shower stall, but should transfer to the mat outside the shower, remaining in a sitting position. This crawling technique keeps the client close to the floor and provides a steady base of support, reducing the risk of falling. The same principle is applied to getting out of a tub. The client never stands, rather he assumes a kneeling position in the tub; using safety bars, he lifts his legs, one at a time, and arms, over the side of the tub onto the floor mat. What he is doing is sliding over the side of the tub, rather than standing and stepping over the tub. As with the exit from the shower, the client is providing himself a broad base of support and keeping his center of gravity close to the floor. Although these techniques are very important when in an oil bath, they certainly are applicable to all baths and showers for the older adult, whether at home or in a long-term-care facility.

Proper rinsing after emollient baths. Because the cutaneous layer of the older adult flakes to a greater extent than a younger person's, attention must be paid to proper rinsing after an emollient bath. Often the oatmeal, cornstarch or oil cling to the body, causing unsightly clumps of flaking skin on body surfaces and pubic hair. Have the client remain sitting in the tub while the bath water is draining. Keep the drain open and run fresh warm water into the tub. The client then uses a plastic pitcher, shower hose, or Water Pik extension shower to rinse the flaking skin off his body. If the client is at home and is responsible for cleaning the tub himself, it is convenient to have him take a towel and wash off the sides of the tub before he gets out. The bath additives do leave a greasy ring on the tub walls. If the client cleans it immediately, he doesn't have to bend, stoop, and reach in order to clean it later.

DAILY HYGIENE MEASURES

Most older adults do not take a full tub bath or shower daily. Daily hygienic measures should consist of at least partial baths in the morning and evening care. In the morning, the client should have mouth care before breakfast. At his choice, the rest of the partial bath should be done either before or after breakfast. The partial bath consists of washing the face, hands, axilla, and genital area. Many clients do not wash their faces with soap. The hands, axilla, and genitals should be washed with a mild soap and rinsed thoroughly with tepid water. Dry these areas completely by patting with a soft cotton terry towel. Deodorant, cornstarch, or talc may be applied to the axillae. The need for deodorant in the older adult is diminished because of reduced gland secretions. However, the habits of many years prevail, and most older adults continue to use these products. Many men and women use talc in the genital area and find it refreshing. It is not uncommon to find that the older adult prefers the stronger, more flowery scents. As the olfactory acuity diminishes, the threshold for fragrance identification rises.

The talcum powder absorbs the moisture in the genital area. Baby powder may be preferred because it is a finer talc, and has a smooth, soft texture. When applying talc, the client should be taught not to shake it liberally on his body as it disperses in the air and is inhaled into the respiratory tract and becomes an irritant. A small amount of talc should be placed into the palm of the hand and rubbed or patted on the desired area.

Bathing at the sink

In order to keep the care in the long-term-care facility as homelike as possible and to avoid hospital routines, the client should be encouraged to do his partial bath in the morning and evening at a bathroom sink. Usually bathrooms are set up ideally for this type of activity. Have the older adult keep his toilet articles in a closed cabinet or vanity area. If several clients share a bathroom, each client should have an area labeled with his name or a container kept in his bedside cabinet for the toilet articles. By keeping all his articles in a box, he saves needless trips back to the bedside. Safety is observed because none of the articles are left out when not in use. They do not pose a hazard to a confused person who might inadvertently drink some of the mouth care or lubricating solutions, or cut himself with a razor or nail scissor. If the client tolerates activity and full mobility, then he can stand and wash at the sink. For the client who cannot stand at the sink, the toilet adjacent to the wash sink can serve as a seat. Cover the lid with a towel, so the client is not sitting on the cold hard surface. This towel is later used to dry the perineal area after genital care. Put another towel over the client's lap and fill the basin with fresh water. He can wash his hands and face, axillae, and genitals in this position. If the client voids and has a bowel movement at this time, the perineal area may be cleansed while still on the toilet. If the toilet is too far from the sink, a bath chair or straight back chair can be brought to the sink. Bathing at a sink is a more practical routine than the traditional in-bed partial bath. With the sink bath, the client gets out of bed and can meet his elimination and toileting needs in an independent style. Mobility and purposeful activity are achieved. In-bed hygiene care connotes illness or lack of independence and discourages mobility. The maintenance of the older adult's independence in self-care and mobility are a priority for all older adults. This procedure also saves the staff time. While the client is washing in the bathroom, the bed can be made and housekeeping duties completed. Before the client dresses, the nurse can provide back care and do an assessment of the integument.

The bath at the sink technique is also well suited for the older adult at home. Even in the home environment, independent daily hygiene practices benefit the client both physically and psychologically. It is goal-oriented behavior, and it stimulates and refreshes.

Eyes

A frequent eye hygiene used by older adults is an eye wash or irrigation with a boric acid and water solution. This might be a danger to the client because it is toxic if absorbed from any open skin area. Boric acid also has a low saturation level, leaving many undissolved crystals in the irrigating solution. These crystals act as foreign bodies in the eye, causing abrasions. Health teaching regarding eye hygiene should include this information, because the practice is so wide-spread in the older adult population.

The nurse should emphasize the importance of clean hands before beginning any care of the eye. *Staphylococcus aureus* and *Escherichia coli* are common sources of infection that are easily eliminated with handwashing after toileting. Demonstrate to the client the method of cleaning the eye lashes and eye lids using separate corners of a clean face cloth or tissues for each eye, wiping from the inner canthus out. This method reduces the risk of introducing discharge into the naso-lacrimal duct, which drains the eye. Frequently, the older adult experiences dry crusting material on the eye upon awakening, which can be a result of excessive tearing, windy weather, or the glare from sun and snow. If such tearing or crustiness occur, cleanse the eye with tepid water.

Eyeglasses. A great majority of the older population wear eyeglasses. The nurse should teach the client to include eyeglass care as a part of daily hygiene. Often the older adult's eye sight is diminished further because of heavily soiled or poorly fitting eyeglasses. Each morning the glass and frames should be cleaned with cool running water or glass-cleaning solution and dried with a lint-free cloth. Using hot water can cause plastic frames to warp. Using tissues can scratch plastic lenses. Glasses should be cleaned over a towel, so if dropped, they will not break. If the client does not wear the glasses continuously, they should be kept in a case, glass caddy, or hung from the neck with a chain or ribbon. Glasses not protected become scratched, further distorting the client's vision. The client should routinely place his glasses in a particular location, so he can find them quickly when needed. This practice reduces the risk of losing the glasses when a food tray is removed or when bed linen and clothing are changed. The client's name should be marked on the frame. The

method of identification depends upon the size of the frame and material from which the frame is made.

Both glare and windy conditions in the outdoors cause irritation and diminished acuity caused by tearing and squinting. Although not suitable for all older adults, nonglare sunglasses are helpful to many. These glasses can be made up in prescription lens as well as a clip-on model for regular glasses. An alternative outdoor eye protection device is a broad-brimmed hat or a hat with a sun visor.

Contact lenses. Many older adults now wear contact lenses, particularly after cataract surgery. Contact lenses are particularly useful for the older adult because they provide correction of peripheral vision which glasses do not. Nursing intervention should include a demonstration of aseptic technique and proper handling of cleansing solution. The nurse should also verify that the client removes his contact lenses each evening before retiring. Sleeping in contact lenses can predispose the older adult to corneal abrasions. The cornea receives oxygen not from its own blood supply, but takes oxygen from the atmosphere and tears. Since the metabolic rate of the cornea increases when a client is wearing contact lenses, it needs the oxygen available during the night hours when the lenses are out.

Adequate moisture in the air can prevent dryness in the eyes. The nurse should adjust environmental conditions so that the relative humidity range is between 30 and 60 percent. For the client whose home is very dry, the nurse can suggest a cool water humidifier or dishes, containers, or cans of water placed near the radiator as aids in humidification of a room.

Ears

Accumulated cerumen in the ear of the older adult client is a frequent cause of reduced auditory acuity. The packing of cerumen in the ear can be minimized through daily ear hygiene. When cerumen softens and flows out of the ear, it collects in the auricle. The auricle should be cleansed with warm soapy water and dried with a towel. A small edge of the towel is gently inserted, never pushed, into the external auditory canal. Water and cerumen are drawn out by capillary action. Any attempt to cleanse the area with a cotton swab simply forces the cerumen back against the tympanum in a hard, packed mass. Health teaching includes instructing the client not to insert hairpins, paper clips, or any other objects into the ear in an attempt to clean it. Some sources recommend irrigations of Water Pik spray to remove cerumen. However, caution should be taken before undertaking such a procedure. Excessive cerumen accumulation can be caused by irritating dust or from fungal or bacterial infections in the ear. A perforated ear drum can produce hard, cerumenlike discharge. When the nurse, using an otoscope, observes packed cerumen, the client should be referred to a physician.

Hearing aids. When the client wears a hearing aid, care of the instrument should be included as part of daily hygiene measures. The ear mold and receiver are separated and washed with warm soap and water. Because cerumen can accumulate in the cannula, it is checked for patency. If cerumen is present, the cannula is cleaned and dried with a pipe cleaner. Before the instrument is inserted into the ear, batteries are checked for functioning. Have the client keep an extra set of batteries available for quick replacement if the old battery begins to decline in power. The volume switch should be in the "off" position as the hearing aid is placed in the client's ear. The tubing or cord should be straight, with the ear mold hanging free. Turn the switch on, and adjust the volume. When the volume is too high, the client hears distorted sounds. Often an audible squeal can be heard. If the instrument does not appear to be working, remove it and check to see if the switch is on and if the battery if working.

When the hearing aid is removed, the client should store it in its own box, away from sources of heat and direct sunlight. To preserve battery power, it is taken out when the appliance is not in use. Extra batteries retain their freshness longer when stored in the refrigerator.

Nose

The same rules for nasal hygiene that apply to other age groups apply to the older adult. The one area that might present a difference in hygienic care is the grooming of nasal hair. Older adult males in particular often have large amounts of nasal hair, some of which extend beyond the nares.

For those cultures that consider nasal hair unsightly, trimming of nasal hair becomes a necessity. The client should have at hand a mirror, tissues, blunt-end nasal hair scissors, and the procedure should be carried out in a well-lighted room. Only those hairs that extend beyond the nares are trimmed, and much care must be taken not to nick the skin of the nose itself. Instead of a scissors, some men prefer to use the large straight-edge toenail clipper. They find it safer and easier to handle. These hairs should never be tweezed because of the risk of infection at the hair's root inside the nose.

Care of mouth and teeth

Teeth in good condition offer the opportunity for eating pleasure, adequate first-stage digestion in mastication, and body image. If the client is to be well nourished and have opportunities for communication, sociability, and the sensation of taste, oral hygiene and good dental care are a must. As for all other age groups, the older adult should have an orientation to health maintenance of the teeth. Prevention of decay and loss are the goals. Most older adults today lived in an era when problem teeth were pulled rather than treated. Complex dental surgery and root canals were not available. Most older adults share the mistaken belief of the general population that it is natural to lose all your teeth, just as loss of hair and hearing are manifestations of aging.

Prevention of tooth decay should begin as a primary focus for basic primary hygiene care for the client. It is unfortunate that dental care is such an expensive and costly item in an older adult's budget. Because there is little or no money available for oral preventive care, the older adult is often denied the right of health maintenance.

Prevailing attitudes mistakenly believe that oral disease is present only when you have toothache or bleeding and swollen gums. Very often chronic low-grade dental disease smolders for a long time without overt symptoms. A complete oral cavity assessment should be performed at least once a month while the client is under the nurse's care. All older adults should have oral hygiene care a minimum of once a day.

The smell and appearance of the mouth are a great part of the client's social acceptability.

A clean, fresh-tasting mouth is very pleasant and comforting no matter what setting the client is in—home, hospital, or long-term-care facility.

Evaluate the client's living style and how it would affect the routine of oral care. A person who is outgoing and has many social commitments will be attentive to his teeth or dentures and the condition of his mouth. Elderly women who wear makeup and lipstick regard their mouth and lips as a part of their overall style.

Oral hygiene and nursing care. Teach the staff the importance of routine oral hygienic care as a part of the daily care. If oral hygiene care is delegated to nurse assistants, the nurse should check to see if these tasks are done satisfactorily. As a point of in-service education, the nursing assistants should be reminded of the importance of oral hygiene. Have the staff brush one another's teeth. This exercise gives the staff the sense of how it feels to be the client dependent upon them for hygienic care. Often an assignment of not brushing his own teeth for the first 3 hours after he gets out of bed is enough to convince a staff member of the fundamental comfort level affected by oral hygiene.

Motivate both the family and the client toward good hygiene. The client as well as the family should be taught how to do an assessment of the mouth. Bad breath, bleeding, or receding gum lines, and inflamed or swollen tissue signal the client's need for dental care. Any discomfort or pain when chewing or talking, intolerance to hot or cold fluids, or crusted thickened saliva also indicates a particular need for oral hygiene. Nutritional level and condition of the oral cavity are intimately related, particularly for the older adult. If an older adult's appetite decreases, or there is evidence of an apparent weight loss, one area of investigation should be the mouth. The older man or woman often resorts to a diet of tea and toast, eliminating other food from the diet, when eating or chewing is painful.

The gums are particularly vulnerable to infection; yet it may be difficult for the client to ask others about his oral hygiene. The nurse should take the first step and ask questions regarding comfort and hygiene. Dental examinations should be part of semiannual or annual routine of health maintenance for the older adult. A visit to the dentist or having the dentist come to the long-term-care facility as part of overall services makes it available to the client.

Providing privacy and assistance. While preparing to address the oral hygiene needs of the client, recognize that it is a sensitive and personal procedure. Provide privacy and be considerate of the person's feeling of self when dentures are removed from the mouth for cleaning. Provide abundant running water, dentifrice, the brush, wastebasket or bag, and extra tissues. When doing care for the client or when teaching the client proper oral hygiene, emphasize that the tissue is sensitive and one must be gentle while doing hygiene measures. If the client has a right-sided or left-sided weakness, do check for food left in the mouth on that side. In addition, if there is recent memory loss because of a neurological problem, the client may forget if oral hygiene care was done. It is up to the nurse to follow through and assist him as necessary.

If the client's hands are unsteady or weak, it is useful to provide toothbrushes adapted for these situations. Often electric toothbrushes are useful, and although each client has his own attachment, the base of the appliance can be shared by a number of clients. When electric toothbrushes are used, the brush part must be changed more frequently and each should have an identifying name tag.

Oral hygiene must be done as a routine part of care. It should not be left until the end of the bed bath, because then it is often forgotten. Oral hygiene is not a frill to be left until there is some extra time, but a necessity basic to the client's physical and emotional health.

Gums and mucous membranes. Saliva both serves as a part of the digestive process and has a bacteriostatic action as it washes across the gums and teeth. In the older adult, it is not uncommon to have decreased salivary activity. A combination of decreased fluid intake, the presence of dentures, such drugs as reserpine, chlorpromazine, cholinergic blocking agents, antihistamines, and radiation to the head and neck all cause the saliva to become thicker. It works less as a cleaning mechanism for the mouth and actually can cause dentures to slip. With the thickened saliva, a brownish crust forms called *sordes*. These foul-smelling crusts present a complicated nursing problem. Useful remedies include increasing the client's fluid intake, increasing the humidity in the room, and lubricating the client's mouth and lips. Irrigations and swabbing with half-strength peroxide (USP 3% peroxide) help remove food organisms and epithelial waste material. Additional nursing actions include offering the client sugar-free sodas to sip or other carbonated beverages such as ginger ale or Seven-Up. The carbonated action of the sodas seems to thin out the salivary secretions and have a very comforting effect on the client's mouth. Sour candy balls help stimulate salivary activity and relieve the dryness. Always encourage the client to rinse his mouth more frequently with water or a pleasant-tasting mouthwash. Eating and drinking more frequently also help decrease the discomfort from the diminished salivary volume. All gum and mucous membrane care should be gentle. In the older adult, sensitive tissue can be damaged from coarse textured foods and too vigorous oral hygiene measures.

The older adult on antibiotic therapy is particularly vulnerable to fungal or *Candida* infections (moniliasis). Drugs used as anticonvulsants such as phenytoin (Dilantin) can cause hyperplasia, an excessive formation of gum tissue.

Often, because of dryness in the air from central heating or poor intake of fluids, the older adult suffers from dry, cracked lips. An application of lanolin, cocoa butter, or petroleum jelly is very effective and comforting. These creams act as softening agents and keep the tissues pliable. Their effect is produced by decreasing the water evaporation from the tissue of the lips. Mouthwashes are a refreshing conclusion to oral hygiene. Warm, plain tap water is often a very useful and inexpensive mouthwash. Avoid strong medicinal mouthwashes and salt or sodium bicarbonate for those clients on a low-sodium diet.

Water jet spray appliances are not recommended for the older adult, particularly those with cardiac disease. Bacteria can be forced into the bloodstream as placque is being loosened, causing bacterial endocarditis.

In the hospital, hydrogen peroxide or milk of magnesia is used for mouth care. Research studies demonstrated that hydrogen peroxide is better for the over-50 population, and the milk of magnesia is better for the under-50 population.

Hydrogen peroxide has an effervescent, oxidizing action. It debrides accumulated material and reduces the anaerobic microorganism colony count in the mouth, the cause of bad breath or halitosis. If hydrogen peroxide is used as a mouthwash, it must be rinsed thoroughly. Hydrogen peroxide should not be used orally for a prolonged period of time. It can leave the gums spongy and sometimes can cause decalcification of tooth surfaces.

Remedies for dry mouth. After mouth care, have the client apply a plain or favorite-flavored oil—not mineral oil, but a vegetable-based oil. Mineral oil is not absorbed and can cause pneumonia. Often flavored rinses with a little bit of peppermint or lemon juice are effective. Glycerin and lemon juice are not recommended. This combination was found to be hypertonic, which dehydrates and irritates the gum mucosa. When tested, the glycerol and lemon solution was found to be far more drying than a plain sodium chloride solution.

Adjusting to dental prosthesis. Often the older adult does not realize the necessity of having a missing tooth replaced. When a natural tooth is lost, its absence changes the mechanical and biological system, which gives balance and function to the mouth. Adjacent teeth slip over and trap debris underneath, and placque forms that cannot be removed. The remaining teeth move out of alignment as they slip to fill in the missing space. The stress on gum and supporting tissue increases dramatically, and the appearance of the face changes. The cheeks become hollowed, and the bones of the jaw and mandible become prominent.

Speech is affected by the loss of a tooth. Pronunciation of sounds is more natural when the tooth is replaced. If it takes longer than a few days for the client's speech to return to normal, recommend that he be checked again by the dentist.

Missing teeth are replaced by a prosthetic appliance known as a bridge. The bridge substitutes for the missing teeth, reduces stress on adjacent teeth and prevents bone loss around the natural teeth. This mechanical action prevents additional weakening on the natural teeth and makes chewing easier for the client.

A partial denture replaces several missing teeth

and makes contact with gum on both sides of the mouth. Like a bridge, it preserves the remaining teeth. The nurse's role in the use of dentures lies in helping the older person understand the use of dentures, get referral to a dentist, and adjust to the new prosthetic appliance.

Often a feeling of bulk in the new dentures is very disconcerting to the older person. Even if lightweight material is used, the increased difference in texture and size takes a few days to get used to. The client may complain that the tongue feels too large in the mouth, and with tongue action, the denture may be pushed out of the mouth. The nurse can instruct the client to use the muscles of the cheeks and the tongue to hold the denture in place while speaking or eating. One exercise that is helpful in learning how to use the tongue and cheek muscles is to have the client read aloud to the nurse or into a mirror. This slipping of the denture happens particularly with the lower denture when the partial denture is supported by gum rather than by a clasp to the natural teeth.

Encourage the client to begin eating small amounts of soft food. He should take small bites and chew the food slowly and thoroughly. Day by day he can return to his usual diet, eating more coarse foods. Hard foods and foods that have a sticky consistency should be avoided until the client is completely familiar with the dentures. This avoids accidents and embarrassment.

Cooking techniques should be adapted so that the client can be provided with tender food that requires less chewing power. Cooking the foods for longer periods at lower heats and adding more water produces softer, more chewable food. Keep in mind that the biting and chewing capacity of normal teeth is about 300 pounds per square inch and is reduced to 50 pounds per square inch, or even less, when dentures are in place. If clients are uncomfortable with raw vegetables, fruit, or coarse grains, have them eat cooked fruits and vegetables and softer cereals until they are more familiar with the dentures. All care is geared to reducing mouth infections, because with infection the mouth becomes sore, and communication and eating are restricted.

The positive supportive approach of the client's family and nurse is a great help in having the client accept the denture. By wearing the new denture routinely and getting used to its care, the client can enjoy the social, digestive, and communication advantages it affords. If the client does not wear the denture, or if the client is having difficulty with pain and sores in the mouth, investigate the reasons why.

Care of complete dentures. Dentures should be taken out every night. This gives the tissue an opportunity to rest, and the saliva washing over the gums has a bacteriostatic action that will reduce the incidence of mouth infections in the older adult. The gums can be cleaned with a gauze pad. Dentures left out longer than just one night cause the gum tissue to swell. Edema causes poor fit and irritations of the margins of the denture.

Tobacco stains and collected food can lead to tartar formation, just as on natural teeth. The dentures should be brushed and rinsed with cold water after each meal. The mouth and tongue may also be brushed with a soft nylon brush and rinsed with warm water.

When taken out, dentures should be placed in water in a covered receptacle labeled with the client's name. The denture water should be changed daily. The water prevents them from being warped and brittle. Essence of peppermint in the water creates a pleasant taste when dentures are replaced. However, tap water, saline, or commercial preparations are satisfactory too. Do not put dentures in cups or dishes that are used for eating. It is unappetizing and unaesthetic. Avoid transparent containers for the teeth for the same reasons.

Encourage the client to put the teeth back in every morning. If the teeth are left out for too long, the gumline changes. During acute illness the teeth are taken out during different therapies. As soon as possible, the nurse should encourage the client to begin to use the teeth again.

Keep in mind that dentures are fragile and quite expensive. Provide for their safety. Avoid dropping the teeth; chips and breakage occur easily. Vulcanate is porous and absorbs food odors and debris and deteriorates. With a breakdown of the material, a sour odor and taste is produced in the client's mouth.

Stains on dentures can be cleaned only by one of these solutions:

1. One teaspoon of ammonia in 8 ounces of water.
2. One tablespoon of white vinegar in 8 ounces of water.
3. One tablespoon of Clorox and two tablespoons of Calgon detergent in 8 ounces of water.

For hard deposits on the dentures, soak them overnight in white vinegar; brown vinegar will stain the pink base.

Those dentures made of chromium, cobalt, or nickel alloys cannot be cleaned with a Clorox solution. Some family toothpastes discolor the plastics from which dentures are made. Plastic dentures are better than vulcanite because they are lighter and less porous.

Care of natural teeth and partial dentures. The partial denture serves as a brace or splint for the mobile teeth, and it helps the formation of bone around the roots of the tooth. It is imperative that as part of the oral hygiene plan, the nurse include basic principles of cleaning the natural teeth as well as the dentures. Keeping the natural teeth and gums in healthy clean condition is essential to protect the integrity of the tissues of the mouth. When the natural teeth that support the partial denture are lost, the dentist may have to recommend complete dentures.

The natural teeth should be brushed and flossed. Have the client give special attention to the areas under the metal clasps of the partial dentures. The placque formation promotes decay in these areas. Often the older adult thinks that partial denture clasps lead to decay, but this is not the case. It is the placque and debris formation under the clasp that cause tooth decay and loss of the adjacent teeth.

In addition to the usual flossing and brushing routines recommended in nursing textbooks, encourage the client to rinse his mouth first before brushing. The natural teeth should be brushed first, using a soft, round-bristled brush and short vibrating strokes by the tooth margin. By all means, encourage the older adult to use a fluoridated toothpaste on his natural teeth. It will encourage the integrity of the enamel.

When cleaning the partial dentures, brush gently and thoroughly. Use a dentifrice, hand soap, a commercial cleanser, or even bicarbonate of soda. The partial denture can then be soaked in an effervescent cleanser; however, they must first be brushed to get rid of the debris and plaque formation.

Identifying dentures. All dentures should have a permanent identification tag. Have the client request that his name be embedded in the plastic denture material when it is being manufactured. If this has not been done, the nurse can write the client's name on a thin piece of onion skin paper and put it on the denture, and then coat it with three coats of clear nail polish. Commercial tapes are sold that can be marked with the client's name and glued onto the denture.

Repairing broken dentures. Repair of full or partial dentures at home is strongly discouraged by the American Dental Association. Any reforming or reshaping of the metal clasps at the ends of the partial dentures damages their power to support adjacent teeth. Improper filing or relining the base of the denture causes uneven pressure on the gum line and often increases the rate of bone absorption. The added irritation to oral tissue causes pressure sores and even oral cancer. Any complaints of soreness or ill-fitting dentures should be reported to the dentist. The client who complains of a sore or irritation in the mouth for more than a week or two must be referred for examination.

Inserting and removing dentures. To insert dentures, have the client stand over a basin half-filled with water with a towel placed at the bottom of the basin. The water and towel act as cushions and protect the denture if it should be dropped. Apply even, gentle pressure on both sides of the mouth. Use a direct action over the metal clasp, not at the bases of the denture. Explain to the client that he should avoid biting down to set the plate in place. It is much easier to insert a denture when it is wet. A good bond forms between the denture and the gum.

To remove the upper denture, grasp with thumb and index finger, move up and down to break the suction. To remove the lower denture, retract the cheek, turn the cheek slightly to the side, and remove the lower denture at an angle. Rinse with cold water and replace.

Fingernail and hand care

Manicure. The nails of the older adult tend to be ridged, grooved, thickened, and brittle. They grow at a rate of 0.5 mm per week, half the rate of a young adult. In view of the nails' fragility, special nursing intervention is warranted. Weekly manicures, followed by daily care, are recommended.

Equipment for manicure
Towel
Emery board
Q-Tip
Orangewood stick
Cotton
Small basin, bowl, or plastic container, deep enough to submerge fingers
Cold cream, baby oil, petroleum jelly, or cuticle cream
Hand cream or lotion

All nail care should be done in a well-lighted room, so the client can see what he is doing. Some clients with diminished vision will need assistance in doing nail care.

Procedure	Rationale
1. Wash hands under running water. Use pointed end of orangewood stick to clean under nails. Rinse orangewood stick off.	Using a metal instrument to clean under the nails roughens the nail and makes it easier to collect dirt.
2. Dry hands thoroughly.	
3. Massage nails and cuticles with choice of softener rubbed into the sides of the nails and the area where the nail extends over the fingers.	Massage stimulates circulation to the nail beds, promoting strong nails and, thus, preventing thickened nails. Keeping the skin area soft on each side of the nail prevents callous formation. Emollients massaged on cuticles help prevent hangnails. Cuticle separation from nail bed allows organism invasion and chronic paronychia, a frequent problem of older adults.
4. Soak the nails for 3 to 5 minutes in warm, soapy water.	
5. Push back the cuticles gently with a Q-Tip or orangewood stick with cotton or soft towel wrapped around the blunt side.	Harsh rubbing or poking at cuticles causes them to split into hangnails and predisposes the nail bed to infection. Never cut with a clipper or scissors.
6. If the cuticle is torn, cut off the loose flap of skin only.	Cutting into the cuticle itself causes it to thicken and become infected.
7. Shape the nails into an oval with the fine side of the emery board held at a 45-degree angle to the nail. Use a one-directional stroke, rather than a sawing motion.	Cutting the nails tends to make them brittle. A sawing motion leads to rough edges on the nails.
8. The nail should not be filed too close to the sides of the finger.	This prevents injury to the cuticle and skin around and nail.
9. Apply base and nail polish and sealer, if desired.	
10. Apply hand cream.	

The weekly manicure keeps the nails attractive and in good condition. Daily care should also be given to the nails. A moisturizer should be massaged into the nails and cuticles. If no nail polish is used, buffing can be done daily. This encourages circulation to the nail beds. A number of brands of nail polish contain ingredients such as nylon that strengthen the nail and prevent breaking. The older woman might find the softer tone polishes such as mauve, light pinks, or clear polishes most flattering to her hands. Bright red polishes pick up the redness and skin discolorations prevalent in older skin. Older men are often not familiar with a manicure. But it is recommended that older male clients use the same manicure technique as women to protect their nails and cuticles from tears and infections. A clear nail polish on a man's nails gives his hands a well-groomed appearance. Teach the client to keep his hands out of water as much as possible. Nails soaked in water for longer than 5 minutes become very soft, and they break. The client should wear cotton-lined, rubber gloves when hands will be submerged in water or working with harsh chemicals. The skin on the back of the older adult's hands is particularly delicate. The client should always wear gloves when going out in cold weather to prevent chapping and loss of body heat. Gloves should also be worn when gardening and working with cleaning solutions.

Leg, foot, and toenail care

Client mobility is related to foot comfort to such a great extent that shoe and foot care are an important part of nursing intervention. In addition, diminished peripheral circulation in the older adult makes special attention to his legs and feet a necessity. Prophylaxis is the key. All sources of bruises, abrasions, and infection should be eliminated. Some general rules for protecting the legs and feet of the older adult follow.

1. The knees should be padded when doing gardening or other work requiring kneeling.
2. Tight bands or clothing around the waist, legs, or feet, such as tight belts, tight undergarments, garters, elastic top socks, and knee-high stockings should be avoided.
3. Closed-toe slippers and shoes should be worn.
4. Shoes should fit correctly with no areas of pinching, binding, or rubbing the skin.
5. New shoes should be broken in over a period of days. New shoes should be worn for no more than 30 minutes at a time while breaking them in.
6. Stockings and socks should be changed each day. Socks should be made of 100 percent natural fibers, cotton or wool.
7. Shoes should never be worn without socks. Shoe or sneaker liners should not bind or constrict the toes.
8. For cold feet at night, bed socks should be worn. The bed should be warmed with an electric blanket rather than a hot water bottle or heating pad.
9. Shoes and slippers should be worn at all times to avoid injury to the foot and to reduce the risk of athlete's foot.
10. The water temperature should *always* be tested before immersing feet. Start with cooler water, and add warmer water as needed.
11. Heavier leg coverings should be worn during cold winter weather (wool slacks, snuggies, long-leg underwear, cotton stockings, and knitted or fiber-filled leg warmers).
12. Legs should be crossed at the ankles, not at the knees.
13. The legs should be elevated for 15 minutes periodically throughout the day to prevent venous stasis.

The older adult's feet are prone to corns and callouses. In addition to causing pain, they are a hazard to mobility. A corn is a keratosis resulting from friction and pressure on the bony prominences of toe joints. The corn penetrates deep into the soft tissue, and sometimes even into the bone. Corns can be prevented from forming by massaging the foot and toes to increase circulation and avoiding pressure areas from footwear. Teach the client the characteristics of changes in bone with age. Changes in the bony spine, such as osteoporosis and kyphosis, alter the center of gravity and change the distribution of the body weight across the feet. Although the length of the foot does not change, the contour of the toes change as bone overgrowth at the joints, or lipping, progresses. Contour changes occur also as a result of arthritis. A condition called *hammer toe* is prevalent in the older adult also. The weight of the body falls on the second toe, and it is elongated. The tendon does not grow proportionately, forcing the joint to contract, causing callouses to form on the toe superiorly.

Shoe styles worn by the older adult should accommodate their changing foot contour due to weight loss, atrophy, and swelling. It is recommended by orthopedists that shoes have a "(1) straight inside line, (2) adequate space for the forefoot without undue spreading, (3) sufficient length to prevent pressure on the ends of the toes, and (4) a low heel as broad as the foot itself" (Henderson and Nite, 1978). The shoe should have a reinforced shank and counter, and enough room for each toe to bear weight and turn in walking. Lower or midhigh heel shoes distribute the body weight evenly across the foot. Higher heeled shoes throw the center of gravity of the body forward, causing added weight on the toes. The front of the shoe should be rounded enough to accommodate the toes in proper alignment.

If the client experiences foot edema, the width

of the vamp should be sufficient enough to accommodate the foot. Clients with edema whose feet size vary should choose a loafer or slip-on wedge rather than an oxford. Sneakers and playshoes do not offer enough protection for the older adult and are discouraged. A cushioned inner sole and the natural ventilation provided by leather or calfskin rather than manmade materials offer added comfort.

Foot discomfort affects general health and mobility; pain is felt locally as well as in other parts of the body; the client tires easily, and he has an abnormal gait. In addition to assessing the client's feet and shoes, the nurse should teach him body mechanics in sitting, standing, and walking. In special cases, the nurse may refer the client to an orthopedic shoe store or have a representative from the store visit the client at home or in the agency. These stores are able to apply special shoe padding, and have steam and other equipment for adjusting leather shoes to the contour of the client's feet. On occasion, a consultation with a podiatrist will be required. Molded arches and other shoe appliances may be prescribed. The nurse should inform the client that Medicare partial reimbursement is available for the older adult's visit to the podiatrist. Those clients on Medicaid can often get physician or podiatrist foot diagnostic services paid for according to the state program. When foot ailments are diagnosed and treated early, the extent of the damage is limited and client mobility is preserved.

Treatments at the podiatrist's office can be very pleasant for the older adult. The feet are soaked in a whirlpool bath, then the corns and callouses are treated, and lubricating lotion, mole skin, or corn plasters applied. Thickened toenails require the podiatrist's special instruments for cutting. Most long-term-care facilities have a podiatrist as a consultant. The diabetic client should receive special instructions and care regarding the feet.

Foot hygiene

Foot hygiene is very similar to the hygienic care of the hands and fingernails. The nurse can demonstrate the foot care procedure to the client and his family. After a return demonstration, the client can then carry out his own foot care at least once a week. Because the legs and feet are often difficult areas to reach, assistance can be given by the nurse as indicated.

Equipment for pedicure

A plastic or metal basin half filled with warm, soapy water at 88° F to 95° F (31.1° C to 35° C) and large enough for complete immersion of the feet

A straight-edge toenail clipper

Orangewood stick with the tip wrapped in cotton

Nail buffer

Pumice stone

Towel

Cuticle cream, petroleum jelly, or mineral oil, lubricating lotion or cream

Optional

Nail polish

Nail polish remover

Clear base coat polish

Polish sealer

Dusting powder or spray cologne

Foot hygiene procedure

1. Under good lighting, inspect the feet including between and under the toes for signs of redness, cracking, abrasions, lacerations, scaling, corns, callouses, hammer toes, ingrown toenails, skin color, temperature, presence of hair on the toes, blanching of the nail beds, thickness of the nails, and mobility of the nail at the base. A check of the pedal pulse quality and rate can be made also.

2. Have the client soak his feet in the warm, soapy water for 10 minutes.

3. While the feet are in the water, have client wriggle his toes, stretch his foot, flex and extend his toes and ankles, and bring the foot and toes through a full range of motion.

4. Rinse the feet, pat each foot dry, include the areas between each toe.

5. Massage the selected emollient preparation onto the feet and nails.

6. Use the pumice stone to remove dry, dead skin on the heels and sides of the feet.

7. Razors or other sharp instruments should never be used to shave off calloused or horny skin.

8. Clip toenails straight across. If the nails are pitted, discolored, fungus-infested, ram-

shorn shaped, painfully inverted, or badly ingrown, a podiatrist should cut them.

9. Do not clip nails too short on clients with circulatory insufficiency or probe in the nail groves.

10. The thick deformed nails of the older adult sometimes adhere to the skin and turn inward. To prevent this, use an orangewood stick under the nail to loosen the skin adherence. After clipping the nails straight across, place a wisp of cotton or lamb's wool with the orangewood stick under each corner. This encourages the nail to grow outward. The cotton or lamb's wool should be changed daily.

11. Rub cuticle cream, petroleum jelly, or mineral oil into the nails and cuticles.

12. With a cotton-wrapped orangewood stick, push back the cuticles gently.

13. As an anticipatory guidance measure, discourage the client from using harsh irritants (which may break the skin and cause a dermatitis) such as corn nostrums, medicated plasters, silver nitrate, or tincture of iodine over an inflamed bunion, corn, fissure between toes, nail grooves, or ingrown toenails. Moleskin, lamb's wool, and emollients are the safest preparations to use on the feet. Encourage the client to seek professional help and discourage self-diagnosis and treatment of foot ailments.

14. Apply body lotion, cologne, or dusting powder to feet.

15. Wipe off excess lotion with towel. Put on clean socks or stockings and shoes or slippers.

After foot hygiene, clients often state that they feel very relaxed and clean. Foot hygiene can be counted as one of the most valuable comfort measures that nursing can render. For the older adult, pain-free, well-cared-for feet are a prerequisite for an active life-style.

First aid care for the feet. Until a podiatrist can be seen, the nurse can suggest or render the following foot first aid care.

Painful corns and callouses. Apply petroleum jelly or cold cream and dress lightly. Avoid wearing the shoes that are causing the friction or pressure on the toe.

Suppurating soft corn. Apply a continuous cold wet dressing of either saline (1 teaspoon table salt in 1 cup of water) or boric acid (1 teaspoon of boric acid crystals to 1 cup of water).

Athlete's foot, itching, and burning. Spray with aerosol merthiolate or apply a fungicidal powder. Cover foot with tubular gauze number three or white cotton socks.

Fissure between toes. Swab with peroxide, alcohol, or mercurochrome. Place cotton or lint square between the toes.

Painful metatarsal head. Make a 2 inch × 2 inch × ¼ inch pad from a foam rubber make-up pad or chamois. Place the pad inside the sock or stocking on the sole of the foot.

Burning and itching (without rash). Rub with witch hazel or a mentholated preparation. Wear light-weight cotton stockings or socks. Nylon hose are hot and irritating, obstructing air to feet and causing an itching and burning sensation, especially in warm weather.

Abrasion or blister. This demands immediate attention. Dress lightly with ½-inch gauze, lamb's wool, absorbent lint bandage, or narrow tubular gauze.

Profuse perspiration and foot odor. Swab feet twice daily with rubbing alcohol or witch hazel. Dry thoroughly, and dust feet with a foot powder or antiseptic powder. Wear white cotton socks, and change twice daily to keep feet dry.

Hair hygiene

An individual's appearance makes a statement about how he feels about himself. Because depression occurs at a high rate in the older adult population, the nurse should note any changes in the client's personal appearance, particularly in the hair care and clothing.

Nursing intervention addressed to hair cleanliness and style assists the older adult personally as well as socially. Grooming of the hair encourages the older adult to extend himself to present a neat and atrractive public image.

He should brush and comb his hair every day. These actions stimulate scalp circulation and distribute the natural oils to the ends of the hair shaft. Once a week the hair should be washed with mild shampoo. The hair of the older adult is often dry, and shampoos designed for dry hair can be suggested. Baby shampoos are useful because they are mild and cause no irritation if soap gets into the eyes.

It is convenient to wash the hair as a part of the shower or tub bath. Some older adults with arthritis or osteoporosis find it uncomfortable to bend over a kitchen or bathroom sink to wash their hair. Sinks equipped with a spray hose attachment are suitable, because the spray enables the older adult to rinse the shampoo out completely. Once a month, older adults should condition their hair with a warm oil treatment. Corn oil is better than olive oil because it penetrates the hair shaft. A teaspoon of corn oil is warmed and then is combed through the hair. The hair is wrapped in a warm, wet towel, and after 30 minutes, the hair is shampooed thoroughly. This treatment helps prevent the hair ends from splitting and adds a sheen to the hair.

When the client's hair is very fine, have her blot her hair dry with a towel and then apply a setting lotion. The hair will hold its set longer and be easier to comb. The types of rollers or clips used to set the client's hair depend on what type of curls the client desires and how much dexterity she has with hands. Friends or family members can make hair care a social time by setting each other's hair. Many older women enjoy having their hair washed and set by a beautician in a hair salon. Reduced rates are often available for older women on a midweek day. Most hospitals and long-term-care facilities have barber and beautician services available.

The older adult's hair should be cut at least once every 8 weeks. A style that is simple and flattering helps the older adult present a well-groomed appearance without undue work. A style that has a soft edge (less geometry) and waves or curls is becoming. A hair style that lifts the hair off the temples makes the face appear softer. When the older adult's hair becomes thin and fine, a cut that is rather short looks fuller and frames the face. Longer hair has more weight, which causes a flat look at the crown. If at all possible, the haircut should be done by a professional haircutter. It looks easy to cut a simple short style, yet it requires complicated sectioning to give a good styling. The haircut is the basis of a well-groomed look.

The hair should be covered when going out in cold weather. Freezing temperatures can cause the older adult's dry hair to become brittle and split. If static electricity is a problem, a wide-toothed aluminum comb is helpful. Permanent waves are preferred by many older women. When care is taken to keep hair conditioned, permanents reduce the time needed to keep hair in an attractive style. A client who uses hair spray should be advised to apply it only in a well-ventilated room and to cover the eyes and nose while spraying. The aerosol mist can be aspirated and cause lung irritation.

The loss of hair with age exposes the scalp to danger of sun burn when the client is out of doors. Both older men and women should wear a cap or hat while in the sun. Male hair loss is almost always at the temple area where the skin is thin and especially sensitive to sunburn. A sunscreen lotion or cream should be applied daily. This area of skin is a very vulnerable one to the development of keratosis. The nurse should assess for these precancerous lesions as she inspects the integument.

Wigs, chignons, and toupees. There are times when older adults (male and female) express concern over the thinning and loss of their hair. Many of these clients opt to purchase hairpieces. In addition to these, other older adults buy hairpieces to have hair care convenience and the fun of having the selection of hair styles. Because the hairpiece affects the hygiene of the hair and scalp, the nurse should offer anticipatory guidance in both the purchase and care of a hairpiece.

Choosing a hairpiece. When choosing a hairpiece, the client should look for a base with loose lattices of flexible ribbon or meshwork that will permit air circulation to the hair and scalp. The client's eye color and skin color are considered in the selection of the hair color of the hairpiece. The style should be flattering to the shape of the client's face. The basic shape and arrangement of the hair in a synthetic hairpiece cannot be changed because it is styled into the hair. Some simple modifications can be made to suit the individual client's preference by cutting bangs or softening curls. However, fit is final, and the client should be satisfied with it before leaving the store. The hairpiece should be tested and proved comfortable enough to stay in place during a vigorous head shake and tilting of the head. It should feel comfortable and secure on the client's head.

When putting on the wig or toupee, the client should hold it in the front, place it over the forehead, and work it over the back of the head, similar to putting on a swimming cap. The client should observe himself in a full-length mirror to get the total effect of the hairpiece. A hand mirror may be used to observe the look of the back of the head.

Wear and upkeep of a hairpiece. If the client has short hair, it is tucked in and under around the bottom of the wig with the tail of a rat tooth comb. The client may prefer combing the sides of her hair back and securing it with a bobby pin. Long hair may be parted into sections and pinned down into side, flat pincurls, rolled into a flat chignon, or gathered in the back, turned up and pinned flat against the back of the head. It is recommended that a wig be worn for no more than 5 or 6 hours at a time. Wigs of any weight cause the scalp to perspire more than normal, and continuous wear can cause dandruff and other scalp damage.

Wigs are kept cleaned and styled by brushing with a Denman-type brush. If worn frequently, a wig should be washed once a month in cool water with a wig cleaner or Woolite and rinsed with cool water. Hang to dry over a towel rack away from direct heat. Brushing when wet will remove the curl. Have the client wait until the wig is dry, shake it to fluff it up, then style with a brush. It may be stored on a wig stand or in a drawer or box. Avoid crushing the wig tightly, because the headband and hair can become mishapen. Chignon and toupee care is similar.

Removing facial hair. Changing hormone balances frequently cause hair to grow on the face of older women. If these hairs cause embarrassment, they can be removed by tweezing, waxing, depilatory, or electrolysis. If the client does not find facial shaving too masculine, it is a quick way to remove these hairs. Contrary to popular belief, shaving does not make hair grow in faster or coarser. Never pull a hair growing from a mole. If the hair is to be cut, care must be taken not to cut the mole.

Eyebrows change in thickness with aging. Men's eyebrows become fuller and coarser. If they appear too unruly, a man can brush or comb them in one direction for a neater appearance. Women's eyebrows thin out, often becoming very sparse in the outer third. A light gray or charcoal colored eyebrow pencil can be used to contour the brows. Loss of the outer third of eyebrow hair can be a sign of thyroid disease. The nurse noting such a loss should assess the client for presence of additional signs of thyroid dysfunction.

Hair care for black women. Here is some baseline information regarding a black older adult's hair:

- Hair is normally dry.
- Dry shampoos aggravate dryness.
- Oils applied to the scalp and hair prevent dryness and breaking at the follicle and splitting of the ends.
- Hair is usually curly and subject to matting and tangling.
- Mineral oil lessens the degree of dryness.
- Discuss with the client her usual hair care practice.
- Well-cared-for, attractive hair meets a physiological need.
- Cultural hair styles enhance the client's self-concept and self-esteem.

Method A (natural hair)

- Shampoo hair and apply a cream rinse, then apply oil, and style or set. An alternate method of cleansing follows.
- Check scalp for cuts.
- Ask the client about allergies to oils and alcohols.
- Secure the client's permission for type of hair care preferred.
- Mix 1 ounce of alcohol with four ounces of mineral oil together in a labeled bottle. Warm by immersing bottle in warm water. Shake mixture vigorously to emulsify. Pour slowly onto the scalp and hair to thoroughly massage into the area, making sure it penetrates the ends of the hair.
- Comb saturated scalp and hair by starting at the front and combing toward the nape of the neck using wide-tooth comb (Afro-Comb).
- The natural direction of combing is from the nape of the neck forward for client in a sitting position. This assures that no matted hair is overlooked.
- Support the hair next to the scalp to prevent pulling while freeing tangles.
- When tangles are free, towel dry the hair.
- Apply warm olive oil, baby oil, or usual lubri-

cant to hair (alcohol will have removed oils from the hair and scalp in cleaning process).

- Massage oil gently into scalp and hair until it is less dry.
- Remove excess oil with a clean towel.
- Women with Afro hair styles may use a hot blow-out comb to make the Afro fuller.
- Recomb hair and style in usual manner, then roll on curlers or braid to prevent matting and tangling.

Method B (chemically treated hair). Many black older women prefer a permanent relaxer applied to their hair approximately 20 to 30 minutes before shampooing. Companies such as Ultra Sheen, Black & Lovely, and L'Oréal make permanent relaxers that leave the hair easy to manage. After this type of treatment, the hair will only require shampooing, oiling of the scalp, and setting. Application of these relaxers is needed approximately every 60 to 90 days depending on the texture of the hair. To shampoo hair, simply use any regular shampoo, and apply a cream rinse, such as Tame, Wella Balsam, or similar products.

Another preference of black older women is the use of a hot pressing comb. These clients may use a Vigorol relaxer, which is applied to the hair using the same procedure as mentioned above for permanent relaxers.

Vigorol detangles and "loosens" the texture of the hair, which leaves it more manageable to enable easier usage of the hot pressing comb. Pressing combs are either electric or made of metal to allow for heating on the stove. The hair is sectioned and the warm comb is run through it to straighten the hair. Care should be taken not to burn the scalp. Hair can then be worn in a straight style, set in rollers, or braided to the client's preference. A Vigorol treatment should be applied once monthly, or when coarseness begins to return.

A wide-tooth comb, Afro-Comb, or stiff-bristled brush should be used on a black clients' hair. These items will prevent pulling and tugging of the hair, which could cause scalp irritation.

If the client does not use a commercial pomade product, get permission to use either mineral oil, olive oil, or white petroleum jelly.

Hair care for black men. Older adult black men usually prefer the natural hair style. A regular shampoo and conditioner detangler is used. Several commercial companies such as Afro Sheen manufacture a full line of hair care products, which include shampoos, conditioners, oils, and sprays. After oiling, some older black men with slightly longer hair braid it. It is combed out later with an Afro-Comb to make the Afro style fuller. These men may also prefer a hot blow-out comb, which is used in a similar manner to a woman's electric pressing comb.

For older adult black men who prefer a permanent relaxer, there is a special mild cream relaxer on the market for men called Sta-Sof-Fro Style Kit. It leaves the hair soft and lustrous looking for blow-outs, and curly, wavy, or straight styles. Men, too, have a choice of hair care products that best suit their individual preferences for a style that reflects their personality and self-concept.

Cosmetics

When morning hygienic care is finished, many older women apply facial cosmetics. These ageless beauty rituals are a part of the woman's social self-image and play a positive part in self-esteem. The nurse should encourage her client to continue these grooming practices knowing that when a woman feels good about herself, her health is optimized. Admission to a long-term-care facility should not be a cause for a decline in the woman's physical appearance.

Knowing the characteristic changes of the skin with aging, the nurse is in a good position to help the older woman keep her cosmetics tastefully applied and flattering to her skin. When assisting the client in bathing, the nurse shares with the client the benefits of well-cleaned and moisturized skin.

Before any makeup can be applied, the face should be cleaned thoroughly. After cleaning, moisturizing is the most important skin care activity. A moisturizer acts as a protective layer to the skin. It does not penetrate the skin, but protects it like a film of plastic wrap, so that moisture is held within the skin and dryness is reduced. Conversely, when moisturizers are applied, air impurities and makeup do not penetrate and the skin is protected. Older women may be familiar with glycerin and rose water creams and soaps. The nurse should discourage use of these products because they draw water to them and out of the skin.

Creams containing estrogens and other hormones are of questionable value and are potentially dangerous. Older skin does not necessarily have to have a thick, heavy moisturizer, but it does benefit by a good amount of light moisturizer. Moisturizer is applied to clean, damp skin. This helps to spread it smoothly with less drag on the skin tissue. The client should apply the moisturizer from breasts to the hairline in gentle upward strokes, paying particular attention to the throat and delicate tissues around the eyes. These areas have little sebaceous gland activity in youth and even less in the older woman. Any remaining moisturizer on the hands should be applied to the elbows and feet—why waste it? If commercial moisturizers are too expensive for the client, she might have soy oil or almond oil in her kitchen. Both will go a long way to moisturize dry, parched, flaking skin.

The nurse can explain that with age the skin becomes thinner and so a sheerer foundation is needed. Heavy or dry foundations accentuate wrinkles and further dry the skin. Many older women are used to using powdered rouge. Light liquid blushers blend smoothly over the tissue-like skin of the older woman and give a soft, translucent glow to the skin, rather than a dry spot of color from powdered rouge.

The older woman should avoid drawing a hard, definite line with the eyebrow pencil. A soft, feather stroke with a light colored pencil or brush will accent the eyes without a harsh look. Use an eyebrow brush to fluff up thinning, light colored brows by running it across the eyebrow in the opposite direction of the growth of the hairs. Brush the eyebrows again from the inner aspect out. Any color used around the eye or eyelid to shadow or highlight the eyes should be light-textured liquid. Powdered eye shadows accent the crepe paper folds of the eyelids. Avoid pearlized, frosted makeup and face powder because they give older skin a hard and caked look.

Lipsticks in the more subdued tones, rather than the fiery reds are usually more becoming to the older woman. Lip gloss is a must; it gives lips a soft luxurious glow. Lipstick also has a therapeutic use of keeping the lips soft and moisturized, which prevents chapping. Clients prone to cracked lips and chapping may use Chap Stick, lanolin or Vaseline on their lips.

The goal of making up the face is to have a soft, dewy look. The goal is not to have the older woman look like a teenager, but rather to present a mature yet contemporary look. A woman who uses the same makeup she used 30 years ago looks dated. By taking advantage of the technology of the cosmetic field, she can treat her skin to moisturized makeup that flatters her new complexion. Cosmetics need not be expensive; many good brands can be bought in drug stores, supermarkets, and department stores. Encourage the client to try the tester bottles available at cosmetic counters. Advise the client to buy small bottles of makeup rather than large ones. The cosmetics themselves do separate with time or dry out. Clients should feel free to explore new colors and brands as the seasons change, because complexions will vary and makeup should vary accordingly.

If the client is interested in learning the "tricks of the trade" in applying cosmetics, she can have the cosmetologist select the correct shades for skin color and facial contours.

Makeup should be removed with an oil or a cream, then the face is washed with soap. If possible, the client should apply a skin freshener that removes the last traces of makeup and soap. The client should then apply a moisturizer as she did in the morning.

It is fun for the clients in a long-term-care facility or day-care center to have a makeup demonstration day or even an entire course on hair care and makeup. Revlon and Mary Kay Cosmetics are two of many cosmetic firms that present such demonstrations.

Basic list of makeup. Purchase items in small sizes and keep in a waterproof plastic zippered bag to prevent clutter in the bathroom or bureau drawer.

Two liquid eye shadow colors
One mascara wand
One child's toothbrush (for eyebrows)
One tweezer
Six cotton balls
One lipstick brush
Two lipsticks
One lip gloss
One liquid foundation
One blusher
One skin freshener

One moisturizer
One small bottle baby oil
One emery board
One cuticle cream
One perfume spray

Cosmetics for black clients. The older adult black woman has several cosmetic houses that manufacture makeup in warm tones and a variety of skin care products. Fashion Fair is one of the leading companies whose products are especially created for the black woman. It is available at the Fashion Fair counter in leading department stores. Moisture lotion and deep rich warm tones such as Ebony Brown Glo Creame Foundation, Royal Red Blush, Burgundy Brown Eye Shadow, Dark Orange Lip Liner Pencil, and Cinnamon Crush Lipstick are samples of the colors available to promote a naturally, freshly, glowing skin for the older adult.

Another company called Honey and Spice manufactures face makeup (pressed powder, liquid makeup, blusher, eye shadow, mascara, lipstick) and nail polish at reasonable prices. The Honey and Spice line of cosmetics may be purchased in a drug, variety, or discount store.

Ambi Skin Cream with Moisturizers is another trade name product manufactured for the black older adult skin. Within 3 to 5 weeks, it is supposed to "fade the darkness that appears in wrinkles and laugh lines and uneven color blotches in mature skin."

The same general guidelines in makeup application may be used by the black older adult.

Facial care for the older male

As much as attractively applied cosmetics enhance the self-esteem of the older woman, so does attention to facial grooming add to an older man's good feelings about his appearance. During daily hygiene, the nurse should encourage the male client to shave his face and trim his mustache, beard, and/or sideburns. The older male's skin is dry and thin, as is the older woman's. Although aging thins hair on other parts of the body, a man's facial hair is usually the same quantity into advanced older age. His thinner skin, however, is easily damaged by a razor that is too sharp. Bacteria enter and infect the deeper layers of the skin. Lather creams that are applied with a shaving

brush are recommended for the older man, because the mechanical action of the brush stands the hair up, permitting the soap to penetrate the shaft of the hair. Softened facial hair permits the razor to glide over the skin without injuring it. Have the client stretch the skin as he is shaving. This will flatten out wrinkles in the skin and prevent nicks. Inadvertent cuts can be treated with a styptic pencil or small piece of facial tissue applied to the area. The black client may use a rougher cleansing agent such as a Buf-Puf before shaving. The buffing action will help free ingrown hairs that cause razor bumps. This helps reduce blemishes that can lead to scarring.

The client may require assistance in shaving if his hands are unsteady. If the nurse does assist with shaving, it should be done daily. Often by the time the agency barber makes his weekly rounds, some of the older male clients who are unable to shave themselves look totally unkempt.

Moisturizers are also beneficial for the skin of older men. As with women, the moisturizer keeps the skin supple. Any moisturizer suitable for women can be used by men. In fact, manufacturers of moisturizers usually sold to women are bottling the same creams and lotions in "masculine-type packaging" and giving them macho-sounding names. A stimulating after-shave lotion serves as a skin freshener. The scent of the after-shave lotion can serve as a signature for the man as a perfume does for a woman. An after-shave lotion serves as part of a sexuality message for the older man, as it does for a younger man.

Clothing

Availability of clean clothing provides the older adult with a source of dignity, pride and individuality. The older adult living in a long-term-care facility usually has laundry services as part of the basic service cost. When the client lives at home, nursing intervention should include an inquiry into the client's ability to buy, repair, and launder his clothing. When clothing and laundry services are not available, it can become the first step away from attention to personal appearance, and client regression can occur. Consider the emotional consequences to Mr. Clark, 74 years old, when he wears the same food-stained suit day after day. Because he is embarrassed about his appearance, he does not extend himself socially. Wearing the same clothes is one example of a nonstimulating environment. Mr. Clark's community health nurse was attentive to his needs as a total person, and she inquired into his feelings regarding his mode of dress. He stated he had limited money to buy clothes. After assessing the situation, she made the nursing diagnosis of insufficient knowledge of available sources to purchase or obtain clothing. The nurse suggested that he might purchase clean and mended used clothing at several local voluntary agency thrift shops. If transportation is available, she might suggest special factory outlet and discount stores that sell "irregulars" or "seconds" at marked savings. In addition, his nurse recommended that he purchase wash-and-wear shirts, sweaters, and trousers that he can rinse out in his kitchen sink and drip dry.

Unfortunately, it is often difficult for the older adult to find clothing that fits well. Physiological changes alter the body proportions. The distribution of body fat changes, which causes the waist, hips, and abdomen to expand, and legs become thinner. Ready-to-wear clothing is cut in standard sizes, which are geared to the young and middle adult proportions.

Poorly fitting clothing impedes movement, causes discomfort and makes the client feel unattractive. Clothing has a therapeutic value. It can be a source of compliments and can make an occasion seem special. In addition, the act of choosing what one is to wear for the day is an expression of the client's control over his own life. "New clothes can also be a link with the outside world and convey a sense of the future rather than the past" (Phipps, 1977, p. 21).

Some of the considerations older adults have when purchasing clothing relate to the comfort, ease of putting on and taking off, and attractive styles and colors. Older women often prefer one-piece dresses in a shift or semifitted waist style and A-line skirts. Some also prefer lower neck lines and short raglan or straight sleeves without cuffs. A further convenience is a garment with front closure, with a zipper or large button fasteners. Large patch pockets are an added feature they also appreciate. Bright colors and shades of red such as rose, wine, or pink, are particular favorites. Various shades of blue or green are also popular.

Fabrics made of cotton or wool blended with polyesters make laundering easier and less expensive. The nurse might suggest to the client that all-polyester clothing is often uncomfortable to wear and irritating to the skin. A better choice might be a blend of at least a 50 percent natural fiber. Knit fabrics are a particular favorite with the older adult, because they are soft, warmer in the winter, and have stretchability. Dressing for the weather is important for the older adult in order to prevent loss of body heat through chilling in the winter and loss of fluid and electrolytes through perspiration in the summer. Layering of clothing is useful. The basic physiological need for warmth and protection is met by the client himself by adding or removing a sweater or jacket as the temperature indicates. The nurse should keep in mind that the older adult's perception of room temperature and discomfort from wind drafts from windows, doors, fans, or air conditioners may be different from her own, because of changes in skin sensitivity and decreased layers of adipose tissue. The slower moving adult generates less body heat and so will be more sensitive to lower room temperatures.

Bed wear. Bedtime clothing should also be a source of comfort and protection for the client. The client's preference for pajamas or nightgown should be respected. Many men have worn their underwear to bed as night garments for years, and their preference should also be honored. Changing such bedtime attire can cause sleep disturbances. Whatever the manner of dress or undress is preferred, the priority is warmth and comfort. The garment should not bind any part of the body and allow freedom of motion.

Variety in nurse's dress. The dress of the nurse caring for the older adult has an effect on the environment. On one hand, some older adults report that they like the traditional white uniform and cap. They state they feel protected when they can easily identify which person is the nurse. The classic light blue and navy blue uniforms of public health and community health nurses also help reduce confusion for the older adult when the nurse requests entry into the client's home. The older adult is familiar with this symbol of the nurse. On the other hand, a case can be made for uniforms of varying colors and even for street clothes.

Table 10-2. Comparison of causes of decubiti and physiological changes in older adults

Causes of decubiti	Physiological changes in older adults
Immobility	Often immobilized because of arthritis, foot problems, arteriosclerotic disease, general debilitation, depression, and stroke
Diminished circulation	Include venous stasis and decreased capillary and arterial circulation
Irritated skin/abrasions	Skin tissuelike, fragile, and easily damaged
Poor nutritional status	Mastication problems; limited food budget; loss of interest in preparing and eating food; decreased taste buds
Pressure on bony prominences	Decreased adipose tissue reduces padding, bony prominences, decreased muscle mass (Fig. 10-4)
Reduced sensation to pressure and pain	Circulatory impairment; decreased neuron activity; edematous conditions
Incontinence	Loss of bladder muscle tone; stress incontinence; retention with overflow, as in benign prostatic hypertrophy; unable to independently use bathroom or bedpan; diminished mobility in responding to bowel and bladder reflexes; neurological impairment due to CVA; chronic bacteriuria
Debilitation	Seen in the old-old and frail old; depression, loneliness, weight loss, change in bony skeleton
Shearing forces	Fowler and semi-Fowler position in bed, chairs, and wheel chairs; long periods of time sitting in chairs and wheelchairs
Rough, wrinkled, damp bed linen	Friction burns on skin from moving in bed; crumbs from eating in bed; perspiration increase from bedrest; contact dermatitis on dry skin from irritating detergents and starches

Florence Nightingale herself saw the nurses' mode of dress as a way of varying an otherwise monotonous environment.

DECUBITUS ULCERS

Decubitus ulcers are a topic that must be addressed when discussing care of the skin of the older adult. A comparison of the traditionally stated causes of decubiti and the characteristic physiological changes of the older adult is ample evidence of why the older adult is at high risk for skin breakdown (Table 10-2).

A positioning plan is a nursing intervention tool that the nurse may develop jointly with the client. The client's special needs identified on the care plan are considered in the plan's development. The plan will require evaluation on a day-to-day basis by the nurse and client. Each position change includes a lubricated massage over the body prominence and the limbs being put through range of motion. The wheelchair client (Fig. 10-5) is taught how to lift himself off the seat every 20 minutes and massage his sacrum with a cream or lotion. This combination of nursing activities assures adequate circulation to the areas in jeopardy and prevents muscle atrophy and joint contractures. The skin assessment is made at the time of turning. The nurse should note any blanching of the skin over the bony prominences. This pale and white color is the first visible clue that cell damage has already occurred. The ischemia advances to hyperemia, and blood floods the area. It now appears reddened and warm. In the black client, blanching causes a paleness of the skin compared with areas with good circulation. The hyperemic area feels warm upon palpation. At this point, the area is so engorged with blood that gas exchange and nutrient and waste exchange do not occur. If the cause of the pressure is not removed, cell death is inevitable. Studies have demonstrated that deep cell death has occurred before overt signs of ischemia appear. It is very possible that the nurse will not observe these ischemic signs until 2 to 9 days after the cell is damaged.

Prevention is imperative; nursing intervention must be prophylactic. A decubitus that takes a month to heal in a 20-year-old will take 2 months to heal in a 40-year-old, and over 3 months to heal in the over-60-year-old client.

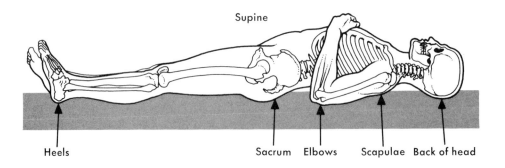

Supine

Heels   Sacrum   Elbows   Scapulae   Back of head

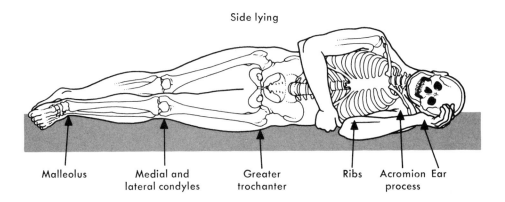

Side lying

Malleolus   Medial and lateral condyles   Greater trochanter   Ribs   Acromion process   Ear

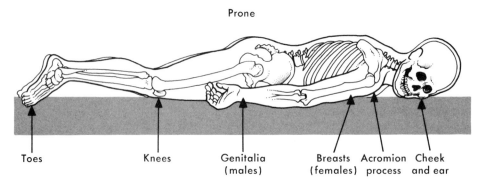

Prone

Toes   Knees   Genitalia (males)   Breasts (females)   Acromion process   Cheek and ear

Fig. 10-4. Areas prone to pressure on bony prominences.

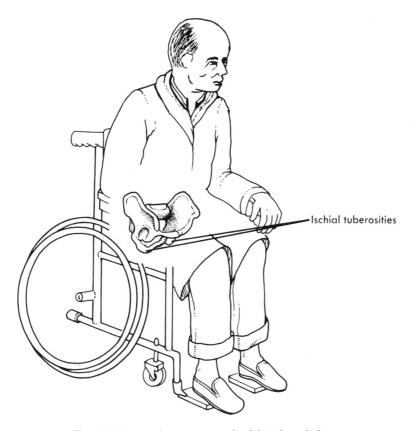

Fig. 10-5. Areas of pressure on wheelchair-bound client.

Preventing decubiti

All nursing intervention is individually planned for the client; however, some general guidelines are useful to the nurse as she carries out her plan.

Promote mobility. Turn and position frequently (Table 10-3). Get client out of bed daily unless absolutely contraindicated. Do range-of-motion exercises as the minimum activity each shift. Have the client use canes and walkers to aid in walking. Apply prescribed braces and prosthetic devices. Do meticulous foot care. Identify early signs of depression.

Increase circulation. Do emollient massages and peripheral vascular exercises. Have client avoid cold environment and wear layered clothes in cold weather. Flannel sheet blankets are warmer than linen sheets. An electric blanket is better than heavy blankets. Teach the client about the vasoconstriction action of nicotine.

Improve nutritional status. Promote adequate dental care, including high protein and vitamin diet, particularly vitamin A, which protects the integrity of the skin tissue, and vitamin C, which forms the matrix of the capillary beds. Vitamin C also prevents fragility of the capillary walls. Keep the client hydrated. Keep menu planning in line with food budget. Share information regarding senior citizen nutritional centers. Provide information regarding the food stamp program and Meals on Wheels. Arrange for social interaction during mealtime. Assist with feeding as needed.

Prevent pressure on body prominences. Turn and position at frequent intervals. Use trochanter supports, flotation pad, plastic foam, natural and

Table 10-3. Change of position schedules

Time	Schedule for wheelchair-bound client	Schedule for bed-bound client	Activity
6 AM-8 AM	Left side lying	Left side lying	Mouth care, breakfast, independently or with assistance, bladder training
8 AM-10 AM	Supine	Supine	Hygienic care, ADL, range of motion by nurse, bowel and bladder training, dress wheelchair client
10 AM-11 AM	Prone	Prone	Back care, increase tolerance of position gradually to 1 hour (turn right side)
11 AM-1 PM	Right side lying	Right side lying	Bowel and bladder training
12 noon	Wheelchair		Lunch
12:45-2 PM	Wheelchair		Therapeutic activities
2 PM-3 PM	Wheelchair		Physical therapy, bladder training
1 PM-3 PM		Left side lying	Visiting, TV, occupational therapist or recreational therapist, bladder training
3 PM-4 PM	Prone	Prone	Range-of-motion exercise by physical therapist or nurse, increase time in position to 1 hour or turn to supine
5 PM-6 PM	Supine	Supine	Dinner independently or with assistance, mouth, face, and hand care, bladder training
6 PM-8 PM	Wheel chair	Right side lying	Visiting, TV
8 PM-11 PM	Left side lying	Left side lying	Century tub bath taken on a stretcher, evening care treatments, bladder training
11 PM-3 AM	Supine	Supine	Sleeping, bladder training as needed
3 AM-6 AM	Right side lying	Right side lying	Sleeping, bladder training as needed

synthetic sheep skins, water and gel pads, foam elbow and heel protectors, foam rubber and lamb's wool, sand bags, alternating air pressure mattress. (NOTE: Cover air mattress with one thin sheet only. Any other linen protectors eliminate the therapeutic value of the mattress.) Use Foster and Stryker frames, and Circoelectric beds. Avoid rubber rings and donuts.

Protect areas of reduced sensation. Identify areas of edema. Assess lower limbs once a shift with careful handling of body parts. Check temperature of bath water, and avoid hot water bottles.

Bowel and bladder training. Cleanse and dry the skin, and change the linen immediately after an incontinent episode. Use protective skin covering such as vitamin A & D ointment, Lubriderm, Keradex, or other emollients. Use soft washcloths and towels. Pat the skin dry; do not rub. Avoid drying agents on the genital area. Implement bowel and bladder training regimen.

Tender loving care (TLC). Use gentle handling, psychological support, understanding, and sup-

portive communications. Ensure a stimulating environment to promote interest. Direct the nursing regimen toward sustaining and supportive care.

Prevent shearing force. Change position at frequent intervals; minimize time in chair sitting; use Fowler and semi-Fowler positions. Increase vitamin C intake to protect capillary beds. Use turning sheet to lift client up in bed. Use foot boards to prevent client from sliding down in bed. Pad the bedpan. Use emollients on elbows and heels, rub in well, and dust with talcum powder or cornstarch to reduce friction.

Assess other sources of pressure. Avoid clothing that restricts circulation or causes edema or tissue damage. Avoid rough clothing. Check seams and wrinkles in clothing, nylon stockings, or bed linens. Avoid wallets and other items in trousers and slacks. Have linen hem smooth side out. Decrease number of layers of bed linen to minimize risk of wrinkles; avoid crumbs, rolled-up tissues, caked powder, and other items in bed. Check heavy seams in shoes and tight-fitting shoes. Inspect braces, casts, splints, bandages, and prostheses for fit and alignment, especially after weight loss or gain.

We have identified the potential risk factors for the older adult's vulnerability to decubitis ulcers. The major nursing responsibility is prevention. This presentation has dealt primarily with anticipatory guidance measures that may be used in intervention to prevent the pain and emotional indignity caused by a decubitus ulcer. Nursing diagnosis and initiation of independent nursing actions of prevention and constant nursing vigilance are essential for the older adult's welfare in the long-term-care facility, the hospital, and his home.

Treatments used for decubiti

In 1968 it was estimated that the average cost of treating a decubitus ulcer was $5,000. The cost of such treatment in the 1980s is likely to be double or triple that. No price tag can be put on the pain and human suffering caused a client with a decubitus ulcer.

When decubiti occur, a potpourri of remedies are used. Many of these remedies are actually preventive measures that should have been done before the ulcer occurred. The pressure from the bony prominences must be relieved, circulation improved, and nutrition promoted. New cell growth does not occur in the presence of necrotic tissue or bacteria. The aim of surgical and chemical debridement is to rid the area of dead cells for new capillary bed formation. Skin grafting is often done after debridement to close the wound. Elase and Santyl are two chemical debriding agents that remove necrotic tissue and encourage granulation and epithelialization.

As much as 50 grams of protein per day can be lost in drainage from a decubitus ulcer. This loss alone is of grave consequence to the older adult, whose normal protein intake needs per day range from 60 to 80 grams. When the client's protein intake is not sufficient to meet both these needs, negative nitrogen balance occurs. The skin is further debilitated by the resulting edema, reduced elasticity, and turgor.

The following remedies are used for decubitus ulcer treatment.

Gel foam
Insulin
Karaya
Maalox
Sugar
Dakins solution
Gentian violet
A & D ointment
Heat lamp
Exposure to air
Wet to dry dressings

The sheer number of these remedies is evidence that no individual one has been proved really effective.

Given the physiological changes in the older adult that leave them vulnerable to decubiti and delayed healing ability, it is imperative that decubitus prevention be a priority in their care.

GENITOURINARY SYSTEM
Incontinence

With increasing age, the capacity of the bladder diminishes, and the older adult has to urinate more frequently. Occasionally, a normal healthy older adult may "spill urine" or have an episode of incontinence. Some authorities feel that the emotional state of the individual is a factor in stress incontinence. Research studies report that incontinence is two times more common in females as a possible result of (1) longevity and physiological changes, (2) confusion, which is two times more prevalent in women than men, (3) physiological differences that permit men to retain a urinal in place and relieve worry about "accidents," and (4) shorter female urethra compared with the longer one in the male. Other studies have found a direct correlation between the morale of the nursing staff and the incidence of incontinence. It was found that the clients who received care from a professional nursing staff had less incontinence than those clients cared for by ancillary untrained personnel. The conclusion was that nursing knowledge and intervention techniques made the difference. Clients who were occupied, out of bed, and permitted to use the bathroom with or without assistance had less incontinence than clients in bed. Little difference was found in the age groups 60 to 70 years and 70 to 80 years and the degree of incontinence. The significant factors contributing to urinary incontinence are (1) organic disease of the nerves, (2) hypertension, and (3) the confused client confined to bed.

Stress incontinence. Stress incontinence is a common disorder in older women. When this problem is identified, the nurse should refer the client for a medical evaluation. Very often the cause of the incontinency is a rectocele or cystocele subsequent to childbearing in her younger years. The simple insertion of a pessary or surgical intervention will frequently eliminate the problem. On occasion, exercises to reeducate the pelvic floor muscles of the woman have been helpful in combating stress incontinence. In addition, the client should be evaluated for participation in a bladder training program.

To prevent the embarrassment caused by stress incontinence, panties that provide added protection may be worn. One solution suitable for a client with only small amounts of urinary drainage is "light day" or "regular" self-adherent sanitary napkins. The client removes the paper strip and attaches the pad to her panties. Some brands of the thinner pads are flushable and others may be discarded by wrapping in toilet tissue and putting in a waste receptacle. These self-adherent pads have an advantage over the belted styles, because they do not ride back and forth as the client walks.

For heavier urinary incontinency, disposable urinary incontinency pants are recommended. These commercially available pants offer convenience and added protection to the client's clothing and bedding. There is a wide variety of styles available, giving the client considerable selection in shape, thickness, and fit, as well as price. Styles with a plastic outer lining should be avoided because they promote perspiration and retention of heat. Special attention should be given to the fit, particularly around the legs, because binding will impair peripheral circulation. It is to the client's advantage if the long-term-care facility stocks several brands of incontinency pants. No one brand is suitable for all clients' needs. The nurse should explain to the client that she understands how difficult the situation may be for her emotionally, as well as physically, but that she will work with her to find a satisfactory solution. When the client understands that several methods of incontinency protection might have to be tried before a satisfactory one is chosen, she is less likely to become discouraged. When incontinency protection is

absorbent, comfortable, and can be discreetly worn under clothing, the client's self-esteem is maintained. The nurses' attitude should be supportive, and communications, both verbal and nonverbal, should be positive.

Baseline data. Research reports a correlation between urinary incontinence and bowel incontinence. Seventy percent of older adult clients who had urinary incontinence had bowel incontinence caused by (1) paralysis, (2) confusion, and (3) bedrest. Urinary and bowel incontinence are problems that can be managed through nursing intervention and a therapeutic bowel and bladder program. The incontinent client needs the understanding and support of the nursing staff while being retrained.

The older adult must be interested in participating in a bowel and bladder program. The client and the nursing staff probably have a good idea how often and when the incontinent behavior occurs. However, there may not be any documentation to substantiate this. Baseline data are the information gathered about the incontinent behavior before intervention can be implemented. It becomes the standard to compare the effectiveness or results of the bowel and bladder program. Baseline data are different from estimating, guessing, or merely observing, in that they are quantitative. It is the result of counting and recording the number of times the behavior occurred. In this case, the behavior is incontinence of bladder and bowel.

Recording system. The recording system should be simple so that the nursing staff will use it. The form must be in an area readily accessible when the behavior occurs, such as the foot of the bed or the bathroom door.

Elaborate recording systems invite the nursing staff to postpone charting and possibly forgetting the incontinent incident. Immediate charting can serve as feedback for the nurse and interested client. The record-keeping system may be tested while collecting the baseline data. Any problems found in forms developed for the system will be uncovered in the baseline phase of the program, before the nursing intervention has been initiated. Corrections are made and the final charting form developed (see p. 209). The pretreatment baseline data helped the nurse document that her intervention brought about a decrease in the client's incidence of incontinence.

Baseline data for bowel and bladder training

KEY: BR = Bathroom
BP = Bedpan
V = Voided
BM = Bowel movement
INC = Incontinent
INC S = Incontinent of stool
INC U = Incontinent of urine

Name _____ Department _____ Date started _____

	Sunday	Monday	Tuesday	Wednesday	Thursday	Friday	Saturday
8:00 AM							
10:00 AM							
12 Noon							
2:00 PM							
4:00 PM							
8:00 PM							
10:00 PM							
12 Mid.							
2:00 AM							
4:00 AM							
6:00 AM							

COMMENTS:

Behavior modification. Behavior modification is exchanging one behavior for another through the use of a reward system. The client's behavior of incontinency is to be exchanged for bladder and bowel control. The reward, called a reinforcer, increases the client's willingness to do the desired or targeted behavior. A positive reinforcer provides those things that the client likes; a negative reinforcer withholds something that the client desires. The nurse who knows her client selects the reinforcers that will encourage the client to perform the targeted behavior. The nurse can determine the appropriate reinforcer by asking:

What kinds of things does the client like to have?
What are the client's major interests or hobbies?
What people does he like to be with?
What makes the client feel good?
What would be a nice present for the client to receive?
What privileges would the client hate to lose?
Mrs. Singer was incontinent four times a day. Her nurse knew that Mrs. Singer's favorite treat was chocolate cake. She explained to Mrs. Singer that each time she voided in the commode, she would receive a small square of chocolate cake. After a 2-week period of reinforcement of the tar-

geted behavior, she was continent of urine. The reinforcer was continued for 4 more weeks, until the pattern of continence was firmly established. The reinforcer was then gradually withdrawn.

Program design for bowel and bladder training

PURPOSE: To establish bowel and bladder continency.
PRETRAINING STEPS

1. Select client who is able to understand and cooperate.
2. Screen out clients who have a limited possibility of successful training, such as those who exhibit:
   a. Inability to cooperate
   b. Severe confusion
   c. Established habit of incontinence
   d. Loss of sphincter control
   e. Urinary or bowel obstruction
   f. Chronic bladder distention
3. Take a bowel and bladder history (see example on p. 211).
4. Discuss the plan with the client's physician, and obtain specific orders for diet, physical activity, and/or catheter removal.
5. Discuss the program with each client, explaining what, why, and how. Include the client in goal setting and recording activities. The client and the nurse select the reinforcer. It is essential that the entire nursing staff on all shifts work together. They should plan to train only one or two clients at a time, until a pattern is established. Avoid beginning a training program when the client is disturbed, distressed, or some other condition interferes. Accidents should be expected to occur during the learning process. Do not show anxiety or frustration.

BLADDER TRAINING
Method A

1. Keep a detailed record of incontinence for 1 week to collect baseline data and establish a pattern. Check every 2 hours for incontinence, and record time, amount, and characteristics (see p. 209).
2. Provide proper diet and fluids.
   a. Include in the menu high-fiber foods.
   b. Give at least 2000 ml fluids per day, unless limited by a physician's order.
   c. Push fluids from 6 AM until 7 PM. Divide fluid intake evenly, about 300 ml/hour.
   d. Avoid carbonated beverages, since they seem to irritate the bladder. Vary fluids, because milk's high calcium content promotes formation of stones and fruit juices alkalize the urine and affect bowel consistency.

3. Make a training plan.
   a. Collect a bowel and bladder history.
   b. Analyze baseline data to develop plan. Identify the times of the day when the client is incontinent, any activities that may contribute to incontinence, and distinguish between bowel and bladder incontinence. Does the client void in small, moderate, or large amounts? Does he receive a prior urge to void? Is there an urgency when he feels the need to void and cannot get to the bathroom fast enough? Does client dribble between voidings? Identify the frequency of voidings. NOTE: Keep client clean and dry for esthetic and physical reasons.
   c. Develop a plan with the client's assistance, and make sure he understands it.
   d. Take the client regularly to bathroom or place him on the commode, bedpan, or offer urinal at time intervals determined by step 1 baseline data.
   e. If tolerated, client should use toilet or commode.
   f. Position as close to a semisquat as possible.
   g. Provide privacy, warmth, and comfort. If successful, reinforce behavior by giving reinforcer.
4. After 20 minutes, if the client is still unsuccessful, say "Try again next time."
5. Document results on recording system kept on bathroom door.
6. Keep accurate intake and output record. (IMPORTANT: Allow the client to help keep I & O if possible.)
7. Increase the physical activity of the client, as tolerated.
8. Dress the client in clean street clothes, including underwear, shoes, and socks.
9. Discontinue diapering. A protective panty may be worn by the client under clothing, only if needed.
10. In the beginning, periodically evaluate the program every 3 days by reviewing the recording system. Adjust the training schedule as necessary.
11. If possible, give the responsibility of the program to the client gradually.
12. Persistent regularity is essential to the success of the program. Take the client on schedule to the bathroom or commode, and always reinforce successful behavior immediately. Use bedpan or urinal if indicated.
13. All nursing personnel *must* support the program and encourage the client.

Suggestions for stimulating voiding

1. Run water slowly.
2. Give the client a glass of water to drink.
3. Have the client blow bubbles with straw in glass of water.

Bowel and bladder history

Bowel

1. What time of day do you have a bowel movement?
2. How often do you have a bowel movement? ☐ Daily ☐ Other (specify) _____
   Number of times _____
3. Do you have any awareness before or during a bowel movement? ☐ Yes ☐ No
4. Do you have any suggestions regarding your bowel habits?
5. Do you take a laxative, suppository, enema or use other measures to stimulate a bowel movement or change stool consistency?
6. Do you eat fresh fruits and vegetables? ☐ Whole grain cereals ☐ Bran ☐ Bread ☐ Fruits/vegetables
7. How much fluid do you drink a day? ☐ Milk ☐ Water ☐ Tea ☐ Coffee ☐ Soda ☐ Soup ☐ Fruit juices Estimate amount _____
8. What do you normally do when you are on the toilet? ☐ Read ☐ Smoke Other _____
9. Do you drink prune juice or eat prunes each day? ☐ Yes ☐ No ☐ Prune juice ☐ Prunes
10. Do you have to strain to have a bowel movement? ☐ Yes ☐ No
11. Would you be interested in having a bowel training program explained and participate in one? ☐ Yes ☐ No (explain) _____

Bladder

1. Approximately how many times a day do you urinate?
2. Do you have to get up during the night to urinate? ☐ Yes ☐ No How many times? _____
3. Describe the color of your urine.
4. Do you have dribbling or leaking of urine right after you have finished urinating? ☐ Yes ☐ No
   Do you have it between episodes of urinating? ☐ Yes ☐ No
5. Approximately how many times a day are you incontinent of urine?
6. When are you incontinent? Specify approximate time. ☐ In the day ☐ At night
7. Do you urinate in ☐ Small amounts ☐ Moderate amounts ☐ Large amounts?
8. Is there any particular activity that you are engaged in when you have an episode of incontinence?
9. Do you spill urine or lose urine when you cough, laugh, or lift something? ☐ Cough ☐ Laugh ☐ Lift a heavy object ☐ Other (explain) _____
10. Are you aware of a need to urinate? ☐ Yes ☐ No If yes, what kind of sensation or sign do you have to alert you to go to the bathroom?
11. Do you have a sense of urgency when you have to pass your urine? ☐ Yes ☐ No
12. Do you get to the bathroom in time? ☐ Yes ☐ No
13. Do you have any ideas about the cause of the incontinence? ☐ No ☐ Yes (explain) _____
14. Do you have pain when you pass urine? ☐ No ☐ Yes (explain) _____
15. Do you have to strain to urinate? ☐ No ☐ Yes (explain) _____
16. Do you wear any kind of protective panties or shorts? ☐ Yes ☐ No
17. Would you be interested in having a bladder training program explained and participate in one? ☐ Yes ☐ No (explain) _____

4. Pour warm water over the perineum of the client.
5. Dabble the client's hands in water.
6. Put feet in warm water.
7. Lean forward slightly.
8. Lightly press on bladder area.
9. Tickle certain "trigger points," such as inner or outer aspects of thighs, navel, hips, buttocks, abdomen, sacrum, or coccyx.

RETENTION CATHETER REMOVAL
Method A: with physician's order
1. Clamp off catheter at 1-hour intervals or until client has discomfort or distention. Do this during the day; allow continuous drainage at night.
2. Increase clamp-off time to 3- to 4-hour intervals, 24 hours a day, if possible.
3. Remove catheter.

4. Encourage fluids to 2000 ml/day, 7 AM to 7 PM, unless contraindicated.
5. Continue offering toilet, commode, bedpan, or urinal at same intervals that catheter was allowed to drain. Reinforce successful behavior immediately. Say, "Try next time" if unsuccessful.
6. Increase physical activity if possible.
7. Bladder irrigation, rather than catheter irrigation, helps maintain muscle tone, but should be done only with a physician's order. Unless contraindicated, Crede technique may be used to manually express urine from the bladder.
8. Do not assume that the bladder is paralyzed when patient has suffered a cerebrovascular accident.

Method B: with physician's order

1. Starting at breakfast, give the client 200 ml of liquid every hour for 3 hours.
2. Remove catheter, and encourage the client to void normally; use reinforcer. If unsuccessful, say, "Try again next time," and repeat in ½-hour and 1-hour intervals. Reinforce successful behavior immediately.
3. Document results, and note any incontinence between voiding attempts.
4. Use aids to stimulate voiding.
5. Look for signs of a need to void, and make client aware of them: restlessness, headache, chill, flushing, perspiration, and a vague feeling of fullness.
6. Reinsert catheter if voiding has not occurred within 3 to 4 hours.
7. Check for residual urine after voiding. Insert Foley catheter and measure the results. Authorities recommend less than 100 ml for a spastic bladder, and less than 50 ml for a flaccid bladder. Physician may order catheter to remain in place if results are unacceptable.
   a. An alternative method is replacing the catheter at night and repeating the procedure for a few days until the residual is below 50 ml.
8. The Foley catheter is removed when the residual amount is satisfactory. Liquids should be limited, starting at 6 PM. The client is awakened to urinate during the night.
9. Continue to have the client void every 2 to 3 hours during the day, and maintain fluid intake. Document results.
10. Look for signs and symptoms of distention:
    Restlessness
    Perspiration
    Chills
    Distended bladder
    Flushing
    Pale color
    Cold extremities
    Severe headache
    Elevated blood pressure
11. Check residual urine daily in the beginning phase, then twice a week, and then every other week.
12. Incontinent behavior that continues may indicate that the program needs to be stopped for a brief period and restarted in a week or two.
13. Bladder training takes time. Between voidings, there may be dribbling, leakage, or spilling of urine. Urosheaths may be worn by men and protective panties or pads by women if indicated.
14. During the training period if the program has to be briefly stopped, support and encourage the client physically, socially, and psychologically.

SELF-CATHETERIZATION

Method: In the early seventies, urologists reported good results with a clean self-catheterization technique.

1. Candidates for this procedure are clients with neurogenic bladder dysfunction.
2. The procedure is an alternative to surgery, indwelling catheters, and urosheaths.
3. The client or a member of the family is taught the catheterization procedure.
4. Clients using intermittent self-catheterization are usually free of infection and dry.
5. A plan is developed with the client to schedule catheterization throughout the day and night.
6. Fluid intake is adjusted according to the urinary output at each catheterization to prevent bladder distention.
7. Baseline urinalysis and culture are done before self-catheterization is initiated.
8. The client and/or family is assisted with catheterization until the skill is mastered.
9. The nurse periodically observes and supervises the procedure.
10. The nurse, client, and/or family evaluate the procedure and modify the plan as needed.
11. The client and/or family are supported and reinforced for successful mastery of the catheterization skill.
12. A urinalysis and urine culture (if needed) are done after the first week of self-catheterization. The results are compared to the baseline laboratory report. Spot urinary checks are done routinely thereafter.
13. The client usually likes the freedom of planning his own schedule for self-catheterization. His independence and self-dignity are restored by assuming the responsibility for his own care and body function.

BOWEL TRAINING

Method

1. Review the bowel history with the client.
2. Determine if the client has the "laxative habit" and needs reeducation through health teaching. Stool consistency is important. It should be fairly firm, but soft. A loose stool is difficult to control and makes training impossible.
3. Do abdominal palpation and rectal examination to determine existence of fecal impaction unless contraindicated. (IMPORTANT: This will be done by a physician or an RN *only*.)
4. If impaction is present, follow the physician's orders for removal. A small oil retention enema followed by a cleansing enema in several hours is usually preferred to manual removal.
5. Establish the client's elimination pattern from step 1 baseline data. The best time schedule is after a meal, when the gastrocolic and duodenocolic reflexes are activated. A change from a day to evening schedule or vice versa takes 2 to 3 weeks to establish the pattern. A 1-, 2-, or 3-day schedule is permitted for a bowel movement.
6. Give the client proper diet and fluids, and encourage physical activity as for bladder training.
7. Take the client to the bathroom or commode, or offer the bedpan at the same time each day, every other day, or every third day, as established in step 3 of bladder training.
    a. Have the client sit erect, if possible.
    b. Provide privacy, warmth, and comfort.
    c. Allow the client to read or smoke, if this has been a habit.
    d. Do not hurry the client.
8. Follow steps 4 to 13 of the bladder program.
9. Give a laxative, suppository, or enema according to physician's order if diet and fluids are not adequate to encourage elimination. Know the pharmacological action of the laxative. Administer to promote a bowel movement at regular intervals, eventually discontinuing use of medication as a pattern is established.
10. Insert a suppository, if ordered, approximately 10 minutes before breakfast (this may be done before lunch or dinner, if it is better suited to the client's pattern).
11. Record the length of time between the suppository insertion and defecation. This will provide you with a defecation time frame for the next treatment. Time varies with clients, anywhere from 15 minutes to 45 minutes.
12. Encourage the client to exercise, unless contraindicated. Walking and moving about improves muscle tone and aids elimination. Bed clients may use passive and active exercises to promote elimination, such as bending knees and pressing thighs against abdomen.

Suggestions for stimulating bowel movement

1. Use a circular massage on the client from right to left and down abdomen.
2. Have the client do push-ups sitting on the toilet seat.
3. Have the client lean slightly forward.
4. Have the client place his feet on a footstool.
5. Wearing a finger cot or rubber glove, touch or circle external sphincter of rectum of client.

Training program results. It is most important that the nurse enter into a bowel and bladder training program with the cooperation of the client. Her philosophy must be a positive one, and realistic, attainable goals must be established jointly with the client. Patience, endurance and mutual support on the part of the nurse and client will help ensure success. Nursing intervention and anticipatory guidance are geared to the individualized needs of the client. The work is well worth the effort, and the success and satisfaction shared by the client and nurse are a great reward. The client's control over his bladder and bowel will enhance his self-esteem.

General catheter care

On occasion the older adult has an indwelling catheter in place. Care must be taken to prevent infection. The catheter is usually changed every 2 to 4 weeks and only irrigated upon a physician's order. A closed, sterile drainage system is maintained. Care is taken to prevent irritation in taping a catheter to the skin. It is taped on the inner thigh, just below the femoral area in a female and on the abdomen in a male, to minimize pressure and irritation by increasing the penoscrotal angle.

Male clients in the prone position should have the penis positioned laterally, toward the drainage system. Ambulatory clients may attach the catheter with straight drainage to a leg bag. The sterile drainage system's recommendations should be followed for changing the system and leg bags. They are cleaned, deodorized, and disinfected daily.

Male and female cleanliness in the urethral area is most important, because this dark, moist area is perfect for microorganism growth. The male penis is washed with mild soap using firm strokes. The uncircumcised male foreskin is retracted, the glan and prepuce washed and dried to prevent accumulation of smegma, and the scrotum is gently bathed.

Accumulation of debris in the female perineal area is removed with toilet tissue before bathing with a mild soap and rinsing thoroughly. Any noted excoriation is treated; otherwise the area is kept clean and dry.

While cleansing around the catheter and urethral area in the male and female client, inspect for leakage and correct catheter size. Finally, the anal area and rectum are bathed, rinsed, and dried carefully. The client may be taught to participate in his catheter care.

Perineal/genital hygienic care

Common terms that the older adult uses to refer to his genitalia are "my privates," "private parts," or "crotch." Most cultures cover the genitalia, and exposure is embarrassing to the person. In addition, the older adult grew up during an era of conservative fashions, which covered most of the body.

Diminished natural cleansing lubrication in the older woman's vagina and a higher vaginal pH can lead to a dry and uncomfortable sensation in the perineal area. Furthermore, these changes alter the normal flora, which increases leukorrhea and its accompanying symptoms of irritation to the vaginal mucous membrane. Some older women treat these frustrating symptoms by douching or spraying with one of the over-the-counter preparations on the market. Men, too, use the spray preparations indiscriminately in an attempt to control genital odor. If the woman is used to douching or must douche, an acid vinegar douche made with 3 tablespoons of pure white vinegar to 3 liters of water is recommended by most gynecologists.

Alkaline douches are not recommended for the older adult woman whose vaginal pH should be from 6 to 7. Physical injury to the vaginal tissue is possible as the older woman douches. Rugae normally found in the younger vagina are absent, and the walls are far less elastic. Therefore, as the water enters the vaginal vault, the walls can become overdistended and tear. Instructions regarding douching for the older woman should emphasize that the douche bag be no higher than 12 inches

above her buttocks, and that she should not restrict the outflow of water by closing the labia.

Fastidious older adults pay sufficient attention to the genital area as part of their daily hygienic practice. Between showers and baths, the older adult may cleanse the area at the sink or sitting on the toilet, using a soft wash cloth, warm water, and a mild soap.

Some women find it refreshing to have a special plastic dispenser or glass handy in the bathroom to pour lukewarm water over the vulva after using the toilet. Care must be taken to test the water temperature before pouring. As with all age groups, the older adult woman should wipe in a front-to-back motion, discarding the tissue after each stroke to guard against contaminating the vagina with anal microorganisms. One decided advantage of perineal care for the older woman is that it reduces the colony count of those organisms that cause cystitis, a condition to which she is especially vulnerable.

Men and women may cleanse the genital area using Tucks or baby wipes after going to the bathroom. They wash and refresh without water, soap, or towel and are pleasantly scented. They can be carried in the pocket or purse and used when away from the home.

The nurse should discuss with the client his present washing procedure and focus health teaching on the client's individual needs. Some teaching areas may include the collection of secretions, smegma, around the clitoris and labia minora in the female and the prepuce in the male, the potential for bacteria growth, elimination of offensive odors, and proper wiping techniques. The major goal is to prevent excoriated skin in the genital area. Obese clients are more susceptible to this problem, especially in warm weather. Emollients, zinc oxide, Desitin, petroleum jelly, and other protective ointments may be used if excoriation is present. Otherwise, the area should be kept as dry and clean as possible. Some clients prefer talcum powder, baby powder, or corn starch for the pubic hair and inner thigh areas. Care is taken not to shake the powder on the mucosa of the genital area, because it might cause caking and irritation.

Vaginal discharges need to be thoroughly assessed by the nurse. It is not uncommon to misinterpret the older woman's genital manipulation for masturbation when in fact she is plagued by the vaginal itching caused by a *Monilia* infection.

The female client needs to be encouraged to have a Papanicolaou smear every 3 years as recommended by the American Cancer Association and more often as her doctor advises when there are other problems and a history of family cancer. Similarly, the male older adult needs to be examined and tested periodically for benign prostatic hypertrophy and cancer of the genital organs.

Undergarments

The proper undergarments can promote comfort and hygiene. All-cotton underpants provide full absorption for moisture and do allow some air circulation. If excessive moisture is a problem to the client, underpants should be washed in hot, soapy water to rid the garment of pathogenic organisms. Care must be taken to rinse out detergents completely. The legs and waists should fit properly and not pinch or bind the skin. Some older women prefer not to wear underpants and find this comfortable. If panty hose are worn, they should have a cotton crotch. Synthetic slacks and pants increase moisture problems in the perineal area. The nurse can recommend that the older woman wear dresses or skirts and that the older men wear trousers made of natural fibers, such as wool, cotton, or linen.

REST AND SLEEP
Rest

Sleep and rest, although related, are distinct phenomena. Rest is an expression of feelings of tranquility, relaxation, and peacefulness, often connected with a change of activities. For example, a quiet time after a period of exercise or meditation exercises, or hobbies such as reading, watching television, or any change in activity from the day's routine. When an individual has a break or relief from ongoing worries, troubles, or disturbances, that person is described as at rest. Adequate periods of rest are essential for any level of health of an individual. When rest is not adequate, the individual has chronic feelings of tiredness and fatigue, decreased muscle strength, and a general feeling of lethargy and weakness. Also, the attention span is diminished, mental activities are burdensome, and there is an overall decrease in attention and

ability to concentrate. When a person is nervous and irritable, it is frequently the response of lack of rest periods. When a person is well rested, he often has a sense of control over his environment and a sense of organization of his life.

Plan periods of rest intermittently during the day. Rest periods increase the efficiency of the activity coming afterward. It is particularly helpful if the older adult rests for 20 minutes after the noon meal and the evening meal in a reclining position, if possible. Rest does not necessarily mean sleep. Rest can be accomplished by reading or watching TV or listening to a favorite radio show. As the older adult rests, make an observation, and note if the muscular movements seem relaxed. The facial expression should be free from frowning and from wrinkling of the forehead or brow; such nervous activities as tapping of the finger or changing sitting positions frequently while sitting in a chair should be absent. Telling an older individual to "just relax" or "just don't worry" is of little value. If the older adult seems uncomfortable or ill at ease, relaxation can be promoted by helping the client recognize tension patterns and verbally express some of his concerns.

Sleep

Sleep takes up about one-third or one-fourth of a person's life. It is the period of succession of the waking state that enables the body to store and integrate the systems. With the synchronization of the body's activities, sleep enables a person to have a feeling of well-being and comfort. It is the quality and not necessarily the quantity of sleep that determines whether or not the outcome of the sleep is affected. In sleep there is an overall state of muscle relaxation and more or less an ability to respond to the environment.

In the early stages of sleep, a person is easily aroused, but as sleep deepens, arousal becomes more difficult. The sensory system continuously scans the environment for cues. A city person, for example, can sleep peacefully while the sounds of buses and fire engines roar outside, yet be awakened instantly at the sound of a door handle turning or a footstep in the hallway.

Sleep is cyclical in nature. The circadian rhythm is an internal biological clock, which sets the human being's day at approximately 24 hours. Sleep best occurs at the time in the circadian rhythm when body temperature is at the lowest. For most people, this occurs during the night. Such things as the person's age, state of fatigue, presence of acute or chronic illnesses, emotional upsets, and/or the use of alcohol and drugs can alter sleep patterns. Since sleep is as essential for health as is nutrition, any marked change in sleeping patterns will present a serious threat to the health of the individual. During sleep, hormones release the materials needed to replenish cellular constituents and other metabolic repair that help the body prepare for the work of the next day. Psychologically, this period of sleep is a time for the cerebral cortex to reorganize and consolidate its powers of problem solving and concentration. Such reorganization of physiological and psychological systems supports the wellness of the client to use all his assets at peak efficiency. Sleep-deprived persons report feelings of depression, irritability, lower pain threshholds, and confusion. Consider the needs of an older adult whose body systems are already altered as a function of age. The tolerance for sleep deprivation is far lower than in the younger person, and so the older person has a special need to have his sleep requirements met. Whereas stress may increase the wear and tear on body systems, rest and sleep can do a great part in replenishing the resources of the body.

Stages of sleep. Sleep is divided into two categories—rapid eye movement and nonrapid eye movement. During REM sleep, the EEG readings demonstrate wave activity. Although the large muscles of the body are characteristically immobile, there is a rapid darting eye movement. Vital signs reach levels similar to that of the waking state. Respirations alternate between rapid and slow, even with short periods of apnea. The person in REM stage of sleep has an EEG tracing similar to that of someone who is awake, but who is in deep concentration on a particular subject. There is a release of hormones, and blood constituents change. The level of vitality or fatigue and the ability to resist infection are increased. The transmission of neural impulses is also affected by the restorative actions of the body at this time.

REM sleep is a period of active, vivid dreaming. Persons awakened at this time can describe their dreams in color and often with auditory components. It is also during the REM stage of sleep that clients can report angina or other pain episodes; since gastric secretions can escalate, peptic ulcer attacks can occur. One purpose of REM dream stage is to organize past memory traces and store new memory programming. This function serves to coordinate current emotional experiences with similar past memory experiences. Although the REM stage is a large part of the sleep of the young child, its overall percentage declines with age. REM sleep may be necessary for establishing and maintaining neural pathways needed in the coordination of eye movement. In addition, the supply of norepinephrine is restored in the cells, so neurotransmission is protected. Adequate REM sleep, therefore, helps maintain the integrity of the central nervous system, which is particularly vulnerable in the older adult.

REM sleep deprivation occurs when a person is awakened by external stimuli. Particularly, there is REM deprivation when a person can sleep only 3 or 4 hours in a total 24-hour period. Stage one REM sleep deficiencies show clinical signs of an inability to cope with stressful experiences. REM sleep can be made up, but only after any missing stage four sleep is made up.

The non-REM stage of sleep consists of four stages. Stage one is the transition period from wakefulness to sleep. The person experiences a floating sensation, and the EEG has characteristics that are similar to the waking stage. Stage two is called the *door stage,* because it is associated with REM sleep in that it proceeds and follows each REM period. Stages three and four are called *slow wave sleep* because the EEG displays large, low-frequency, slow waves called delta waves. Most of the stage three and stage four sleep is obtained during the first half of the night's sleep. The last one and two cycles of sleep often do not have any stage three or stage four of sleep; REM and stage one and stage two sleep predominate (Fig. 10-6).

Characteristics of sleep in the older adult. There are a number of characteristic alterations in the sleep patterns of the older adult. Data regarding the sleeping patterns of the older adult have been collected either through the use of sleep logs or journals kept by individuals in the studies or with EEG readings in sleep laboratories.

Several aspects of sleep are considered. There is a longer latency or falling asleep time. Up until age 60 there is a latency period of about 10 minutes before the onset of sleep. After 60 the latency increases, reaching a mean of 23 minutes at ages 70 to 79. The old-old adult has a sleep latency of 26 minutes. During the night, there are far more periods of wakefulness, and there is a tendency to require fewer hours of nocturnal sleep. Women report more awakenings during the night than do men, especially during the menopausal years. Men begin to experience more awakenings after

retirement years. On the whole, the older adults go to bed at an earlier hour and awaken at an earlier hour than do youth.

Daytime naps increase in number in the older adult. This might be a function of the return to polycyclic patterns of sleep, or it might be a result of boredom. When the client does not express feelings of fatigue or exhaustion, consider an unstimulating environment as the cause of frequent daytime napping. Daytime naps are associated with particular sleep patterns.

REM sleep predominates during morning naps.

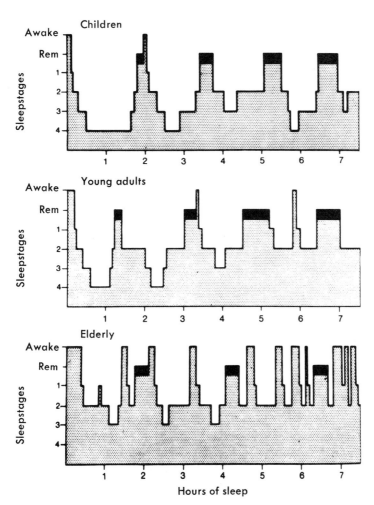

Fig. 10-6. Changes in sleep cycle with aging. (Reprinted from Kales, A., and Kales, J. D.: Sleep disorders, by permission from the New Eng. J. Med. **290:**487, 1974.)

This REM sleep is a continuation of the sleep from the evening before. The client awakens feeling refreshed, because it is a light stage of sleep. In addition, because REM sleep has the purpose of organizing cortex recent memory data, morning naps help the client's ability for lucid thinking. Afternoon naps, on the other hand, predominate in stage four sleep, which is the deepest of all the sleep levels. When the client awakens, he is likely to feel groggy and exhausted. The more stage four sleep in the afternoon, the longer the latency stage or falling asleep stage will be that evening. It might be very useful for the nurse to organize social and recreational activities after lunch. Physical therapy and occupational therapy treatments or shopping trips should be scheduled between 1:00 and 4:00. Such a schedule provides the older adult with ample time to meet hygiene needs and have a rest period before lunch. Purposeful activity in the afternoon prevents boredom and provides the fatigue-producing exercise conducive to evening sleep. Nocturnal sleep latency is correlated directly with the number of hours of prior wakefulness. Clients who have late afternoon naps take three times as long to get to sleep later in the evening.

A useful tool for the client and the nurse is a sleep diary. Have the client log sleep patterns for several days. Included are such sleep and rest activities as naps, time of retiring, estimated sleep latency time, numbers of nocturnal awakenings, reasons for nocturnal awakenings, and time of arising. The data collected during the sleep history, combined with information from the sleep log, give the client and the nurse a base from which to discuss concerns about changing patterns of sleep. The nurse can teach the older adult about sleep theory and the normal characteristic changes found in the older person. A personal sleep log, plus a solid information base, helps the client adapt his sleep habits to obtain optimum sleep.

Planning for wakefulness can be useful. Many sleep researchers suggest that in the presence of wakefulness, the client should not stay in bed, but get up and change activity before attempting to sleep again. Have a bed light near at hand, so books and magazines can be read, or knitting or crocheting can be done in a chair by the bedside. Some persons prefer to listen to a softly playing radio or television until sleep returns. The anxiety produced by the inability to fall asleep is most nonconducive to achieving comfortable sleep. Often minor adjustments in the immediate environment can foster sleep. Change the number of pillows, or use a pillow, blanket, or quilt from the client's own home. Altering the position of the bed, and improving the room ventilation is often all that is needed to provide a sleep-promoting room.

Record on the Kardex and then follow "sleep rituals" favored by the client. Make arrangements to institute the client's usual bedtime routines. Allow time for the client to perform his usual rituals before retiring. Many older adults have a systematic way of undressing and folding and hanging up their clothes. Often bedtime prayers and other religious activities are part of the ritual. A rushed client who omits one of the procedures from his ritual will be upset and may take longer to fall asleep. The environment itself needs to be supportive of sleep. Room companions should be compatible and retire around the same time. The noise level should be especially controlled at bedtime, and the staff encouraged not to make any unnecessary noises. Care should be taken when checking clients during the night, so that they are not unnecessarily awakened or disturbed. However, underlying causes of observable symptoms, such as restlessness, perspiration, and pain need to be investigated. The client needs to feel secure and have no concerns about his safety. Someone should be readily available during the night if needed. A call or telephone system that is easy to use, within reach, and answered promptly provides the measure of security needed by the older adult. The client should be encouraged to express his fears. Some older adult clients may be fearful that other persons may enter their room or home during the night. The safety of their personal belongings is often an area of concern and a cause of sleeplessness.

Providing sleep using the nursing arts. Nursing arts should be used to promote sleep as an alternative to sleep medications. Offer back rubs, change and tighten the bed sheets. Close doors if possible. For clients in their own homes, room-darkening shades can block street light and traffic disturbances. Nighttime restlessness and anxiety may be helped by a warm bath, or partial bed bath. Recent evidence supports the theory that a bath or shower is best at night because the body can adjust to the pH skin changes during sleep. A soothing back massage relaxes muscles and gives the client and the nurse a moment to explore the reasons for his wakefulness. Food may be used to induce sleep. A diet rich in protein and a glass of milk before bedtime promote sleep. Warm milk before bedtime has long been the old wives' treatment for sleeplessness. The scientific basis for its action is the protein found in milk, an amino acid, L-tryptophan. Hartman (1974) found L-tryptophan activates the serotonin-containing neurons suspected of causing the onset of sleep. The older adult living at home on a limited, fixed income should be helped to plan a diet that includes dairy foods, legumes, and meat to acquire sources of L-tryptophan.

A simple nursing measure can alleviate such common sleep disturbances as leg muscle cramps and tremors. The nurse can help the client straighten the leg and dorsiflex the foot. In most instances, this will achieve pain relief. In the presence of painful arthritis and peripheral vascular disease, the nurse can suggest one electric blanket or flannel sheets to replace several heavy blankets to provide warmth without pressure.

To summarize, interpersonal relations and communication can help clients express anxiety and worry. Other measures the nurse can provide include the following.

Warm bath
Relaxing back rub
Soiled dressing changes
Sheets tightened
Elimination needs met
Position changes
Sleep rituals respected
Warm cup of milk, no caffeine beverages
Quiet recreation before bedtime
Relief of pain
Environmental control of temperature, lighting, ventilation, and noise

Planning for uninterrupted sleep. A care plan that avoids disturbing the client at night may require special organization of medications and treatments. The purpose and goal of around-the-clock treatments should be reassessed. Medications and treatments should be sequenced to eliminate sleep interruptions. Once awakened, the client must begin the sleep pattern again with latency and progress from stage one. Much REM and deep stage four sleep is lost.

Mr. Judge is a 70-year-old retired accountant newly admitted to a nursing home. He is complaining about being tired, and a sleep log quickly indicates the reasons why.

10:00 PM	Prepares to retire
10:30 PM	Given sleeping pill
11:00 PM	Falls asleep
12:00	Awakened for vital signs
1:00 AM	Nocturia—gets up to go to bathroom
2:40 AM	Asleep
3:00 AM	Nocturia—gets up to go to bathroom
6:00 AM	Awaken—lights on; water pitchers filled; vital signs taken
8:00 AM	Breakfast

When giving his sleep history, he indicated that he usually goes to bed after the 11:00 news and arises at 8:00 AM. The nurse considers also that the diuretic that he takes at 10:00 AM and 10:00 PM might be causing his nocturia. He states that he has no previous history of taking sleeping medications before admission.

Nursing diagnosis

Interrupted sleeping patterns

Client goal

Client will have 7 hours sleep, uninterrupted by nursing activity.

Nursing orders

May watch late evening news using ear plug for TV.
Diuretics will be given at 10:00 AM and 6:00 PM.
Vital signs will be taken at 11:30 PM and 8:00 AM.
No sleeping medication will be offered.
Awaken for breakfast at 8:00 AM. No housekeeping activities in room before breakfast.

Evaluation

After 5 days, Mr. Judge was reinterviewed regarding sleeping patterns. He reported some improvement in hours of sleep obtained. Sleep latency remained prolonged at 45 minutes, but he had only one episode of nocturia during the night and then slept until 8:00 AM. He stated that he was satisfied with the amount of sleep that he was getting. Nurse will reinterview regarding sleep patterns again in one week.

Drugs and sleep. Gerard and co-workers (1978) studied the sleeping characteristics of a group of young-old (65-74), old-old (75-98), and young adults (16-39) living at home.

He found no significant differences in the sleep habits of the two older adult groups other than the old-old retired earlier and went to sleep faster. However, both groups arose at about the same time. The young group had as many spontaneous nighttime awakenings as the two older groups. Females in both older adult groups woke up earlier and more frequently during the night, and were less able to return to sleep. Hypnotics were a common practice for 58 percent of the older adults. They took sleeping pills almost every night. A larger proportion of young-old adults, 41 percent, took hypnotics compared to old-old, 28 percent. Those who took hypnotics rated sleep quality worse than those who did not.

The term *sleeping medication* is a misnomer. Few sleeping drugs produce an unaltered pattern of sleep. Almost all will affect the older adult's sleep cycle, and some will even alter behavior during the waking period the next day.

Various drugs suppress REM activity in varying degrees, from as little as 2.6 percent as in flurazepam hydrochloride (Dalmane) to 100 percent as seen in tranylcypromine, an MAO inhibitor. Some drugs, such as glutethimide (Doriden) and pentobarbitol (Nembutal) suppress stage four sleep, particularly in the older adult. Even after short-term use, there are significant withdrawal symptoms after the drug is stopped. A client recovering from a REM-suppressant drug can expect prolonged REM stages for the first week. Clients report vivid nightmares, restlessness, and insomnia. Sleep disturbances without the drug seems worse than before it was taken. (It is not un-

Table 10-4. Pharmacology and the stages of sleep in man*

REM		Stage IV
Decrease REM time		**Decrease Stage IV time**
Ethchlorvynol (Placidyl) 500 mg.	Morphine	Glutethimide (Doriden) 500 mg.
Glutethimide (Doriden) 500 mg.	Heroin	Pentobarbital sodium (Nembutal)
Secobarbital sodium (Seconal)	Alcohol	100 mg.
100 mg.	Thiopental (Pentothal)	Diazepam (Valium) 10 mg.
Pentobarbital sodium (Nembutal)	Nitrazepam (Mogadon)	Reserpine 0.14 mg./kg.
100 mg.	Dextroamphetamine	Heptabarbital
Methyprylon (Noludar) 300 mg.	Imipramine hydrochloride (Trofanil)	Chloral hydrate 1.5 gm.
Methaqualone (Quaalade) 300 mg.	Amitriptyline (Elavil)	Depression
Diphenhydramine hydrochloride	Methadone hydrochloride (Dolo-	Hypothyroidism
(Benadryl) 50 mg.	phine)	Dextroamphetamine and pentobarbi-
Scopolamine 0.006 mg./kg.	Meprobamate (Miltown) 1200 mg.	tal
Monoamine oxidase inhibitors (MAO)	Amobarbital	
	Heptabarbital (Medomin)	
Allow normal REM time†	**Increase REM time**	**Increase Stage IV time**
Chloral hydrate 0.5 gm., 1.0 gm.,	Reserpine	Moderate to vigorous exercise carried
1.5 gm.	LSD	out several hours before bedtime.
Flurazepam hydrochloride (Dal-		Antidepressants in the presence of
mane) 30 mgm.		depression.
Methaqualone (Quaalude) 150 mg.		
Chlordiazepoxide (Librium) 50 mg.		
Diazepam (Valium) 10 mg.		
Caffeine		

*Copyright 1971, American Journal of Nursing Co. Reproduced with permission from the American Journal of Nursing, December, Vol. 71 No. 12. Bibliography for table available on request.
†These findings are only for the specific dosages listed.

common to have a significant increase in depression, anxiety, and fear.) These periods of uncomfortable withdrawal symptoms lead the client to request more drugs. The hazards of suppressant hypnotics are not limited to psychological manifestations. With the use of REM-suppressant drugs, there is an increase in nocturnal angina pectoris attacks and an increase in hydrochloric acid secretions in clients prone to duodenal ulcers. Given the long half-life of some hypnotics, particularly flurazepam, and the slower excretion time in some older adults, the effects of these drugs can extend into the next day as confusion and grogginess. These symptoms may be viewed as changes in behaviors for the older adult and treated with other medications, compounding the problem (Table 10-4).

Sleep loss as a sign of organ dysfunction. All altered sleep patterns reported by the client should be taken as meaningful by the nurse. When the sleep history and sleep log indicate obvious sleep disturbances that cannot be remedied through nursing measures, some organ dysfunction should be considered.

Congestive heart failure is one example of a systemic disorder whose symptoms are manifested at sleep time. Mrs. Jenkins is a 72-year-old woman who was casually telling her nurse neighbor how she plans to buy some extra pillows at the next department store sale. She goes on to say that she has been using her guest pillows for herself at night in order to sleep. Even in this informal setting, the nurse realizes that Mrs. Jenkins is relating an important component of her sleep profile. The nurse explains to Mrs. Jenkins in layman's terms that she is experiencing three-pillow orthopnea, very possibly related to congestive heart failure. Mrs. Jenkins is referred to her family physician.

Sleep interruptions are seen as nocturia in benign prostatic hypertrophy and diabetic mellitus. An older male adult who normally voids once during the night now states he has to get up three or four times during the night. Referral to a physician is indicated for this client.

Insomnia, early morning awakening, or inability to get out of bed are classic signs of depression. (Depressed individuals have a lower level of serotonin and catecholamines such as norepinephrine.) Because depression is widespread in the older adult population, the nurse must be alert to these alterations in sleep patterns.

NUTRITIONAL CONSIDERATIONS FOR THE OLDER ADULT

The nutritional needs of the older adult are similar to those of all other age groups. What changes are the availability of food, the ability to eat and

Table 10-5. The basic four groups assessing nutritional needs of older adults

Milk group
Two or more servings. One serving includes: 1 cup fat milk, buttermilk, or dried milk powder equivalent; 1 ounce unprocessed cheese, or ½ cup cottage cheese.

Meat group
Two or more servings. One serving is:
2 to 3 ounces of beef, veal, pork, lamb, poultry, or fish; two eggs, 1 cup cooked dry beans, peas, or lentils; or 4 tablespoons peanut butter.

Bread/cereal group
Four or more servings (whole grain, enriched, restored). One serving includes: 1 slice bread, 1 ounce ready-to-eat cereal or ½ to ¾ cup cooked cereal, cornmeal, grits, macaroni, noodles, rice, or spaghetti.

Vegetable/fruit group
Four or more servings a day (½ cup or one piece of fruit equals one serving) and should include:
One vitamin A source
　Broccoli
　Carrots
　Greens
　Beet greens
　Chard
　Collards
　Dandelion greens
　Squash (winter)
　Sweet potatoes
　Apricots
　Cantaloupes
　Papayas
　Peaches (dried)
One vitamin C source
　Cantaloupes
　Citrus fruit
　Strawberries
　Broccoli
　Brussel sprouts
　Peppers
Two or more other vegetables and fruits, including potatoes.

absorb food, and the social milieu conducive to good appetite, food preparation, and eating.

A nutritional assessment of the older adult, using a 24-hour food recall or intake log, is useful in determining the client's nutritional status. A typical day's intake is evaluated with the client to determine if each of the four basic categories has been included every day (Table 10-5). When the client's diet has a deficiency in one or more of the basic four food groups, the nurse can do a more in-depth nutritional history. An inquiry into the client's dietary habits, food preferences, and shopping and food preparation arrangements can reveal nutrition-related problems that should be addressed. The older adult's eating patterns are long established and reflect his social, economic, cultural, and health history. Nutritional patterns of many years should not be expected to change to any great extent. The nurse can offer nutritional information and make recommendations for modifications and adaptations of dietary practices in a way that will build on the client's nutritional assets.

The need for calories decreases at a rate of 5 percent per decade from age 30 to 50, and 7 percent per decade after 70. The rise in weight is often an undramatic one, one or two pounds a year. A man at an ideal weight of 160 pounds at age thirty can be an obese 190 pounds at age 60 with no added calories in his daily diet. With age, the caloric intake should gradually decrease while the protein, carbohydrate, lipid, vitamin, and mineral intake should remain the same. There is little room in the diet for foods with no nutritional value (empty calories).

Protein needs

The need for protein remains at approximately 1 gm per kilogram of body weight as needed in youth. A 72-kilogram (160-pound) man needs about 72 gm of protein a day to meet his body needs for tissue growth and repair. A balance must be struck between too much and too little protein. The aging kidney has reduced filtration capacities and is at risk in the presence of high nitrogen levels as a result of protein metabolism. A ratio of 1.5 gm of protein per kilogram of body weight will overload the aging kidney, and some protein is excreted in the stool. Lower than 0.7 gm per kilogram

of body weight protein ratios are inadequate to meet the growth, protection, and repair mechanism usually carried out in the body. Protein intake can be measured easily by using the following rule of thumb estimates:

  8 gm protein
    Milk, 8 oz
    Meat, fish, or poultry, 1 oz
    Hard cheese, 1 oz
    Cottage cheese, 3 oz
    Peanut butter, 2 tbs
  6 gm protein
    Egg
    Fruit or vegetable, ½ cup
  2 gm protein
    Bread, one slice

These protein foods are also very good sources of other vitamins and trace minerals. The older adult with a chronic poor protein intake, as often seen with the typical tea and toast diet, will complain of muscular weakness and even muscle wasting. In such cases, the body's ability to repair disease or injured cells is severely restricted. An adequate protein intake assists the older body to keep the pH of the blood stabilized. In addition, the high molecular weight of the protein molecule stabilizes the fluid balance in the tissues.

Fat needs

Fats are essential components of the older adult's diet. They serve the older adult particularly well because they are the satiety component of food. Feeling full offers a sense of well-being and security. This is particularly true in many ethnic cultures, which relate food to love and satisfaction. Fats are useful in improving the appetite, because they add flavor and texture to many dishes. Fat aids in digestion by reducing gastric emptying time, which permits hydrochloric and other enzyme action to be exerted to their fullest extent on the food. The completeness of these early digestive processes ensures a higher absorption rate in the lower digestive tract. Fat is also essential in the absorption of the fat soluble vitamins A, D, E, and K. Vitamins A and D, frequently deficient in older adults, are critical elements in the integrity and repair of skin and bones. Vitamin K is an essential factor in the blood clotting mechanism. Fatty pads are important to protect body organs from injury. In the older adult, fat intake must be adequate in order to protect the fat pads that hold the kidneys in place on the walls of the midback. Fat layers in the body serve as ready sources of energy and act as insulation against colder air temperatures.

Carbohydrate needs

Carbohydrates are energy sources for metabolic needs as well as the sources for many vitamins and minerals. When carbohydrate calories are obtained from unprocessed foods, they serve the older adult well. However, too often the carbohydrates are obtained from sugars and starches totally stripped of any nutritional value. The so-called convenience foods, which are readily available and easy to prepare and eat, are often of this "empty calorie" variety. The money and time expended in the use of these foods decrease the money available for those foods that go into a varied and well-balanced diet. Although overt clinical signs of malnutrition may not occur, subclinical malnutrition is frequently manifested in the older adult and is seen as confusion, depression, and weakness.

Carbohydrate intolerance is most prevalent in the form of a lactose deficiency. Lactose intolerance is culturally associated with the inability to digest milk. It affects 10 percent of American white adults, 80 percent of American black adults, and 95 percent of American Orientals. After drinking milk, these persons will complain of abdominal distention, flatulence, and watery stools. The calcium normally obtained from milk sources can be obtained from nuts, beans, vegetables, and fish sources. The nurse can suggest these alternatives:

Almonds
Asparagus
Cabbage
Kale
Canned salmon
Peanuts
Beet greens
Collards
Spinach
Oysters
Coconut
Broccoli
Dandelion greens
Turnip greens
Sardines

The older adult on a limited food budget can use carbohydrate to his best advantage by buying whole grain cereals and breads. These carbohydrates contain the B complex vitamins, iron, and fiber. Processed breads and cereals sometimes have these substances added; however, the rate of absorption of these additives into the body is questioned.

Culture and geographic areas influence the form in which carbohydrates are consumed. Familiarity with the carbohydrate dish can spark food interest and appetite in the older adult. Some carbohydrate preferences of specific heritages follow.

Black American
Corn fritters
Baking powder biscuits
Corn bread (served as crackling bread hotcakes, hush puppies, and spoon bread)
Hominy grits
Rice

Jewish
Bagel
Blintzes (thin pancakes filled with cottage cheese or fruit served with sour cream)
Bulke (yeast roll)
Challah (braided bread)
Farfel (noodle dumpling for soup)
Kasha (buck wheat groats)
Matzo (unleavened bread)

Puerto Rican
Rice
Corn meal mush
Oatmeal

Mexican-American
Corn
Rice
Macaroni
Spaghetti
Atole (corn meal gruel)
Sopapillas (deep fried dough)
Tortilla (thin unleavened cakes)

Italian
Pasta
Polenta (a cornmeal mush served in a casserole with sausage or cheese)
White crusty bread (made with high protein flour and little fat)

Near Eastern
Bourglour (cracked whole wheat bread)
Rice

Chinese
Rice
Noodles
Millet (a small grain cereal grass)
Irish
Potatoes
Bread
German
Potato pancakes

When an older adult is transposed from his ethnic environment, one of the principle losses is his traditional foods. It would be ideal if the long-term-care facility could serve entire menus consistent with ethnic preferences. One alternative is to focus variety on the bread and cereal groups.

Because breads and cereals are the relatively inexpensive part of a meal, ethnic preferences can be respected using the breads and cereals. Mr. Pedona has had pasta every Tuesday, Thursday, and Sunday for 70 years. After admission to a long-term-care facility to convalesce after surgery, he simply could not understand why he has to eat baked potatoes or rice. To him, a meal is incomplete without the pasta and tomato sauce. After a consultation with the dietician, Mr. Pedona was able to receive pasta three times a week. His family was also permitted to bring in his favorite pasta weekly.

Although it is not feasible to have all types of breads and cereals available, the nurse and dietician can be guided by the ethnicity and cultural patterns predominent in the client population. The long-term-care facility serving a geographical area will have certain cultural groups represented. These familiar "just like home" foods stimulate the appetite and are a positive reinforcement with ethnic and cultural identity. The nurse involved in Meals on Wheels programs, nutritional centers, and community health agencies can make similar recommendations regarding adding variety to the client's meals through the bread and cereal group.

Vitamin needs

Vitamin deficiencies constitute one of the most serious health threats to the older adult. Nutritional surveys have demonstrated widespread inadequate intakes of vitamins A, C, D, and K. Fruits and vegetables are the most common sources of vitamins, but they are seasonal and can be expensive and difficult to prepare. Nutritional requirements of these essential vitamins are the same as for a younger person. Those elderly adults who are chronically ill or on various medication regimens that alter vitamin absorption or use need higher levels of vitamins. Canned and frozen fruits and vegetables offer the client a convenient and less expensive source of vitamins.

Vitamin A needs. The condition of the client's skin, eyes, and mucous membranes lining the mouth, stomach, intestines, respiratory, genital, and urinary tracts reflect the client's intake of vitamin A. The skin and mucous membrane protect the body against bacterial invasion. An intact skin and mucous membrane surface offers the older adult a barrier against upper respiratory tract colds and sinus conditions and lower respiratory tract bronchial infections and pneumonia. Night vision requires adequate levels of vitamin A for the retina pigment.

Because vitamin A must be taken with fats in order to be absorbed, the nurse should suggest that the client eat the vitamin A vegetables with a small amount of butter, margarine, or oil. Salad greens and tomatoes should be dressed with a small amount of oil-base dressing. Fruit and fruit juices rich in vitamin A can be taken at a meal that has a fat component either in milk, meat, or butter.

Mineral oil taken orally as a laxative inhibits the absorption of fat-soluble vitamins. To prevent fat-soluble vitamin deficiencies, anticipatory guidance should include instructions to the client to take the mineral oil well after meals, preferably at bedtime.* Debilitated older adults should not use mineral oil because of the danger of aspiration and lipid pneumonia.

B complex vitamins and folic acid needs. The vitamin B complex group is needed for the proper function of cell metabolism, particularly in the nervous and digestive systems. Inadequate intake of meats, vegetables, and whole grain breads and

---

*NOTE: The nurse can encourage alternatives to cathartics. Some measures the nurse can suggest are dietary bulk, adequate fluid intake, exercise, sleep, and privacy in meeting elimination needs. These health-promoting activities aid in proper bowel functions.

cereals causes a high incidence of chronic B complex deficiencies in the older adult. Many drugs, such as hypotensive agents, used by the older adult increase the body's need for the B complex group.

Anemia occurs at a high rate in the older adult population. In the age group of 65 to 74 years, 7 percent of men and 11 percent of women are found to have anemia. In the age group 75 years and older, these rates rise to 20 percent in men and 23 percent in women. The low hemoglobin rate (below 12 gm/100 ml) causes the client to feel weak and irritable and often to have insomnia. Stomatitis (cracks and sores at the side of the mouth) and dermatitis may be related to the anemia also. Pyridoxine (B_6), considered an anemia-preventing agent, helps relieve these symptoms. Vitamin B_{12} deficiency related to the diminished hydrochloric acid gastric secretions of older adults is also a cause of anemia. Injections of B_{12} help relieve the symptoms of pernicious anemia.

Folic acid is associated with anemia of the older adult population also. A number of studies have shown that up to 80 percent of this group have folic acid deficiencies. "Low serum folate levels have been correlated with mental disorders. It has, in fact, been suggested that folic acid deficiency may be the cause of certain mental disorders rather than the result" (Mead Johnson Laboratories, 1975). Folic acid is found in fresh green vegetables, especially lettuce, and liver.

Anemia should never be ignored. When the dietary iron intake and absorption are good, cancer is often the cause of an unexplained anemia.

Vitamin D needs. Vitamin D influences the absorption and use of calcium and the mineralization of bone. A deficiency in vitamin D causes an adult onset of rickets called *senile osteomalacia*. The skeleton decalcifies, and the client has neurological impairment of the nerves in the spinal column.

There are few dietary sources of vitamin D, so the nurse should recommend that the client get sufficient exposure to sunlight. Except during the cold winter months, the older adult should have his skin exposed to the sunlight for a few minutes each day. Those clients in long-term-care facilities should have sun decks or walkways available for outdoor strolls or sunbathing in the early morning or midafternoon. Exposure to fluorescent lights is adequate for vitamin D production when the client is unable to go outdoors.

Vitamin C needs. Ascorbic acid deficiencies are frequently seen in the older adult as subclinical scurvy when cuts, surgical wounds, or leg ulcers have delayed healing times. Review the client's vitamin C intake. Bleeding gums, sheet hemorrhages of the legs, and slowed hair growth are also signs of low serum ascorbic acid.

Vitamin K needs. Vitamin K is essential to the body as a factor in the production of prothrombin. It is available in large amounts in those deep green leafy vegetables that are also abundant in vitamin A. Like vitamin A, it is also fat-soluble. Vitamin K is also produced by the normal flora in the large intestines. The purgatives taken routinely by the older adult can reduce the vitamin K, producing bacterial flora in the large bowel. Vitamin K is also available in citrus fruits, bananas, and chocolate.

Vitamin E needs. Vitamin E is an antioxidant agent that accentuates the use of vitamins A and C in the body and maintains the integrity of cell walls. In addition, it promotes the production of red blood cells in the bone marrow. These functions are of value to older adults because of their reduced metabolic rate and need of support of new cell production.

Mineral needs

As with all nutritional components, the older adult's need for minerals is, on the whole, the same as for younger persons.

Restriction of sodium in the presence of congestive heart failure is often one important limitation in the older adult's mineral intake. Any accumulation of fluid adds an overwhelming burden to the pumping ability of the heart. Hypertension and decreased filtration ability of the kidneys, both common in the older adult, also limit the amount of excessive fluid tolerated as a healthy state. Because sodium is a water-holding mineral, its elimination from the diet reduces fluid transport problems for the older person.

Potassium is an essential body mineral that is lost through normal metabolic activities. It must be replaced daily in the dietary intake. Up to 50 percent of older adults have an inadequate potassium intake because of overall limited variety of foods eaten and because often they take diuretics, which increase potassium excretion. A low serum potassium level will cause muscular weakness and mental confusion, both frequent symptoms erroneously associated with "normal aging." A client who eats a variety of fruits, vegetables, and nuts each day will have a sufficient potassium intake.

Iron deficiency is also a common nutritional problem for the older adult. Complaints of fatigue and breathlessness are associated with anemia. Iron is available in so many meats, vegetables, cereals, and nuts that the older adult has a wide selection. Cream of Wheat cereal is an excellent source of iron. It is inexpensive, stores easily, and is quick to prepare. A 1-ounce serving provides 50 percent of the minimum daily requirement. Liver, dried fruits, organ meats, and molasses are also excellent sources of iron. Clients using daily aspirin in the treatment of arthritis can have a significant enough blood loss through gastric irritation to cause anemia. Supplemental iron preparations are not recommended, because they can mask low-grade chronic bleeding from a malignant lesion.

Adequate serum zinc levels are necessary for wound healing and taste activity. There is atrophy in many taste buds as an individual ages. Older adults who use canned fruits and vegetables exclusively are at risk for zinc deficiency. Considerable zinc is lost during canning, so the nurse should suggest that some fresh fruits and vegetables be taken each day if at all possible. Studies of persons with decreased taste acuity improved when given oral zinc. The potential for optimum taste acuity for the older adult can be provided by sufficient foods containing zinc, such as fish, chicken, liver, peas, spinach, cabbage, and potatoes.

Water needs

The body's need for fluid remains at 2500 to 3000 ml during the older adult years. During illness, the older adult needs even more fluids than a younger counterpart. The older kidneys need dilute fluids in order to filter efficiently. Fluids that are concentrated damage the nephrons and further reduce kidney function. Clients who are on bedrest or who have markedly reduced mobility require up to 4 liters a day to flush the renal pelvis and prevent stone formation.

Fiber needs

Dietary fiber or bulk aids gastrointestinal motility and produces soft and easily evacuated stool. Older adults frequently rely on laxatives and cathartics, which can cause vitamin and trace mineral loss. When constipation or laxative dependency is part of a client's history, health teaching should include instruction regarding dietary fiber. The client should substitute for refined bread and cereal servings the following whole grain breads and cereals:

Breads	Cereals
Whole wheat breads	Oatmeal
Whole rye rolls, breads, and muffins	Rolled oats
Bran muffins and breads	Bran flakes
Graham crackers	Granola
Rye-Krisp crackers	Grape Nuts
	Shredded Wheat
	Wheat flakes
	Brown rice
	Bran

Anticipatory guidance should include an explanation that some flatulence and mild cramping will occur as bowel functioning improves. These signs of gastrointestinal activity should encourage the client, and he should continue the improved fiber intake. After a few days, the defecation urge will be vigorous and the stools will be soft and easy to pass.

For the client wishing to reduce his laxative dependency, the nurse can recommend this bowel stimulating routine. Upon awakening, drink 8 ounces of water. At breakfast eat a bowl of All-Bran cereal with milk and sugar, 4 ounces of orange juice, grapefruit juice, or prune juice, and a cup of tea or coffee. Within an hour, sit on the toilet and try to move the bowels. *Never ignore the sensation to move the bowels.*

Social nutrition

Food habits are closely related to emotional and social events. The brain's arousal system must be stimulated in order to maintain a good appetite. Rituals associated with eating are deeply ingrained and are difficult to change. Social interaction is the most common expectation of the eating situation. In the day-to-day situation, eating alone is the most frequent cause of disinterest in food preparation and diminished appetite. Special occasions are always marked with food. Holidays, birthdays, weddings—even the seasons of the year—are events that have special food traditions. A client with a poor appetite can be encouraged to eat with others. A recent widow who no longer eats properly because she doesn't like to cook just for herself can be referred to an "out of residence" food service.

These local clubs, nutrition centers, churches, and senior centers prepare and serve well-balanced and inexpensive meals. Many of these facilities are funded as part of the Older Americans Act of 1965. Any person over 65 is eligible to participate in the nutritional, educational, and social programs at these centers. Five hot meals are provided a week, and each meal supplies at least one third of the older adult's nutritional requirements. There is a modest cost for the meal, but no older person is denied a meal because of inability to pay.

Long-term-care facilities can promote healthy appetites at mealtime by using colorful, properly prepared, and varied diets. A dull looking tray will quickly dull the client's appetite.

One facility organizes an International Night once a month. The dining hall decorations, menu, and recorded music are coordinated to the country being celebrated. Each resident is expected to dress in his best clothes and can invite a guest. The excitement generated by this once-a-month activity keeps the residents active and interested for weeks. Often the residents themselves assist the dietician in the menu planning and give their old country recipes a try once again. Because it is such an important social event, everyone takes extra care in his appearance, and both the residents and the staff enjoy the evening.

Meals on Wheels

Meals on Wheels, an international volunteer program, has been providing home-bound persons, including many older adults, with nutritious meals for many years. Lunch and supper are provided five days a week. The midday meal is a two- or three-course hot meal, and supper is a prepackaged sandwich or salad meal that is placed in the client's refrigerator. The volunteers are trained to interview the client in person and to discuss the client's appetite. Any difficulty in delivering the meal is reported at once to the supervisor. This program provides not only the nutritional service, but also is an opportunity for social contact for the client. Often prevention of institutionalization and crisis intervention are some of the stated goals of these organizations.

SHELTER

Shelter is listed as a primary needs in Maslow's hierarchy. *Shelter* protects a person from the elements, provides an area of privacy and personal belonging, and gives a person a feeling of safety. The place of residence of the older adult is of particular importance for him, because the physiological changes of aging reduce his skills to interact with the larger, more complex world. Nursing intervention often includes counseling clients and their families regarding options in living styles. Knowledge of housing accommodations and community resources suitable to the needs of the older adult permits the nurse to discuss alternatives to institutionalized care.

To a greater or lesser extent, the client's place of residence is the center of his personal care and recreational and social activities. The older adult can participate in a wide range of activities if they are convenient. The selection of housing for the elderly should have accessibility as a priority consideration.

The federal government recommends that public transportation be available within ⅛ mile (2 ½ city blocks). Within the same radius, there should be a food store, preferably one that handles some medication. It is further recommended that the following facilities be located within a half mile (10 blocks) comfortable walking distance:

1. Medical clinic or doctor's office
2. Shopping center
3. Park or recreational area
4. Restaurant with carry-out food service
5. General entertainment area
6. Library
7. Houses of worship
8. Hospital

A neighborhood offering such facilities provides the client with easy access to support services needed for food, clothing, health care, recreational, and spiritual needs. Ready access to other people of all age groups helps the older adult have social contacts and relieves boredom. The combination of a safe, private dwelling place and accessible services will keep the older adult independent. The federal government reports note that these housing site recommendations regarding accessibility to stores and other facilities are usually only found in the urban and more developed suburban areas. The housing reports also state that the older adult prefers these shopping and recreational conveniences and the independence they offer to the quiet natural beauty of remote rural areas. "The living environments of older people have decisive impact upon aspects of their life styles and well-being, which are reasonably subsumed under 'quality of life.' " (Donahue, 1977).

The importance of housing to the older adult can be measured in the time he spends at home. The older adult spends more time at home than almost anyone else over the age of 5, and because of this, more of his life satisfactions are related to his sense of home. Likewise, many of his problems are home-generated. Other than his spouse and his health, his housing accommodation is the most important element in the life of the older adult.

Usual living arrangements of older adults

Studies have indicated that some generalizations can be made regarding living arrangements of the older adult.

1. Older adult couples prefer to live independently of their older adult children. Most couples report contact with the children at least once a week. Only 9 percent of older adults actually live in the household of their adult children.
2. Those older adults who move after retirement move to Florida, Arizona, and California. Of those who remain in their own state, many moved from small towns to larger metropolitan areas.
3. The percentage of older adults living in urban centers has been increasing, because they remain in the city when the younger adults move to the suburbs.
4. Considerable numbers of low-rent, public housing projects have been designated for the older adult population.
5. Single-room occupancy (SRO) accommodations found in hotels and apartment houses

are more frequently being used by adult widowers and widows.

Given these data, the urban community health nurse can expect the older adult to be represented as a large population within her catchment area. The concentration of older adult clients in certain geographical areas does have an advantage for planning health-related projects. Voluntary agencies have designed day-care centers for the older adult that provide recreational, occupational, and nutritional services.

Churches and synagogues with many older adults in their congregations can have active senior citizens' groups. These groups organize day trips, vacations, clubs, hobbies, and consumer action committees. Over 79 percent of older adults attend their house of worship at least every week or two, and 71 percent define religious affiliation as very important in their lives. These voluntary agencies, health centers, and religious groups should be the nurses' focus for health screening projects. Health teaching and illness screening programs for common age-related illnesses, such as glaucoma, diabetes, hypertension, cancer, tuberculosis, and emphysema should be done annually by the nurse. The community health nurse visiting the client in his home can recommend the client's participation in these local programs. Frequently, these agencies also provide home-bound assistance in the form of friendly visitors, pastoral counseling, transportation, and Meals on Wheels.

EXERCISING, VITALITY, AND FLEXIBILITY

A 10-year longitudinal study correlating health practices and incidence of illness in persons aged 60 to 94 has found that, of inactivity, obesity, and smoking, inactivity was the most damaging to the health of the older adult. The older clients with little locomotor activity were hospitalized, had surgery more frequently, and died sooner than actuary tables expected, as compared with the more active groups. Exercise strengthens the cardiac muscle, normalizes the blood pressure, stimulates deep and efficient breathing, and is an outlet for nervous tension. The key to successful exercising is regular and moderate exercising habits. The older adult must avoid competition in conditioning workouts. Isometric exercises are not suitable for the older adult. The nurse should encourage the client to choose sports and activities that develop skill and coordination, rather than speed, strength, and endurance. Also, activities that require sudden starts and stops or cause strain on the lower back or legs should be avoided. It is recommended that persons of all age groups be given a physical examination before starting a new program of vigorous exercises. The older adult should have an electrocardiogram (ECG) in addition to the physical examination. The client should be aware that any signs of breathlessness, pounding heart, dizziness, tightness or pain in the chest, nausea, or loss of muscle control are signs that he is overtaxing his body. Slow warm-up periods enable the muscles to reach peak activity by distributing the blood flow in an easy and uniform manner. The heart is spared the burden of having to supply blood on a sudden demand. The cool-down period after exercise serves a similar purpose. It permits the return of blood to the central veins at a moderate rate and lets the muscles gradually decrease their need for oxygen.

Initiating an exercise program

The nurse should build on the client's assets. Often, when a nurse is discussing exercise, the client will state that he never exercises. The nurse should point out that for the older adult, daily hygiene and dressing practices, as well as light household chores, such as dusting or folding laundry, are counted as part of light exercise. Moderately strenuous activities such as gardening, light household painting, and walking are listed as moderate exercises. By making these points, the nurse demonstrates that the client can build on his normal pattern of daily activities. For those clients who are not interested in formal exercise classes, the nurse can suggest wake-up stretches and walking as the exercise program.

Clients in the over-60 age group who are interested in sports, golf, swimming, stationary cycling, and walking are encouraged to continue these activities. Strenuous sports, such as jogging, handball, basketball, squash, and singles tennis are usually not recommended. The nurse can further build on the client's assets by reviewing the client's social history. Many older adults can relate stories of a very active childhood, not in sports per se, but in walking miles to school, bicycling, doing farm and household chores and heavy industrial labor. Women in the days before modern household appliances exercised vigorously when

Table 10-6. Level of exertion of activity for the over-50 adult

Light	Light to moderate	Moderate	Heavy
Billiards	Archery	Archery	Bicycling (briskly or uphill)
Fishing	Badminton	Badminton	Handball
Quoits	Bicycling (easy pace)	Basketball	Tennis (singles)
Shuffleboard	Boccie	Bicycling	Walking (upstairs, uphill)
	Bowling	Cross-country skiing	
	Canoeing	Curling	
	Croquet	Deck tennis	
	Dancing	Fencing	
	Darts	Golf (without cart)	
	Golf (with cart)	Paddle tennis	
	Horseback riding	Rowing	
	Horseshoes	Skating	
	Putting	Swimming	
	Rowing	Tennis	
	Sailing	Tennis (doubles)	
	Shooting	Walking (briskly,	
	Skindiving	level ground)	
	Volleyball		
	Walking (slow pace,		
	level ground)		

scrubbing floors, doing laundry by hand and line-drying it, beating carpets, or carrying coal or wood for the stove to prepare meals. Well-meaning friends and family do the older client a disservice by providing low shelves that prevent the older person from reaching and stretching and denying them household duties that would be sources of exercise for them (Table 10-6).

The sedentary client might start an exercise program with only stretching exercises before getting out of bed in the morning. Just as a cat stretches his body and limbs to their full length, the client can move his arms, trunk, and legs slowly and enjoy the feeling. A mere 5 minutes of ROM exercises a day will prevent joint immobility and muscle wasting. The client can then exercise his eye myscles by shifting his gaze on near and then distant objects. If constipation is a problem, the client can be taught to strengthen the anal sphincter muscle by contracting and relaxing buttocks and thighs. These can all be done before the client even gets out of bed in the morning.

The client might prefer walking as an exercise. Walking can be called the best of all exercises. It is free and requires no expensive clothing; it can be done alone or with others; and it is an excellent cardiac and respiratory tonic. Walking can be adapted to include the client's interests. If the cli-

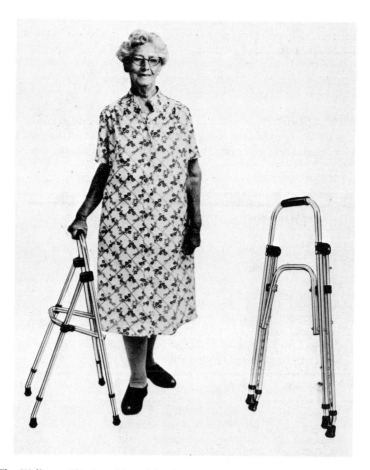

Fig. 10-7. The Walkane. This broad-based fourfooted cane is lightweight and can fold for storage. (Courtesy Lumex, Inc., Bayshore, N.Y.)

ent likes nature, he can walk through a park or by a lake. If he prefers activity or window shopping, then a walk along a main street will be stimulating.

For the eclectic older adult, Tai Chi Chuan is recommended. This Far Eastern form of dance is suited for the older adult. It is a slow-paced series of movements that flow together in a dance. Correct posture, concentration, breathing, and balance are developed without strain or pain.

Breaking the fatigue cycle

The less you do—the less you want to do
The less you want to do—the less you do
The less you do—the less you are able to do
The less you are able to do—the less you do
Helping the client break the fatigue cycle is a challenge for the nurse. The choice of exercise and where the client will do the exercise will depend on the conditions and desires of the client. There is no one set of exercises that is best. Any

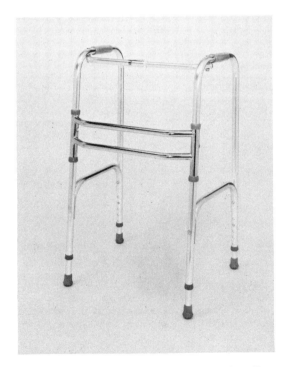

Fig. 10-8. Older adults who need support while walking find a walker gives them a feeling of security and safety. (Courtesy Lumex, Inc., Bayshore, N.Y.)

activity, ADL, sports, or calisthenics will enable the client to break the fatigue cycle and feel more vigorous. The exercises in the selected reading, Life Is Movement (pp. 232-240), for good posture, flexibility, kinesthetics, relaxation, and cardiorespiratory tone are some suggested movements that the client may do by himself or with a group.

Aids to walking

The older adult's inclination to walk depends to a large extent on his perception of the safety of his gait. Aging is manifested in such things as poor vision, vertigo, proprioceptive inadequacies, and skeletal changes. Each of these factors causes the older adult to feel unsteady and unsuited for walking. Walking aids are valuable when they provide the client with a sense of safety and stability. Walking with a standard or tripod cane can be taught to the client by the nurse or physical therapist. The cane is the simplest and most uncomplicated walking aid that is used to help the client with his balance. It widens the base of support, giving the client a sense of security from falls. A rubber safety tip prevents the cane from slipping by providing a secure hold on the floor (Fig. 10-7).

Walkers without wheels are recommended for older clients (Fig. 10-8). An exception to this is the client with a neurological disease such as Parkinson's disease, who does not have the hand grasp needed to lift the walker. Four-legged walkers are suitable for those clients whose gait has changed significantly enough to require a broad base of support. The walker does not encourage the client to develop independent balance, and an abnormal gait pattern is needed by its use. However, for those clients who would be immobile or chairbound, the walker is a very useful aid. Clients have expressed their feelings of security with the walker, because its metal frame surrounds them on three sides (Fig. 10-8).

REFERENCES

Barckley, V.: How to eat on $1.18 per day, Geriatr. Nurs. **1**:50, May-June 1980.

Bortz, W. M.: Effect of exercise on aging—effect of aging on exercise, J. Am. Geriatr. Soc. **28**:49-51, February 1980.

Brower, H. T., and Tanner, L. A.: A study of older adults attending a program on human sexuality: a pilot study, Nurs. Res. **28**:36, January-February 1979.

Coroman, S. C.: The elderly patient: a dental thought, Age Ageing **7**(2):65-7, May 1978.

Donahue, W. T., and others, (editors): Congregate housing for older people: an urgent need, a growing demand, DHEW Publication No. (OHD)77-20284, 1977.

Fass, G.: Sleep, drugs and dreams, Am. J. Nurs. **71:**2316, December 1971.

Feldman, R. S., et al.: Aging and mastication: changes in performance and in the swallowing threshold with natural dentition, J. Am. Geriatr. Soc. **28:**97, March 1980.

Gerard, P., Collins, K. J., Dore, C., and Exton-Smith, A. N.: Subjective characteristics of sleep in the elderly, Age Ageing Suppl:55, 1968.

Giambra, L. M.: Sex differences in daydreaming and related mental activity from the late teens to the early nineties, Intl. J. Aging Hum. Dev. **10:**1, 1979-80.

Hartman, E.: L-tryptophan: A possible natural hypnotic substance (editorial), J.A.M.A. **230**(12):1680, December 23, 1974.

Henderson, V., and Nite, G.: Principles and practice of nursing, New York, 1978, MacMillan Publishing Co., Inc.

Kalchthaler, T., and Tan, M. E. R.: Anemia in institutionalized elderly patients, J. Am. Geriatr. Soc. **28:**108, March 1980.

Kales, A., and Kales, J. D.: Sleep disorders. Changes in sleep cycle with aging. N. Engl. J. Med. **290:**487, 1974.

Kelly, M.: My long term patient, Geriat. Nurs. **1:**56, May-June 1980.

Malone, M.: Old and on the street, Aging **291-292:**20, January-February 1979.

Mead Johnson Laboratories: Nutrition and the aged: nutritional perspectives, No. 6, 1975, Evansville, Indiana.

Nollker, L., and others: Aged excluded from home health care, Gerontologist **18:**37, February 1978.

Phipps, C. A.: Clothing design for handicapped elderly women, J. Home Econ. September 1977, p. 21.

Pomerantz, M. A., Solomon, J., and Dunn, R.: Permanent gastrostomy as a solution to some nutritional problems in the elderly, J. Am. Geriatr. Soc. **28:**104, March 1980.

Reynolds, C. F. III, Coble, P. A., Black, R. S., and others: Sleep disturbances in a series of elderly patients: polysomnographic findings, J. Am. Geriatr. Soc. **28:**165-170, April 1980.

Roberts, I.: The elderly: a challenge to nursing—planning care at home, Nurs. Times **74:**154, 26 January 1978.

Roslaniec, A., and Fitzpatrick, J.: Changes in mental status in older adults with four days of hospitalization, Res. Nurs. Health **2:**177, December 1979.

Spangler, R.: Small Business Administration Program. Keep retired executives active, Geriatrics **33:**21, March 1978.

Teaff, J. D., Lawton, P., Nahemow, L., and Carlson, D.: Impact of age integration on the well-being of elderly tenants in public housing, J. Gerontol. **33:**126, January 1978.

Vir, Sheila C., and Love, A. H. G.: Anthropometric measurements in the elderly, Gerontology **26:**1, 1980.

Wolanin, H. J., and Putt, A.: The long road back from stroke, Geriat. Nurs. **1:**34, May-June 1980.

Yen, P. K.: Nutrition, Geriat. Nurs. **1:**64, May-June 1980.

SELECTED READINGS

Life is movement

Committee on Physical Fitness of Elders*

BASIC SITTING POSITION (GOOD POSTURE)

1. Find a chair low enough to allow both feet to be firmly placed on the floor.
2. The seat should be flat or slightly raised in front.
3. The back should be straight.
4. Place hands in lap. Sit with

*Reprinted with permission from: Connecticut State Department on Aging, 1979. *Authors' note:* Illustrations have been added to help clarify some of the exercises.

weight evenly divided between both legs.

5. Imagine that your spine is an accordian held vertically. One handle is at the top of your head, the other at the base of your spine. Lengthen your spine by stretching the handles away from one another. Make sure your shoulders and chest stay down and that your chin stays parallel to the floor.
6. Your abdominal muscles press back toward your elongated spine.

7. Allow your breath to flow in and out easily.
8. To relax and rest, slowly curve your back allowing your head to bend towards chest. Let your shoulders, arms and hands hang loosely at your sides or on your lap.

FLEXIBILITY EXERCISES— SITTING

All these exercises should be done slowly. Remember to stop if discomfort appears. Try these exercises five times each to start, gradually increasing the number of repetitions.

Warmup

Sitting in chair with good posture, raise arms over head, hugging ears, try to reach for ceiling! Then stretch your right side up, then stretch your left side up. Relax, bringing arms down. Try to inhale as you lift arms and exhale when dropping them.

Abdominal breathing: Breathe in and out slowly, expanding abdomen as you inhale. Slowly exhale, pulling abdomen in.

Exercises for each part of the body
Eyes

Flirting: Good for your eye muscles. Look to the left—look to the right—up, down and all around, without moving your head.

Neck

Head roll: To relieve stiff and tense neck and shoulder muscles: In comfortable sitting posture, close eyes and *slowly* allow head to come forward, resting chin on chest if possible. Slowly lift head, stretching chin to ceiling. Return head to normal position. Turn head slowly from one side to the other. Also, try moving your head so one ear drops toward your shoulder. Now do the other side. Keep shoulders down throughout the exercise (Fig. 10-9).

Arms

6-count movement: Start with hands in lap (Fig. 10-10, *A*). When doing the exercise, keep arms straight. On the count of:

1—Raise your arms in front of chest
2—Slowly move arms to the sides of your body, shoulder height
3—Raise arms over head (Fig. 10-10, *B*)
4—Return arms to sides of your body, shoulder height
5—Bring arms to front of chest
6—Return hands to lap

Then pretend you are swimming!

Use your arms to do the crawl or the breaststroke.

Arm circling: Extend arms out to side, keeping them straight. Circle them moving first in one direction then the opposite. Make large circles, then make small ones (Fig. 10-11).

REST AND BREATHE DEEPLY.

Shoulders

Do the shrug: Raise your shoulders up toward your ears (Fig. 10-12). Lower away from the ears as much as you can.

Roll your shoulders: Slowly move your shoulders forward, up, back and down. Repeat going back first, then up, forward, and down.

Fingers

Wrist and finger stretcher: Clasp hands in front of chest. Turn palms away and stretch arms forward keeping hands clasped. Return to beginning position. Place arms out in front of chest, keeping arms straight. Open and close palms with fingers. Try palms up, then palms down. Try squeezing a soft, crocheted or foam rubber ball. Loosen your fingers and play an imaginary keyboard; from left to right, right to left.

Wrist

Circles: Extend arms forward to a comfortable position. Rotate hands downward, sideward, upward, sideward. Do motion clockwise, then counterclockwise.

Shake: Loosen hands and shake from the wrists. Sure helps get the old stiffness out!

Back

Beginning with your hands on you lap, bend forward, dropping hands toward the front of your body, trying to reach the floor (Fig. 10-13). As you return to your sitting position, slowly bring arms up over your head. (Try to touch the ceiling!) Return to original position. (If you have high blood pressure, do not drop head down when bending.)

Waist

Sit straight in chair. Raise right arm. Reach toward ceiling. Continue reaching, (arm stays near ear) leaning head and torso toward the left side. Make sure right hip stays down in chair. Do the opposite side.

Stomach and legs

Knee lifts: Slowly raise bent knee—return and then raise the other. Raise bent knee, straighten leg forward, bend knee, return to place. Repeat other side.

Raise bent knee, place hands under thigh, draw knee toward chest. Simultaneously bend head and torso forward. Straighten and return to original position. Relax.

Foot and ankles

Ankle flex: Extend leg forward. Flex ankle. Stretch toes up toward ceiling, down toward floor. Now roll your ankles in circles—clockwise then counterclockwise.

The ol' rockin' chair is good for you! Rock back and forth—to Lawrence Welk or to your favorite radio music. Great for the circulation and the back: remember President Kennedy and his rocker?

REST AND BREATHE DEEPLY

FLEXIBILITY EXERCISES— STANDING
Warmup

March in place: How high can you lift those knees? Now slow your march, purposely balancing one leg at a time.

All the sitting exercises can be done in a standing position.

Some additional standing exercises

Trunk bend: With hands on hips, slowly bend forward as far as comfortable, straighten up, relax. Then try sideways too. Can you bend a little toward the back?

Be a tall man: Stand erect. Slowly raise up on toes and down again. You can hold on to a chair if you need to.

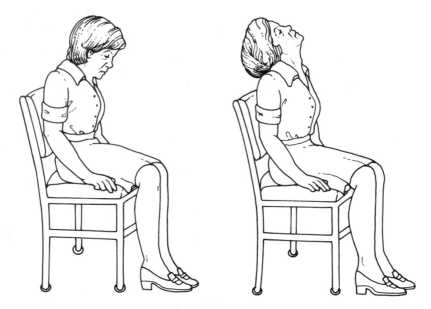

Fig. 10-9. Head roll.

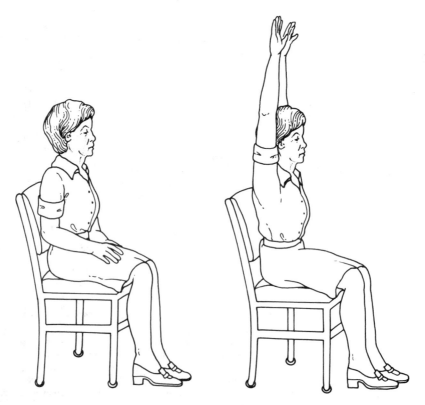

Fig. 10-10. Six-count arm movement.

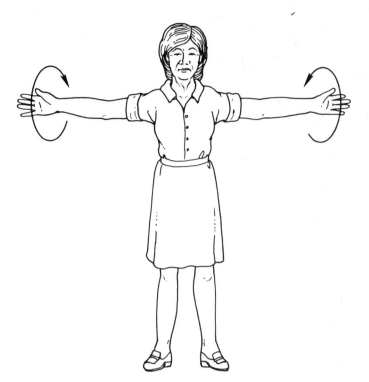

Fig. 10-11. Arm circling.

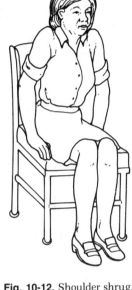

Fig. 10-12. Shoulder shrug.

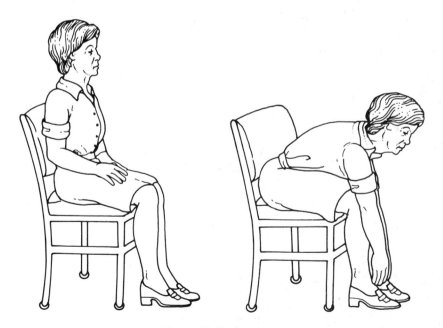

Fig. 10-13. Back exercise.

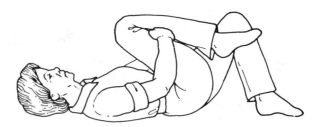

Fig. 10-14. Liver stretcher (knee-chest).

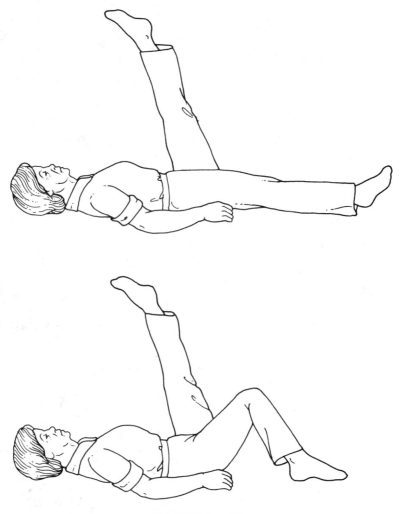

Fig. 10-15. Leg lift.

Crazy walking: Walk on your toes, forward and backward.

Cross left leg in front of right, tapping your toe to the side. Return leg to original position, and then cross your right leg in front of your left. Move forward as you are doing this.

Walk with toes pointed toward each other. Walk with toes pointed away from each other.

Warm-down

March in place, moving quickly at first, then slowing down the pace.
REST AND BREATHE DEEPLY

FLEXIBILITY EXERCISES— LYING ON FLOOR OR ON BED

All exercises from sitting position can be done lying down. Also try these exercises:

Stretching: Start every day by stretching and relaxing, just like a cat. Stretch, relax, change position, stretch, relax. Repeat, changing positions, until the whole body has been treated to a flexing. (Sometimes good for relaxing before sleeping too.)

Liver stretcher (knee-chest): Lying on back, both knees bent, place hands under one thigh and pull your knee toward chest (Fig. 10-14). Hold position as long as it is comfortable. Return to original position. Relax. Now try the other knee.

Leg lift: Slowly raise leg, return, and then raise the other. Always keep one leg bent as you raise the other (Fig. 10-15).

Modified sit-up: Lying on back with both knees bent, raise head, moving chin to chest, hold to count. On next try, if comfortable, slowly lift head and shoulders; hold to count. Relax—lift head, shoulders, and upper body (Fig. 10-16). Then maybe you'll feel good enough to try this next exercise:

Full sit-up: Strengthens abdominal muscles. With arms over head, raise head, moving chin to chest. Start to move shoulders and torso toward knees, slowly bringing arms between the bent knees (Fig. 10-17). Slowly roll back with the end of the spine first until lying flat on back again. The more slowly, the better—it is in the slowness that the muscles are strengthened.

REST AND BREATHE DEEPLY

Canes: Canes or walking sticks can also be used as an exerciser, standing or sitting. They should have a rubber tip at the end for safety.

Hold cane in front of your chest, squeeze the cane with your fingers, release, then squeeze again, relax.

Hold cane in front of your chest, arms straight, bend your wrists, pushing cane up and down.

Hold the cane with the palms of your hands facing upward, resting the cane across your knees.

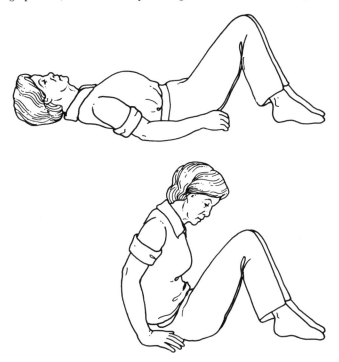

Fig. 10-16. Modified sit-up.

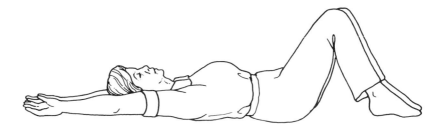

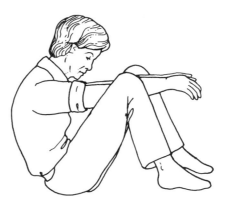

Fig. 10-17. Full sit-up.

Bring the cane toward your chest. Return to starting position.

Reverse your hand position so that palms are facing downward. Raise the cane toward your chest. Return to starting position.

Hold cane across your knees. Bend down with the cane toward the floor. Return to original starting position. Slowly lift the cane up over your head. Return to starting position. Now try bending down with the cane on your left side, then your right side.

Try rowing with your cane!

HOW TO EXTEND THESE EXERCISES CREATIVELY

Stretch your mind and your imagination along with your muscles. Adapt these suggestions to your capabilities:

To loosen up when you are feeling tense or in need of extra energy

Yawn: Take a breath, exhale, rounding your back while sitting in the chair. Let your arms fold across your chest. Start to unfold, stretching your back and your arms out as much as possible. Make a loud oooh sound. Return to original position. Repeat three times.

To get your circulation going

Seated, with one hand pat briskly up and down the opposite arm. Extend that patting to the whole opposite side. Go from arm downward to toes, upward to top of head, patting briskly. Stop, close your eyes, feel that side of you, compare it with your other side. Then do the other side. Feel yourself tingle.

Vary this by gently massaging with the whole hand. Take a dry shower.

Sideways

Be aware of action lines in your body.

Feeling your width: Stretch outward to both sides with your arms as if you could touch both walls with your fingertips; then

Feel yourself narrow: Bring your arms together, press them momentarily against your sides, then release. Repeat these two.

Up/down

Elongating your spine: Feel yourself growing tall, pulled up by an imaginary string attached to the top of your head (crown); then

Give in to gravity, sink down, rounding your back, chin lowered toward chest, feel your weight. Repeat these two.

Open your arms out to sides, stretch, then close arms around you, give yourself a hug. You deserve it!

Walking variations

Walk slowly, eight steps in one direction, stop, change direction, walk eight steps, stop, change direction. Then pick up the speed. Repeat several times. A variation: Somewhere in the sequence, add a pause for eight counts. Hold very still. Try standing in different positions on the hold.

Sidewise walk: Holding table or kitchen counter if you need to, walk sideward crossing one foot in front of the other. Then

Return to the other side, this time crossing one foot in back of the other.

Walk sideward again, this time cross once in back, once in front (the grapevine walk). (You can practice feet crossovers beforehand while seated in your chair. Move left foot over right, return to place. Move right foot over left, return to place.)

More loosening up

Shake hands, then add arms, shoulders, then stop.

Shake legs, add voice and head, and arms again—as if using a jack hammer.

Then stop and relax and breathe deeply.

KINESPHERE

Find *your* kinesphere . . . all the space you can reach with your fingertips from where you are, sitting or standing—above you, below you, in front of you, behind you. Imagine standing or sitting inside a globe of which you are the center. Now stretch to reach all around the confines of that globe. With an imaginary paintbrush in your hand, "paint" the whole inside of your kinesphere. Use one hand, then the other.

Try varying the feeling of the above exercise by actually holding in your hand

1. A thin scarf
2. A leaf
3. A tube from a roll of paper towels
4. A pencil

Open your arms out to sides, stretch, then close arms around you. Give yourself another big hug!

CARDIORESPIRATORY EXERCISES

Walk! Walk around the table, up and down the hall, during commercials on TV—get up and get a glass of water—it cleans the pipes and gets blood moving again. Walk outside when weather is nice . . . around the block . . . to the store . . . to the mailbox . . . in the park; enjoy nature! Walk to see a friend . . . ask your friend to come for a walk. Above all walk a little briskly—enough to cause you to breathe a little deeper! *Excellent* for cardiorespiratory toning.

NOTE: Jogging is for the experts—don't attempt unless you are a regular daily jogger. If you wish to try it, consult your doctor first and then join a physical fitness program, and then attempt only when the trained director feels you are expertly fit and ready!

BRISK WALKING MAY BE THE
TICKET FOR YOU.

Dancing: If you like ballroom dancing and have continued to do it over the years, keep it up. If dancing never was your cup of tea, especially the couples variety, why not try folk dancing. If you are interested, ask your senior center director to organize a group—or get together with a few of your friends, invite someone who knows some folk dances, get a few records and learn. If 20 people get together and request a teacher from your local Adult Education Director, the teacher will be provided at the time and place you indicate. It doesn't have to be evenings—try an afternoon!

Swimming: A great way to exercise too, the water is not only an aid in buoyancy, but can be a great resister. Try moving your arms about under water and feel the resistance on your muscles. Walk or march in water up over your knees.

Water exercises: Learn with a qualified leader from the local "Y" or Red Cross or recreation program.

Floating: On your stomach or back for starters. Add a flutter or frog kick, then a breast stroke until you're

Swimming: Breast stroke with frog kick—a good breathing exercise to increase cardiorespiratory endurance. You may want to try other swimming techniques, one side and then the other. *Don't overdo!* Relax at water's edge when winded; try again if you're feeling up to it.

Social games: Shuffleboard—hand or with pusher, ring toss, beanbag toss, darts, shooting pool or billiards, and croquet.

MUSCULAR ENDURANCE (REPETITIVE ACTIVITY)

All of aforementioned activities, if repeated, could increase muscular endurance. *Do* start slowly with the bending and stretching flexibility exercises. *Don't* do more than you are comfortable doing. *Do* build up to repeating the exercises and adding new ones. Pace yourself. Exercise and activity should be enjoyable. *Don't* force yourself beyond endurance or try for medals!

RELAXATION TECHNIQUES

Too much stress and anxiety is harmful and wasteful of human energy. Below are a few techniques that should help you to relax, for *relaxation is a skill that must be learned and practiced.*

Setting

Practice these techniques in as near a perfect setting as possible.

1. Wear comfortable clothing.
2. Lie on floor that is well padded or sit in a comfortable chair.
3. Place a small pillow under the knees.
4. Have room semidarkened.
5. Use either a metronome or neu-

tral record* (bells, ocean, etc.) in order to dull out disturbing sounds.

Procedure

Diaphragmatic breathing: It will give you a more complete exchange of air and is the most important technique, for it can be easily employed at any time once it is mastered.

1. Lie flat.
2. Place hands on stomach, fingertips barely touching.
3. When you inhale, push stomach out (fingertips will separate).

---

*Records may be purchased from Syntonic Research, Inc., 175 5th Avenue, New York, New York 10022.

4. Exhale, stomach goes in (fingertips will come together). All of this will feel awkward at first but in a few days you will recognize and feel the results of diaphragmatic breathing.

Passive scene: With eyes closed, picture a pleasant passive scene. See yourself in this scene happy and relaxed—spend a few minutes enjoying this scene. This procedure should rest your mind, for it is impossible to be worrying or unhappy if your mind is concentrating on something enjoyable.

Progressive relaxation: (Developed by Dr. Edmond Jacobson) Brief contraction of a muscle (feeling of tension) followed by feelings of relaxation. *Important: anyone over 40*

should not hold the contraction for longer than 3 seconds.

1. Feet and legs: Curl toes downward, tensing until you feel a slight discomfort (no longer than 3 seconds), then slowly and passively let your whole body relax. Wait a few seconds then proceed with all the following in this same manner. Flex foot so toes point to your head. Push heels into floor. Pull legs together and press.
2. Arms and hands: Make a fist. Press palms into floor. Press back of hands into floor. Press arms against body.
3. Shoulders and head: Lift shoulders up to ears. Close eyes tightly. Close jaws.

Sexuality and the aged*

Gerhard Falk □ **Ursula A. Falk**

Throughout history, all human societies have placed strictures on sexual expression.[1] Rigidly supervised and prescribed sexual codes of conduct have served several important functions in society: first, they have provided a form of birth control and, second, abstinence has served as a

---

*Falk, G., and Falk, U. A.: Copyright © 1980, American Journal of Nursing Co., Reproduced, with permission, from *Nursing Outlook* 28:51-55, January 1980.
Gerhard Falk, Ed.D., is a sociologist and professor, and **Ursula A. Falk, Ed.D.,** is a social worker and lecturer at the State University College at Buffalo. They are the authors of a monograph, *The Nursing Home Dilemma,* published in 1976 by R. & E. Publishing Co., San Francisco.

means of disease control. In addition, women have been more easily subjugated by sexual strictures which affect only them, not men. This in turn has led to the exploitation of women in such profitable businesses as prostitution. However, the development of birth control measures and the subsequent rise of self-realization and political and legal emancipation on the part of women have diminished or negated the reasons for some of these strict codes of sexual conduct. In their place has been substituted situation ethics, whereby various forms of sexual expression between consenting adults are both possible and tolerated within society—that is, for everyone but the

aged.[2] For the elderly, society still imposes strict codes of conduct regarding sexuality.

We became aware of the depth and prevalence of society's negative attitudes toward sexuality in the aged during our studies of nursing homes and in private social work therapy. Not only is there a general taboo—almost second to incest—within society toward the appropriateness of sexual expression in the aged, but it is also clearly evident in the attitudes of the children and caretakers of the aged, as well as among the aged themselves. There are many reasons for these attitudes, which we will discuss. To emphasize some points, we have drawn upon our field notes of typical behaviors and reactions we observed in nursing homes and from interviews with aged clients.

VALUES ON YOUTH, NOT AGED

Probably the most important reason is that American culture is youth-oriented and aging is unpopular. The aged person who exhibits bodily signs of age is scorned. For example:

Seventy-eight year old Fay was highly critical of her friend Tanya when the latter wore a bikini to swim at the hotel pool where they were vacationing. "Why does an old wrinkled woman have to make a fool of herself looking like that—is she trying to attract one of the old men? Those dirty old men wouldn't want her anyway—they want the young girls."

Many people believe that aging is a disease, rather than a normal process.[3] This attitude is less related to ignorance than to the hope that age and death can be cured in a scientific society, just the way everything else can be fixed by using a formula, a technique, or a pill. The view that aging is somehow pathological is further underscored in our society by "the national emphasis on older adults who are sick and poor, rather than on the majority who are healthy and active, productive, and even creative."[4]

Sixty-nine year old Mrs. J, observing a group of older people, remarked to a younger woman standing nearby, "I don't know why Annie admires those old men. Who needs those old guys anyway? I had a marvelous husband, may he rest in peace. I wouldn't want to take care of those old cronies. All they do is get sick and I have to play nursemaid. Then I'm stuck. Who needs it?"

"The old are not attractively packaged," says Weinberg.[5] In a society which is very fashion- and package-conscious, the old have lost their appeal. Seldom do the young, or even the old themselves, look at a passing older person. Thus, the old become invisible and therefore also untouchable.[6] Youth is identified with physical love and sex in American culture, and old age with lack of physical capacity of any kind—hence, sexless.

A senior citizen group was out for the afternoon, seeing a popular movie. Although there were some love scenes in the film, it was not pornographic. For instance, one brief scene showed a man and a woman lying side by side in bed kissing. Several of the senior women discussed this afterwards, saying they shut their eyes during this episode and that they should have been better informed in advance about the nature of the film. It was indecent and unfit for viewing by older people who were "not used to this kind of thing and, at our age, we shouldn't see it."

Later, one woman, Mrs. T, who had complained louder than the others, claimed that an older man in her group had rubbed his leg against hers during the movie. She spoke of this alleged incident for days and complained about the inappropriateness of the film's subject matter, retelling her story as well as the sexual version of the movie again and again.

Interestingly, even researchers avoided the topic of sex in people over 60 until recent years, because they thought they would find nothing.[7]

AGE DIFFERENCES IN SPOUSES

The belief that the old are sexless may not be in accord with the facts, but it does have several advantages for those who choose to believe it. This group consists of persons who have no sexual partner, or who never liked sex at any time in their lives, or whose spouses or partners of earlier years have lost their sexual capacity.[8] This belief is in part a result of the traditional age difference between husband and wife in the United States, a factor that affects women far more than men. For instance, the average 70-year-old woman has a 74-year-old husband, but the average 70-year-old man has a 66-year-old wife. Consequently, women's sexual activity is reduced at an earlier age than that of men because of the husband's incapacity.[9] This discrepancy also reflects a double standard that has plagued women for a long time and continues to influence the aged. In a recent article, McCarthy reports that "most married women who have ceased sex relations did so because of their spouses' incapacity—most married men because of their own incapacity."[10]

Mr. and Mrs. S were an attractive couple—he is 78, she 74. Mr. S had confided in his physician that he had extreme difficulty with erections and was unable to perform. His wife was a warm sexual person and adjusted quietly to this condition. In public, Mr. S constantly made derogatory allusions about his wife's inability to sexually perform. He flirted with other available women, creating much anxiety in his spouse. He himself could not accept his current dilemma in our macho culture.

This example clearly indicates that the deprecation of sex in the old creates worse problems for widowed and divorced women than for men. In part, this is due to the longer life expectancy of women and the tradition for women to marry older men. As a consequence, there are three times as many widows as there are widowers, making it almost certain that older women will not be able to find another husband or a societally sanctioned partner.[11] Calculating that women generally marry a man four years their senior and that their life expectancy is seven years greater than that of men, Pfeiffer and Davis conclude that widowhood generally lasts eleven years, and it is therefore protective and adaptive to inhibit sexual activity where so little opportunity for fulfillment exists.[12]

CULTURAL CONDITIONING

If sexual desire appears to decrease among the old, it is not because of the menopause but because beliefs taught in our culture have produced sexlessness with the aid of the self-fulfilling prophecy.[13] Lower expectations, not incapacity or lack of desire, are the principal inhibitors of sexual activity. In short, the whole culture militates against sex by the old, and older persons buy this themselves, since they were once the young who learned that sex belongs only to beautiful bodies or must lead to reproduction.[14] Since reproduction is neither desirable nor possible for the old, this belief further inhibits their sexual expression.

The belief that only the young must be allowed sexuality is widespread and held by young and old alike. Thus, a group of medical students booed and whistled when shown pictures of an elderly couple kissing, while undergraduate students, including nurses from nursing homes, rated three stories related to coitus and masturbation by the old as negative and not creditable.[15,16] This denial of sexuality by the young concerning the old is taught in many cultures whose members are led to believe that there is no parental sexual activity or that, at best, such activity must be ignored and covered up like other unmentionables such as insanity, crime, and alcoholism.

Mary, a 60-year-old mildly retarded woman living in a health-related facility visited a senior day care center three times a week. There she met Jeff, a 65-year-old man who was still active and able to drive a car. The two become romantically involved and he drove her home frequently, visited her at the facility, and brought her little gifts of candy, perfume, and flowers. She was elated and happy. As soon as Mary's brother and sister-in-law learned of this situation, they visited the health facility and squelched the relationship between Jeff and Mary by expressing their disgust. They let the personnel know that if they continued to allow Jeff's visits, they would insist on Mary's removal from the institution.

CHILDREN FEAR FINANCIAL LOSS

Inhibiting sex in the elderly serves the younger generation in several ways. First, it insures them their possible inheritance. Thus, the reaction of many adult children to the idea of their parents' remarriage is often greeted with such comments as, ". . . they ought to know better," because they fear loss of possible financial gain after death of their single parent.[17]

Louis had had a poor marriage for 50 years when his wife died in a mental institution. Within the year he found Amy, a friendly, emotionally strong widow his age who was delighted to accept his attentions. They went dancing together at many senior citizen functions, vacationed in Florida together in the winter, and enjoyed each other as they had not been able to do with their respective spouses. They were known as the lovebirds, since they were often holding hands. Both decided that they wanted to have a more permanent union. When Amy announced her intentions to her sons, they placed a great deal of pressure on her. They used every logical and illogical argument, saying that Louis was old, not absolutely well, could die at any time, would be a problem, and so on. Furthermore, they told her that he was not of good stock, that their friends would talk about them, that she would be better off remaining single. When she tentatively set a wedding date, her three sons visited her with their wives and told her in no uncertain terms that if she remarried they would ignore her from then on. They did not want to lose their inheritance, since she had a great deal of money. Her sons' threats and the subsequent feelings of insecurity caused her to abandon her decision to marry.

Second, the inhibition of sex among the elderly removes them from the arena of sexual competition. Sexual performance by older persons, like all performances by older persons, makes the failure of younger people particularly evident in a youth culture. Third, the celibate state demanded of the old makes it easier for the young to manage them. People who have a sex partner by any label, whether spouse or friend, have an ally. However, our society desires defenselessness in the old,

and sexual deprivation makes them even more dependent on the wishes of the young than they already are. Therefore, nursing homes notoriously practice a form of sexual "fascism," totally denying their residents any sexual expression, not only by the admonitions generally held in our culture but by creating every possible barrier against sexual life.[18]

Mr. and Mrs. K, a married couple, shared a room in a nursing home. They were a fairly healthy couple who enjoyed engaging in intercourse on a fairly regular basis. Their normal behavior had become the focus of one of the staff meetings. The nurse coordinator, a 40-year-old divorcee, presented the couple as a problem. She had repeatedly looked through a crack in the door while the couple was making love and believed that Mr. K was "ripping" his wife. She subsequently spoke of Mr. K as a "filthy old man" and claimed that Mrs. K was too old and frail to enjoy his advances. Other staff members were encouraged to become voyeurs and they in turn were in total agreement with this nurse's opinion about the situation. Objectively, Mrs. K was much less tense after intercourse and seemed to enjoy the activity. Nevertheless, the nurse coordinator interfered, asked many questions of Mrs. K, and frightened her into feeling embarrassed and inhibited. A physician was drawn into this situation, and Mr. and Mrs. K were moved into separate rooms with roommates of their own gender. Both partners became anxious and morose and a great deal of mental deterioration was seen in these two people.

It is of course evident that this denial of sexuality can have destructive effects, not only upon one's sex life but also upon one's self-image and total interpersonal relationships. Nevertheless, it is a widespread attitude in nursing homes and other institutions for the aged, because it is so common a view outside of institutions. Nursing homes ordinarily restrict contact between the sexes to public lounges, so that the behavior of the residents can be supervised by the staff.[19] This concern for supervising behavior and for preventing and prohibiting the possibility of sexual expressions implies, of course, that those who supervise believe that sexual behavior is in fact possible.

Mrs. S, a widow, and Mr. F, a widower, are often seen in the lounge holding hands. They find comfort in sitting in chairs close to each other. Many comments are made by the personal care attendants of the nursing home—"senile old man, better watch him. Don't let him go into one of the rooms with her—there's no telling what he'll do."

This paradox is evidenced by the fact that while, on the one hand, sex is forbidden in nursing homes, on the other, almost no admission forms to nursing homes ask any questions about sexuality and almost all journals and books on the management of nursing homes ignore the subject.[20,21]

Prevention of sexual expression in nursing homes is thus achieved in three ways. First, it is condemned by society outside of nursing homes; second, it is enforced in nursing homes by lack of privacy; and, third, it is internalized by the aged themselves, since they feel that they are no longer sexually attractive and that any sexual activity on their part stamps them "dirty old man" and "dirty old woman."[22]

Eighty-year-old Edith looked more like 60 with her well-groomed hair, her attractive attire, and her brisk erect walk. Walt, a 60-year-old wheelchair-bound nursing home resident, was very fond of her. The two would sit side by side exchanging loving glances, occasionally holding hands and patting each other's cheek. One day when they thought no one was observing them, Walt placed his hand on her thigh. Residents promptly reported this behavior to the social worker, commenting it was "unfitting." They called Edith a "dirty old lady" and Walt "disgusting." Both were ostracized by the other residents after the episode, and each felt almost criminal for having behaved humanly.

Phrases such as dirty old man reflect fear of ridicule, shame, and embarrassment of the old by the young solely for the aged person's possession of sexual feelings; thus there are no dirty young men in our youth-fixated society because we have persuaded each other that sexual action and even sexual thought are unbecoming in the old. Cameron and Biber, however, found that sexual thought continues throughout the life span, although it varies by sex and age in the sense that it reaches a high point in the teen years and is more frequent with men than women.[23] It is, however, possible that this sex difference is more related to the reporting of female practices than it is to female activity, because in our culture women are reluctant to give factual data about their sexual activity.[24]

In response to the normal concerns of the aged, a New York City nursing home recently integrated its floors and allowed both sexes to live in adjoining rooms.[25] The consequence was most positive. Male residents used profane language more sparingly, were better groomed, and generally became less tense than before. The same changes occurred in the women, although at first they felt obliged to protest the integration and to pretend that the presence of men was objectionable. Since integration led to sexual involvement, it was again the nursing staff that had to be helped to understand the older people's needs and cease their criticism of these activities.[26]

One wonders to what extent the use of tranquilizers in nursing homes would be reduced if nursing homes would allow and encourage sexuality, since it has been found that sexual orgasm relieves anxiety as well or better than tranquilizers.[27] In the future nursing homes will have to permit sexual activity by their patients, since this is a basic human right, restriction and total elimination of which are subject to legal action under civil rights codes of this country.[28]

OTHER DIMENSIONS

The rejection of the old as sexual partners has additional dimensions. While heterosexual people are evidently limited in the satisfaction that is attainable for them, homosexuals are even more troubled in this regard. For while "American society places an inordinate emphasis on youth, the homosexual community, by and large, places a still greater emphasis on this fleeting characteristic."[29] Homosexuals have no wife or husband who will accept their declining sexual attractiveness or children or grandchildren to console them and alleviate somewhat the impact of aging. Instead, many homosexuals find their ability to attract sex partners decreasing even as their need for permanent relationships increases and age overtakes them.[30]

Of course, many elderly people reject each other as much as do the young. In a fascinating study of "Romance in the SRO (Single Room Occupancy)," Stephens describes the sexual behavior of elderly residents of a downtown hotel. She shows that "60-year-old men do not want 60-year-old women," but prefer young prostitutes who arrive at the hotel on the first of each month and earn their pay from the Social Security checks available then. These men evidently prefer the short-lived contacts with prostitutes to involvements with women of their own age, as older women expect male friends to do things for them, an expectation that men view as exploitation.[31] Conflicting demands and expectations of this kind are common in the aged.

The degree of sexual interest for both men and women does undoubtedly decline with age.[32] As people near their sixties, the belief that descent has begun and that erotic capacity should diminish provokes decline of sexual interest. Nevertheless, this decline is inflicted more by our culture and our attitudes than by nature. Rubin found that even the practice of masturbation creates emotional distress among many older women who have no other sexual outlet but have been taught to believe that this practice is somehow sinful or wrong.[33]

In sum, we see that sexuality of the old is condemned, ridiculed, and repressed in our society. It becomes the task of all of us, especially those caring for the aged, to become knowledgeable about the problem and then to find ways to encourage self-expression and freedom of choice governing normal areas of behavior.

REFERENCES

1. Linton, Ralph. The natural history of the family. In *The Family: Its Function and Destiny,* revised edition by R. N. Anshen. New York, Harper & Brothers, 1959, p. 18.
2. Fletcher, Joseph. Situation ethics. In *Perspectives on Sexuality,* ed. by J. L. Malfetti and Elizabeth Eidlitz, New York, Holt, Rinehart and Winston, 1972, pp. 308-309.
3. Tavris, Carol. The sexual lives of women over sixty. *MS* 6:63, July 1977.
4. *Ibid.*
5. Weinberg, Jack. Sexuality in later life. *Med. Aspects Hum. Sexuality* 5:216, Apr. 1971.
6. *Ibid.,* p. 226.
7. Tavris, *op. cit.,* p. 63.
8. McCarthy, Patrick. Geriatric sexuality: capacity, interest, and opportunity. *J. Gerontol. Nurs.* 5:20, Jan.-Feb. 1979.
9. Newman, Gustave, and Nichols, C. R. Sexual activities and attitudes in older persons. *JAMA* 173:33-35, May 7, 1960.
10. McCarthy, *op. cit.,* p. 20.
11. Nobsenz, N. M. Sex and the senior citizen. *NY Times Mag.* Jan. 20, 1974, pp. 87-91.
12. Pfeiffer, Eric, and Davis, G. C. Determinants of sexual behavior in middle and old age. *J. Am. Geriatr. Soc.* 20:157, Apr. 1972.
13. Rubin, Isadore. The 'sexless' older years: a socially harmful stereotype. *The Annals Am. Acad. Polit. Soc. Sci.* 376:86, 1968.
14. Tavris, *op. cit.,* p. 63.
15. West, N. D. Sex in geriatrics: myth or miracle. *J. Am. Geriatr. Soc.* 23:551-552, Dec. 1975.
16. La Torre, R. A., and Kear, Karen. Attitudes toward sex in the aged. *Arch. Sex. Behav.* 6:203, May 1977.
17. Rubin, Isadore. Sex after forty and after seventy. In *An Analysis of Human Sexual Response,* ed. by Ruth Brecher and Edward Brecher. Boston, Little Brown and Co., 1966, p. 251.
18. Kaas, M. J. Sexual expression of the elderly in nursing homes. *Gerontologist* 18:372-378, Aug. 1978.
19. *Ibid.,* p. 373.
20. Horn, Patrice. Problems of a not so gay old age. (Newsline) *Psychol. Today* 8:35, Oct. 1974.
21. McCarthy, *op. cit.,* p. 20.
22. Kaas, *op. cit.,* p. 377.
23. Cameron, Paul, and Biber, Henry. Sexual thought throughout the lifespan. *Gerontologist* 13:144, Summer 1973.
24. Newman and Nichols, *op. cit.,* p. 33.
25. Silverstone, Barbara, and Wynter, Lolita. The effects of introducing a heterosexual livingspace. *Gerontologist* 15(Pt. 1):83, Feb. 1975.
26. *Ibid.,* p. 83.
27. Horn, Patrice. Rx: sex for senior citizens. (Newsline) *Psychol. Today* 8: 18, June 1974.
28. Downey, G. The next patient right: sex in nursing homes. *Mod. Health Care* 1:56-59, June 1974.
29. Laner, M. R. Growing older male: heterosexual and homosexual. *Gerontologist* 18(pt 1):496, Oct. 1978.
30. *Ibid.,* p. 496.
31. Stephens, Joyce. Romance in the SRO (Single Room Occupancy). *Gerontologist* 14:280, Aug. 1974.
32. Vorwoerdt, Adrian, and others. Sexual behavior in senescence: changes in sexual activity and interest in aging men and women. *J. Geriatr. Psychiatry* 2:163, Spring 1969.
33. Rubin, Isadore. The 'sexless' older years a socially harmful stereotype. *The Annals Am. Acad. Polit. Soc. Sci.* 376:86, 1968.

11 Modifying nursing approaches for the older adult: psychosocial needs

This chapter continues through the fifth level of Maslow's hierarchy. Environmental safety is presented first, followed by community acquired illnesses, community communication services, love and belonging, self-esteem, and self-actualization. Nursing intervention modified for the special characteristics of the older adult will help the client fulfill the psychosocial needs of each level.

ENVIRONMENTAL SAFETY

The nurse who visits the client in his home or sees the client in the hospital or long-term-care facility is responsible for maintenance and care of the immediate environment of the client. By being aware of environmental needs, the nurse addresses both the comfort and safety aspects of the client's care. Because the nursing actions are designed to elicit a safe environment from the model of self-care, the client is encouraged to understand the options and risks inherent in his immediate environment. Maslow's hierarchy designates second level needs as *safety* (Fig. 11-1).

Lighting

Lighting is one environmental factor that the nurse should assess. For the older adult, a small light should be left on at night near the bed, bathroom, and hallways. During the day, it is preferable to have several moderately bright lights on, rather than one large light. This arrangement reduces the glare and enables the older adult to see more comfortably. Sheer drapes or stained glass on windows reduces the glare coming in. The furniture should be arranged so that the client's bed and chair do not directly face a bright window. The glare of the bright sunshine dims the client's vision and causes tearing in the client's eyes. Frequently used furniture should be arranged in such a

way that it is in the client's full view. Eliminate clutter on stairs and hallways and around the client's bed and bathroom. Paint stairways in contrasting colors to make them immediately obvious to the client. Painting doors and windows bright oranges and yellows contrasts them boldly against their surroundings and prevents falls for the client whose vision is impaired. When the client is doing close handwork or reading, increase the light to avoid eyestrain. When the client is resting, how-

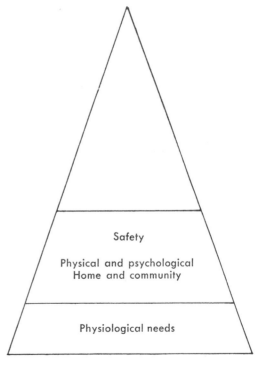

Fig. 11-1. Safety needs—second level of Maslow's hierarchy.

ever, dim the light to a comfortable level. This will foster the comfort and rest needed for sleep. There should be a mixture of natural and artificial lighting in the client's environment. Give some variation to the client's daily activities so that he sees the pattern of a 24-hour day as sunshine, sunset, dark days of rain, and bright skies of clear days. It gives diversion to his environment, and connects him to the outside world if he is indoors most of the time.

Lighting affects the environment and the mood of the client. For instance, proper lighting makes the client look better in most instances. A fluorescent light gives the client's skin a purplish hue. Thus, the new softone lightbulbs such as the pink tones may be better in a dining area for the older client. This type of lighting is more complimentary to the patient's complexion. Full-length windows are being used more by architects because this type of lighting from daylight seems to serve best in most agencies. In the future it is possible that there may be more windows for natural lighting and natural heating from the sun.

The older adult is usually annoyed by flickering lights or changes in the intensity of lighting, especially if going from room to room or traveling through corridors. The same principle may be observed in the home too. In health agencies white uniforms and white sheets on the bed also can create a glare that can cause a discomfort to the sensitive eyes of the older adult. Night lights in the older adult's room help them during the night if they should suddenly awaken out of a sleep. It helps orient them to their surroundings.

General safety

The older adult is predisposed to age-related factors that increase vulnerability to environmental hazards, so extra safety precautions have to be taken. They are aware of the need to rise slowly from a seated position. Their decreased sensory acuity diminishes their ability to interpret their environment adequately. Impaired balance is another factor that causes many hazards within the environment. The center of gravity is moved forward as physiological changes occur. Emotions and their psychological state have an effect; for instance, the client in a state of anxiety or depression will think and react slowly to any environmental stimuli. The older adult may only take in and re-

spond to a certain number of stimuli, and this depends on the individual. The client's orientation and level of consciousness will give baseline information in the ability to respond and perceive hazards within the environment. Older adults who are ill may be weak but unaware of their weakened condition. Medication also causes drowsiness or sedation, and may affect the level of consciousness, or distort the electrolyte fluid balance in the body.

Electric stoves in the kitchen are preferable to gas flames, because of the decreased danger if the person should lean over the stove. With diminished eyesight, often the older adult will try to determine if the flame is on by actually touching the flame. Railings should be placed on all stairways, hallways, bathtubs, and showers. Rubber mats should be used, or nonskid strips should be placed on the tub or shower floor. It is both comfortable and safe to sit on a stool in the shower or tub while bathing. It facilitates transfer and reduces the incidence of orthostatic hypotension.

Fires

Smoke detectors placed in hallways or in bedrooms alert the older adult by means of a piercing siren when smoke, heat, or flames are in the environment. The older adult should be familiar with the alarm and exit plans, and this knowledge should be reviewed at particular intervals. Many smoke detectors do have an intermittent alarm that sounds when the battery is low. The older adult should be aware of the reason for the beeping of the smoke detector and make arrangements to have a new battery installed.

Older adults should have access to telephones, with emergency telephone numbers of friends and services within easy reach. Telephone units are available that do not require dialing, but rather use insert cards punched with computer numbers. The client simply selects the card and puts it into the phone and the number is automatically dialed.

Fire extinguishers should be available in all areas where older adults are living. Review the card on the fire extinguisher to make sure that it has been inspected within the last 6 months. Read the instructions, and review them with the client.

Furniture

A safe environment for the older adult also includes the immediate living area. The floor should be even with a nonskid or no-wax shine. There should be no loose rugs or deep pile carpeting, because these cause the client with an unsteady or slow gait to fall. The windows within the client's home or apartment need to be within comfortable reach and easy to open. Kitchen stove controls should be in the front, so the client does not have to reach over an open flame or electric heating element. Shelves should be low enough to reach needed equipment and supplies, and, if necessary, only a low stepstool with two steps should be used. If a stepstool is to be used, it should be in the best condition. Obstructions around the client's feet such as cords, furniture, or objects should be removed. In the hospital or long-term-care facility, the gatches on beds should be put back into position under the bed. It is also possible that small pets and children can get under the client's feet and become an environmental hazard. Raise the client and his family's consciousness regarding such potential causes of accidents.

Falls and clothing

Falls are the greatest cause of accidents in persons over 70 years of age. Even a small injury may cause immobilization of the client for days. The decrease in muscle strength and reaction time, in addition to decreased visual acuity and decreased balance, makes the client predisposed to falling. Medication causing hypotension is also a cause for falling. Unfamiliar places are often particular problems for older adults. They are taken by surprise by steps and building entrances, and are often confused with escalators that move too fast.

Clothing is often a hazard to the older adult. Ill-fitting shoes or long robes that catch on furniture, door knobs, or cooking utensils can cause the older adult to fall. Heelless slippers, thongs, or poorly fitted shoes often are the cause of the slips.

Older adults must be careful when going out in icy or snowy weather. Protection should be provided against slips and falls in the snow by putting down salt and ashes and by making arrangements to have sidewalks and walkways shoveled.

A fall can cause an older adult physical and psychological trauma. The obvious physical traumas are bleeding, lacerations, fractures, and pain. The immobility during recovery can be a source of protracted discomfort and physical hazard. The loss of confidence and self-esteem and independence

resulting from the immobilization of a fall can be a great psychological detriment to older adults. They feel suddenly old. Family feelings of guilt and anger can arise. Often the family warns the older adult about hazards and risks of falling and, when the fall occurs, blame is placed and bad feelings arise. Fractures mean hospitalization for the older adult and bring loneliness and possible feelings of confusion and rejection. It is better to prevent the fall, rather than treat it.

The nurse is in a good position to help the client modify his environment. On the stairway, fabric or a doorknob on the railing can indicate the level of the steps. Walk around with the client in his environment whether it be a hospital room, a small apartment, or a home. Make sure that all cords are taped down or eliminated entirely. Put throw rugs and place furniture in such a way as to have easily accessible traffic pathways. Particularly, place the furniture on the side of the client's best vision. Make sure there is a smooth surface on the area of the floor where the rug and the flooring meet. Teach the client to scan the environment before proceeding.

Discuss the options available for accident proofing the client's home environment. Of course, in a long-term facility or in a hospital, the nurse is particularly responsible for the environment.

Preventive maintenance

In order to have the physical environment in optimum condition, practical maintenance issues must be reviewed regularly. The nurse should assess housekeeping and plant maintenance on her unit.

Infection control is another important part of the safe environment of the older adult. Having nurses included on infection control committees and abiding by committee recommendations support a safe environment.

Temperature

In addition to the actual physical environment, things that are important to the older adult's comfort and safety are room temperature maintenance, humidity, and noise and dust control. Most older adults prefer the room temperature to be about 72° F (22° C) for comfort. The humidity in a room is the amount of moisture in the air and will affect the moisture evaporation on the client's skin. A combination of high humidity and high (over 85° F) temperatures causes discomfort, especially in the joints of older persons. Air conditioning cools the air and keeps the humidity low. Colder winter weather and its normally lower humidity, combined with dry indoor air, result in excessively low humidity in the room. Low humidity may cause drying of the skin and mucous membranes, especially of the nose, throat, and bronchi. Nosebleeds frequently occur because of the drying of the mucosa of the nose. A water-soluble jelly such as Surgilub or KY Jelly applied sparingly to the nostrils prevents dryness. Air conditioners and furnaces should have humidity control.

Noise

Another environmental aspect that is a part of providing comfort for the client is consideration of the noise level. Sudden loud sounds can be very irritating to a client and create a feeling of fright or disturbance. On the other hand, too much silence can be disturbing also, especially to a client who is used to a city environment, for example. A change from the night sounds of traffic, airplanes, buses and trains and other vehicles to suburban or rural area can affect the sleep patterns of a client accustomed to a much noisier background. Adjust the volume controls on radios and televisions and telephones. The client who has a hearing loss will need a higher volume. Those who do not may prefer a lower tone.

Dust

Dust is an environmental factor that can make a difference in the client's comfort level. Some persons have allergies to dust and will experience respiratory discomfort if the air and furniture are laden with dust particles. Keep in mind that dust particles contain microorganisms that are foreign to the client who is in a new living environment. Damp dusting should be a part of the care of the client's unit. The nurse can teach the client to damp dust the furniture at home. This helps make the room comfortable and clean, as well as keeping dust to a minimum. When sheets on a bed are changed, they should not be thrown into the air and shaken, but rather they should be worked horizontally on the bed as the bed is being made. Keep soiled linen off the floors and in hampers.

This prevents contaminating the sheets with the dust and dirt from the floor and keeps the floors clean if there is any drainage or discharge on the sheeting.

Smoking

Cigarette smoke affects the environment of the client. Even if the client is a nonsmoker, the smoke from cigarettes and cigars of friends and family can fill a room. To a sensitive individual, this smoke can cause headache, throat and lung irritations, and sometimes even allergic responses. In a closed room with many people smoking, often the carbon monoxide level of the cigarette smoke can be raised above the minimum safety level established by the federal government. This puts an unnecessary burden on the older client's cardiovascular and respiratory systems. There is, in addition, the hazard of cigarette ashes igniting pajamas, furniture, couches, or beds if the client falls asleep while smoking. Ashtrays should be large enough to encase the cigarette safely on the inner ring so that, if the person neglects to put the cigarette out, it will burn without falling onto surrounding furniture, but rather into the second compartment of the ash tray. The nurse should keep in mind and advise the client that smoking should only be done in designated areas and not in individual rooms of long-term-care facilities. It is not uncommon for an older adult who has frequent periods of wakefulness during the night to want to smoke a cigarette. It is to everyone's advantage if the nurse encourages the client to go to a designated smoking area and have a cigarette there so the nurse can be aware that he is smoking. An open attitude fosters a more cooperative spirit, rather than risking a client's smoking secretively and falling back to sleep while still in bed. For example, at 2:00 in the morning, Mr. Starks comes to the nurses' station and wants a cigarette; the nurse permits him to sit at the nursing station and have a cigarette. He is able to have an occasional pleasant interlude of talking and having his cigarette even though it is 2:00 AM, and he feels comfortable and relaxed. There is no danger of accidental burns if the guidelines are presented clearly. If the client smokes in his own home, suggest he do so while sitting at the kitchen table, in the bathroom, or some other place where he is not likely to fall asleep. A couch, bed, or settee are not acceptable smoking areas because they are likely to be both comfortable and flammable. In facilities built for the older adult, state regulations mandate designated smoking areas; smoking is not to be permitted in the client's individual room to safeguard both the client and the entire population of the facility. This information should be an important part of the client's orientation on admission. In instances where clients are receiving oxygen therapy, a No Smoking sign should be prominently displayed. In addition, information should be given to the client, other clients in the room, and their families regarding the no-smoking policy. At home, when the client does have stored oxygen for use in treatment of cardiac or chronic pulmonary disease, the family should be aware that oxygen supports combustion. Any flame or spark in the room with an oxygen tank can cause an explosion.

Physical safety

Physical safety includes protection from thermal, chemical, and electrical injury.

Thermal injury. The delicate integument of the older adult has greater thermal sensitivity than that of the middle-aged adult. The temperature of the bath water should be no higher than 105° F. Hot water bottles must be closely assessed for external temperature and covered with a flannelette or terry cloth wrapper. Heating pad thermostats should be checked for correct functioning. Older adults can have a diminished sensory ability in the perception of hot and cold. Note if there is a mixer on the faucets of sinks and bath tubs, so that the water does not get above the 105° F safety temperature.

Chemical injury. Protection from chemical injury mandates that bottles and cups be labeled so that the client will not mistake them for frequently used self-care items. Caustic cleaning solutions or medications should be labeled in large letters, and if they are not to be used by the client, they should be stored away in a cabinet that is not accessible to them. In skilled, long-term-care facilities, federal regulations state that no medication can be left by the bedside and must be stored in a medication closet by the nurses' station. In intermediate-care facilities, the rules are more flexible. Because the needs of the client may vary greatly depending

upon the state of wellness and his progress toward discharge, medications are sometimes left by the bedside. The nurse, however, integrates clear teaching instructions regarding self-medication and evaluates the client so that he understands the regimen of medication care and follows it accordingly.

Electrical injury. Electrical appliances are often a source of injury to the older adult. When visiting the client at home, the nurse should remind the client that electrical appliances are not to be used near water. Radios should not be used in the bathroom or near the kitchen sink. No electrical appliance should be used when the body is wet. An older adult might have a therapeutic measure of warm, moist pack or soak, followed by a heating pad. The skin must be thoroughly dried before applying a heating pad.

As the nurse evaluates the client's home, she should include teaching regarding the dangers of frayed wires on electrical appliances such as irons, coffee pots, and toasters. Also, electrical appliance cords such as on lamps or televisions should not run under rugs. Fraying occurs on these cords. Sparks can be emitted and start fires. In long-term-care or intermediate-care facilities, equipment must be grounded with the three-prong plug system. Because older adult clients often live in older homes and apartments that are underwired for the number of today's electrical appliances, the nurse should also incorporate teaching regarding overloading of the circuits with too many plugs in one outlet.

When teaching activities of daily living skills, the nurse should emphasize the need for safe use of electrical appliances. For example, the nurse is teaching Mrs. Armstrong how to iron at home after her CVA. She observes Mrs. Armstrong using the iron and ironing board. The nurse reinforces the need to turn the iron off and pull the plug out of the socket each time she leaves the ironing board. If the telephone rings, she is to shut the iron off and pull out the plug before she goes to answer the phone. The nurse also reviews the instructions for the proper temperature setting on the iron. Many of the older adults are not used to the synthetic fibers used in today's clothing. They have grown up with natural fibers such as wool, cotton, and linen, and modern acetates and other synthetic fibers used in today's clothing require a much lower setting on the iron. The nurse can instruct the client how to move the different settings and perhaps put a mark or indentation on the medium-to-low setting, if the client is having difficulty reading the small letters on the iron.

Unfamiliar and familiar surroundings

Unfamiliar places can cause difficulty for the older adult. Not being sure where staircases, entrances and exits, elevators, or escalators are can pose a hazard to the older adult. Help the client enter and leave the rooms of the facility until he becomes well acquainted with the physical surroundings.

Consumer safety

Whether the nurse is doing nursing intervention for a single client or a group of older adult clients, it is useful for the nurse to discuss the Consumer Product Safety Commission with programs particularly designed for the older adult. These programs recommend various home structures such as bathtubs, showers, floors, carpets, rugs, and stair design that are particularly safe for use by the older adult. Since most injuries occur on stairways, ramps, and landings, the structural and architectural design that supports client safety should be used when a client is choosing a residence for himself or when a nurse is helping to plan an older adult facility.

Crime

The topic of a physically safe environment is not complete without a discussion of a major threat to the physical safety of older persons in today's violent society. Physical safety is jeopardized by the real risk of violent crimes both to their person and to household belongings. The United States Justice Department Law Enforcement Assistance Administration notes that the older adult is particularly vulnerable to crime. The older adult is not alone in being a crime victim; however, he suffers much physically and mentally the lack of feelings of safety after an incident of violent assault.

COMMUNITY-ACQUIRED ILLNESSES

The older adult is susceptible to influenza viruses and other communicable diseases. Nursing actions can be directed toward teaching the client basic health concepts of dressing for the weather and avoiding very crowded places, such as movies and restaurants, when it is announced that the influenza virus is prevalent. Influenza vaccine programs are offered to vulnerable populations, particularly the ill or weak older adult.

COMMUNITY COMMUNICATION SERVICES

The friendly phone visitor service is a voluntary program run by many churches and community groups. The older adult is called by a volunteer at a specific time each day. If the older adult does not answer, the caller notifies a neighbor or a relative who will go in person to make sure that the older adult is safe and in good condition. The older adult has the security of knowing that he will never be left longer than a 24-hour period and that he has an opportunity for a friendly, even if brief, chat with someone who is caring enough to spend the time to call. It is very useful if the nurse discusses with the client the possibility of giving a key to a neighbor whom the client knows well, or to a family member. This gives the friend or family member easy access to the client in case of need.

LOVE AND BELONGING

As with all age groups, the older adult has innate needs for love and belonging. However, before these can be addressed, he must have satisfied his physiological needs, which are required for survival. Then, satisfaction of safety and security needs ensure the physical and psychological well-being of the older adult. All of these lead to a readiness to expand life energy and resources in fulfilling Maslow's third level, the need for love and belonging. Throughout his life, the older adult has opportunities to give to and receive love from many people, such as his family, spouse, friends, co-workers, neighbors, and pets. Advancing age does not diminish these love and belonging needs. What is reduced are the older adult's opportunities for giving and receiving love. As work and social areas are relinquished, the love network can be limited to the client's family (Fig. 11-2).

Only 12 percent of older adults have no family or close relatives. The great majority, 80 percent, have living children, 75 percent of whom live in the household or within a 30-minute trip away.

The sense of love and belonging transmitted between generations is founded on mutual support and respect, affection, intimacy, independence, and reciprocal giving between the older adult, his family, or significant others. This same foundation and reciprocal interaction between the older adult, nurse, or health care provider can help foster an environment of love and belonging.

Many families of older adults distribute the care and support responsibilities among several members. For example, a son may be responsible for managing the parent's financial assets, or he may assume financial support himself while a daughter is responsible for household chores and meal preparation.

When the older adult is single, widowed, childless, many miles from his family, or the last family survivor, it might be difficult for him to have his love and belonging needs met. Such situations compel the older adult to find new channels and resources for satisfying these needs. Some networks that older adults develop are friendships established within the neighborhood, religious affiliations, and related activities, social groups, clubs, a confidant, pets, and participation in community activities. Individuals who do not have these outlets as support systems may develop a sense of loneliness.

Marriage

A natural relationship for providing love and belonging is through marriage. Those marriages that have survived the postparental years are usually stable. The divorce rate in marriages over 29 years is only 3 percent. Couples who remarry after divorce or widowhood also have relatively stable marriages. The older adult marriage can offer both partners marital love, a deeply rewarding husband-wife companionship, equality, mutuality of interests, open communication, and understanding. Because men die at a younger age than women and are usually several years older than their wives, a woman has a higher risk of losing her

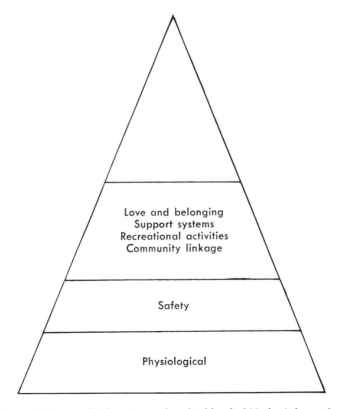

Fig. 11-2. Love and belonging needs—third level of Maslow's hierarchy.

spouse. There are more women than men in the older adult population.

On the death of a spouse, new social networks have to be developed to substitute for the marriage relationship. Often, when an older adult woman and man fall in love and plan to get married, the grown children intervene and discourage the union. The adult children's reason for disapproval may be legitimate concerns for their parent's future or selfish concerns regarding their own sharing of the parent and anticipated inheritance of material goods. The parent who is pressured by his adult children may decide to keep peace in the family and forego the future happiness found in an intimate relationship of a remarriage. Often a couple in such a situation will continue the intimate relationship without remarriage. This may or may not include living together and pooling resources. The couple sometimes finds it easier to maintain the upkeep on one house or one apartment. Many of society's activities and functions are geared to couples. Even packaged vacations and hotel accommodations are less expensive for couples than a single person.

On the other hand, the adult children may be very pleased and happy to have their parent remarry. It may reinforce their belief that the parent is an independent adult who can make his own decisions and lead a life-style of his choice. The parent now has someone to take care of him, and this fact in itself may relieve the adult children of a feeling of responsibility for the parent. The companionship found in the remarriage may relieve the adult children of their function of providing social outlets and supplying recreational resources for the parent. Many remarriages are very satisfying for the older adults and a rewarding experience for the involved adult children.

Some couples find it useful to identify the financial resources of each partner, and have a premarital agreement or wills written before the ceremony. These arrangements help alleviate interfamily disagreements over financial arrangements and inheritance rights.

Widowed older adults

Living through the death of a mate is a great crisis in the life of an older adult. On a scale of life events, the death of a spouse is rated the highest at 100 points (see p. 8). After the initial shock of the death wears off and the grieving continues, the remaining spouse can have feelings of loneliness, isolation, and desolation.

Living through the adjustment to widowhood can be difficult. The grief work helps the client express feelings of anger, guilt, hostility, loneliness, and praise of the deceased mate. During this period, the widowed person needs support from family and friends. Religion is usually a great comfort and sustains the concerned spouse and family.

Some widowers, their families, and friends, react to the situation by interdependence and cohesiveness, whereas others use independence and individual growth to manage the adjustment period. Data support the evidence that an intimate friend or confidant is an asset in maintaining physical and mental health. Grief and personal adjustment must be worked through before new friendships and relationships can be established. In addition, major decisions and commitments should be postponed until the widowed person is emotionally ready. Widowhood brings with it many responsibilities. Decisions must be made regarding finances, investments, living arrangements, household management and repairs, and future roles and obligations to oneself and family.

What can the nurse and health care provider do to help the newly widowed older adult? First, assess the situation, collect and evaluate data that support the significance of the spouse's loss and the effect it has on activities of daily living. Observe the client for signs of depression, mourning, and grief work. Assist the older adult in personal and social adjustment. Listen intently, counsel against hasty decisions, and refer the older adult to the appropriate professional person, local, state, or federal agency for specific help. Most communities have a legal aid center that provides free legal assistance, especially for older persons. Let the client know that he or she is loved and that help is available for problem solving. Direct the client to a local widowed persons program. It is often helpful to talk with other widowed persons who have had a similar experience and who can give new insight to handling the stresses and grieving one goes through. Talking with a friendly and warm clergyman, nurse, social worker, psychologist, or marriage counselor may be all that is needed for catharsis and sharing of problems. Obtain some books from the library for the older adult that deal with bereavement, adjustment to widowhood, and family support systems. Identify specific problem areas such as insurance, housing, Social Security benefits, coping with stress, how to survive, money management, estate planning, household repairs, job-finding techniques, pets, or living with grief. Call the local library and have the librarian research the problem area and reserve the books for the older adult client. Take care that library materials are not outdated, especially those dealing with Social Security benefits and finances. The Government Printing Office has many free booklets that are easy to read and understand, yet are very informative. Additional booklets that address the problem areas are usually available at no cost from local legal aid offices, insurance companies, banks, and savings and loan offices. The local Federal Information Center is available to answer questions and help solve problems related to the federal government's programs for older adults.

From the assessment data, the nurse should have picked up some clues about the client's coping mechanisms. These coping mechanisms may be used to the widowed individual's best advantage to retain his sense of control and help adapt to anticipated changes. As the nurse gets to know the client better, the nursing diagnosis, plan of care, and anticipatory guidance may need to be adjusted. Use therapeutic communication to assess a typical daily profile of the client's activities of daily living. Pay particular attention to subjective and objective symptoms of fatigue, malaise, depression, suicide threats, alcoholism, disorientation, any changes in chronic conditions such as arthritis and diabetes, anorexia, insomnia, and decreases in activities required for daily functioning.

The plan of care developed will address alleviating the symptoms, meeting the needs identified, supporting and encouraging the client, and identifying channels of love and belonging for the client. Encourage family members and close friends to supply the love and understanding needed by the client. They can also help occupy the time that may weigh heavily during the client's day.

In addition, some forgotten hobbies, skills, sports, or activities from the past may now be utilized because there is time available to engage in them. Exercise may be very therapeutic, especially walking, which has been found to be conducive to relieving stress and promoting mental health.

A small circle of family and friends can insulate and cushion the client against further trauma and subsequent hurt. The circle can gradually be enlarged to include other friends and acquaintances. In the beginning, the client's brothers, sisters, or adult children can be more successful in sharing in the client's new life-style and helping him mold a new way of life for himself. They can be influential in getting him to participate in family and other social activities.

There is no prototype for successful bereavement and personal and social adjustment; it is an individual developmental task. The client should not be pressured into stressful situations. The nurse may guide the client, counsel him, identify sources of love and belonging, help him set realistic immediate and future goals, and let him know that he is not alone. The nurse's presence, interest, and therapeutic intervention in the client's problems may be all that the client needs to help him survey his alternatives and provide the impetus for knowledgeable decision making.

Loneliness and isolation

There are times when everyone wants peace and quiet and to be left alone. However, large doses of this over an extended period of time can lead to a feeling of loneliness. By the time an individual has reached adulthood, he has experienced varying degrees of loneliness. Loneliness occurs as a maturational situation and is a lack of personal interaction with another human being. The older adult may experience feelings of loneliness for an adult child who has moved away, a deceased spouse, brother, sister or dear friend. The older adult may experience loneliness and isolation because he is shut in, financially and physically unable to interact, or without access to transportation and thus cut off from peer relationships. Many times loneliness is accompanied by a feeling that no one loves you, depression, and a sense of putting in time before death.

Before discussing loneliness, there are two other terms—aloneness and lonesomeness—that need to be differentiated. Aloneness exists when one lives alone and does not have any company. Aloneness is a state that is required for certain work and recreational activities. Solitaire is a game that is played alone, as are doing a crossword puzzle, reading a book, and painting. Aloneness is usually a chosen state with or without some purpose in mind. Many older adults welcome being alone to think things through, concentrate, finish a project, or just relax. Aloneness may be a safety valve for dealing with day-to-day crises. Aloneness is usually not accompanied by anxiety or discomfort because of lack of company.

Mrs. Carson, who is a resident in a nursing home, has a semiprivate room. She makes arrangements to use the facility's quiet room every day. While there, she reads the morning paper and her book and writes letters. Other days, she reads the new magazines, does her painting, or just relaxes away from all the activity.

Lonesomeness is also being without the company of others. It differs from aloneness in that the older adult wishes to be closer to others and is able to state it in a feeling. The client recognizes lonesomeness because it generates mild to moderate discomfort. Another distinguishing feature is that lonesomeness may occur when the client is with others, as well as being alone. The older adult is able to take the necessary action to relieve the situation and create a more positive situation.

There is no doubt that loneliness is a very personal phenomenon; however, the nurse may intervene in anticipating its potential threat to the health of the client. In addition, the nurse may help the client identify new sources for love and personal interaction.

Mrs. Archer's husband died on Christmas day when he was 69 years old. Since his retirement, they had enjoyed one cruise and a Hawaiian vacation. Another trip was planned for the year he died. Mrs. Archer still feels loneliness, even though it has been 2 years since her husband's death. It is worse in the winter as the holidays approach, and the days seem to drag. Sundays, when they would go for a ride and eat dinner in a restaurant are the worst days. Her married son and daughter have been very supportive. The son taught her to drive the car left by his father. Being able to drive has made Mrs. Archer less dependent on her children. She can visit them when she wishes, as well as

visit her sisters and drive to social functions. The family is now able to face Christmas together. At first, Mrs. Archer's loneliness was a significant problem for her and her children. The family that should be her strongest love and support system instead was caught in the mother's web of loneliness and unable to reduce her anxiety.

A neighborhood nurse helped them work through their feelings and develop strength from the family's cohesiveness. Mrs. Archer found that being extremely busy with holiday preparations was a good coping mechanism for her. She did all the baking for her children's family and the shopping for the toys and gifts. During the day, she enjoyed walking through the malls and having dinner before returning home. She baked, wrote cards, or wrapped presents at night. Her family kept in contact with her daily at this time of the year. Each holiday season seems to become easier to handle as the years pass for Mrs. Archer and her family.

Loneliness reducers. People need people, and when interaction with another person is not available, the alternative outlets include pets, hobbies, television, and radio.

A situation with no interaction can lead to mental deterioration. Recent studies report the therapeutic value of animals as pets for the older adult and isolated individuals. The pet is a living animal that needs the older adult and is the object of mutual love and affection. The pet provides the client with a continuous friend and someone to talk to so that the client can hear his own voice. People who live alone without the opportunity to talk to someone or something may go for a day or longer without uttering a word. Pets have been found to reduce the potential for suicide and improve the person's self-image. The care and feeding that the pet requires may give the client a purpose for living.

When an individual has no animal to relate to, he may turn to other happenings in nature. Isolated persons can fill lonely hours watching spiders spin a web, bees build a hive, and ants transport food. A purchased ant farm for the right client can be a fascinating source of entertainment. Living plants and their care are an excellent means for interaction, not to mention a hobby source. Many clients take pride in having a green thumb and growing a favorite plant, such as African violets, ferns, a small vegetable garden, or just a few tomato plants. The love and affection showered on these plants give the older adult an opportunity to nurture a living thing (Fig. 11-3). The client may start his plant collection with one or two plants or from a transplanted shoot. The client can receive much joy in giving away one of his home-grown living plants or vegetables, symbols of his love.

Inanimate objects that are personal possessions often represent memories of a loved one. The ob-

ject fits somewhere in the time frame of the individual's life. It may trigger reminiscense and pleasant events and be a symbol of past accomplishments. The object possesses an aura of familiarity and makes interaction very easy.

It has been found that daytime television soap operas have served a therapeutic role for the housebound older adult. The client has fictional people and situations to identify with and problems to help them solve. The client often becomes so fa-

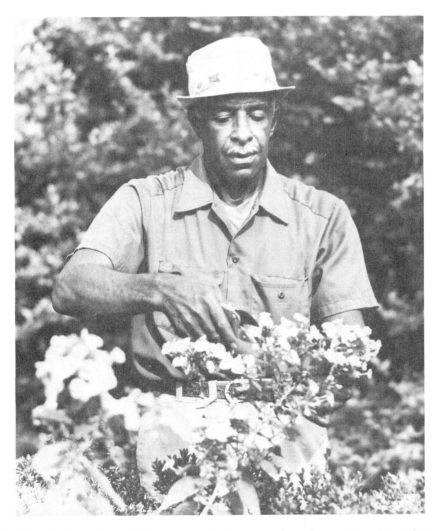

Fig. 11-3. With skill and pride this man prunes his flowers and shrubs. He enjoys his garden as do his family and neighbors. (H. Armstrong Roberts Photo Service.)

miliar with the fictional family members and townspeople that he internalizes the problems, expresses empathy, and has a whole group of new friends with whom to interact and even people to dislike.

The radio is a longtime acquaintance of the older adult. It was the only source of home entertainment before the television era. Many older adults have a favorite station and disk jockeys who provide a source for personal contact. They are able to relate to the disk jockey and feel that he is talking directly to them. Call-in games that include the audience participation allow the client to identify himself as a member of the station's "family." Talk shows also provide a forum for the client to present his views on current issues and topics being aired. There are some stations that play ethnic music and report the news in the client's native language. A radio can fill the void of many quiet hours and is inexpensive company for the client.

There are many sources for interaction for the older adult to overcome loneliness. The telephone and friendly callers have been mentioned with communication in Chapter 9. The nurse and client together can identify his networks for love and interaction.

Suicide. A devastating outcome of loneliness and isolation is suicide. It is estimated that there is at least one suicide every 17 minutes in the United States. Four causative factors have been associated with suicide: hopelessness, suffering, alienation, and search for glory. The statistics for unsuccessful attempts are staggering and range from 350,000 to 500,000 annually.

"Suicide is a maladaptive response to crisis" (Wilson and Kneisl, 1979, p. 257). There is evidence that suicide is low in groups of people in which

1. Hope and optimism are high
2. Ethnic cultures are nurturing, such as the Irish and Italians
3. Religion exercises disapproval, especially the Roman Catholic countries, such as Ireland, Spain, and Italy

Suicide is highest in older adults who are:

1. In discouraging situations, such as inner city dwelling and skid rows
2. Single

3. Married white men who feel hopeless and have given up
4. Having interpersonal, social, and financial problems
5. Experiencing the loss of a love relationship
6. Depressed
7. Terminally ill or have an illness that alters body image and life-style
8. Survivors of previous suicide attempts

The older adult who has not had a satisfactory resolution of Erikson's eighth developmental stage experiences despair over his life. His attitude is a sense of loss and a contempt for others, a feeling of nonbelonging and nonachievement of life desires. He lacks ego integrity and satisfaction with his love. Suicide may surface as a result of an unsuccessful resolution of an identity crisis of the older adult.

The important nursing intervention is to do a suicidal assessment of the client and immediate crisis counseling. Communicate with the client about his concerns and suicide intent. Listen intently, and encourage catharsis of feelings and understanding of the problem. Explore new coping mechanisms and social networks that aid in problem solution. The need for medical assistance, a psychiatric nurse practitioner, hospitalization, or the services of a mental health clinic will become apparent after talking to the client and doing an lethality assessment. The plan of care will depend upon the outcome of identifying whether the client is contemplating using a low-lethality method, such as wrist cutting or a high one, such as a gun. Older adults attempt more violent and dangerous suicidal methods. The evidence that the client has the resources to carry out the method and a plan of action should be explored.

There are different crisis intervention methods that are useful—one-on-one, group, family, telephone, and home visits. The one most appropriate modality for the client's needs should be selected. All crisis intervention is best done by trained personnel. Individual (one-on-one) crisis counseling is usually completed within six sessions. The therapist confines the sessions to the identified issues and with the client, engages in problem solving. Follow-up appointments are made after the crisis is resolved. Group crisis sessions address the issues using group dynamics, strategies, and process.

Each member of the group is experiencing a crisis, and usually the group meets for six to ten sessions. Family crisis counseling is popular for younger families who are experiencing adolescent crisis or midlife crisis. Many older adults who are in a crisis are alone with no family or friends available. However, those clients who do have significant others may include them in the counseling. The family meets for approximately six sessions for counseling. Telephone counseling and home visits are excellent modes of crisis intervention for the older adult. The client, particularly one who is less agile, does not have to worry about transportation arrangements.

Many communities have telephone "hot lines," and some are nationwide such as the one in Garden Grove, California, which can be reached by dialing "NEW-HOPE." The New Hope counseling service is a toll-free number and available 24 hours a day. The philosophy for the service is "An eye that is never shut, an ear that is never deaf, a heart that never grows cold." The crisis hot lines put the troubled older adult in immediate contact with an understanding, helping, specially trained person. The favorable response and success of the telephone hot line programs have increased their adoption and use.

Home visits can be made when the telephone is not available or when the agency is informed about the client by means of a second party, a friend, neighbor, clergyman, or family member. The visit provides an opportunity to assess the home environment, observe the client, and determine if he has the means for carrying out the suicidal threat. The nurse can be alert in preventing suicide and nurturing the client's will to live. The nurse and client together overcome the risk of suicide by setting goals that combat helplessness and hopelessness and address the need for love and self-worth, while establishing an environment of relief from physical pain and support for feelings of discouragement.

Suiciders Anonymous. Suiciders Anonymous is a national nonprofit organization formed in 1978, whose goal is to assist the complete recovery of attempted suicide individuals. The head of the organization is a clinical psychiatrist with expertise in counselling. Its creator was Dr. Robert H. Schuller, founder of the Garden Grove Community Church in California and the syndicated television program "Hour of Power." However, Suiciders Anonymous is not connected with any church, and its members do not subscribe to any one religious philosophy. Its operational framework reflects that of Alcoholics Anonymous, which is recognized as successful in the rehabilitation of the alcoholic. Each small group is anonymous and governed by the members, who share common experiences, support and nurture each other, and set group objectives. The total group maintains order at the meeting, which is unstructured, nonthreatening, and run without a leader or professional help. However, a member may receive outside professional help. A sponsor program similar to that of Alcoholics Anonymous is part of the structure. A sponsor is a person who has recovered and developed inner resources, strength, hope, and love of life that can be passed on to others. Each member is helped to understand and like himself, elevate his self-esteem, and find happiness and purpose in life.

In the short time that it has been in operation, results have been very successful. Even though it is in its infancy, chapters are nationwide. If a community does not have one as yet, one can write to Suiciders Anonymous, Garden Grove, Calif. 92642.

Bridges to love and belonging

Community services. There is a wide range of community services available to the older adult. Finding the appropriate service for the client can be difficult. (The nursing process is the structure to use in making judgments about the pattern of care. Select services to reach the client goal, predict problems, and keep in mind the prognosis, influence of social, environmental conditions, and time balanced against alternative means of help.) After the initial assessment phase and the establishment of a data base, planning evolves as more than one dimension. It is comprehensive and challenging, involving management decisions about the types and kinds of staff and resources needed to meet the expected outcomes.

Day-care centers and day-care hospitals. The day-care center and day-care hospital are two useful ways to help the older adult remain on his own. There are some differences in these two types of centers. The day-care center serves well clients and does not have a primary medical component. The day-care hospital center provides daytime shelter for incapacitated clients having a wide variety of conditions, such as hemiplegia, arthritis, amputation, and organic brain disease. Clients with these conditions functioning at a more independent level may be attending a day-care center. The following are examples of the services offered at day-care centers and day-care hospital centers.

1. Nursing and medical services for health assessment and periodic reevaluations
2. Assessment by other staff members, such as dentist, occupational and physical therapist, optometrist, podiatrist, and social worker
3. Exercise activities
4. Laboratory services
5. Health education classes
6. Continuing education classes
7. Reality orientation and remotivation classes
8. Personal hygiene and grooming classes
9. Social activities
10. Meals

Centers that are sponsored by hospitals usually offer more medically-oriented programs and services.

Many day-care centers are sponsored by nursing homes but operate as a separate entity; others may be sponsored by senior-citizen centers. The availability of client transportation to and from the centers can be an obstacle to the client's ability to attend. When the center provides transportation or the client is able to walk and is within walking distance, participation in center activities is easier. Day-care and hospital-care centers are a necessity and fill a void in the daily routines of many older adults who would otherwise not be able to remain independent in the community.

Home care programs. Home care programs are less expensive than institutionalized care. They are sponsored by a range of providers: government, profit-making, and voluntary agencies and Blue Cross-Blue Shield. The level of nursing care the client receives is determined by the professional nurse and may include clinical nurse specialists, home health aid, and home-making services. Other professional services are delivered in the home to include physical therapy, occupational therapy, and podiatry care. The client's status is intermit-

tently evaluated and adjustments made in the use plan. The time frame for the selected professional and nonprofessional services varies according to the individual client needs. For example, the homemaking service may range from several hours a day to 24 hour, sleep-in services.

In some states, home health aides have to be certified and receive a vigorous training program. The program may be conducted by a community or public health service. The home health aide carries out the same type procedures as a hospital aide. Personal hygiene, vital signs, assisting with physical therapy, and changing simple dressings are examples of aide activities. The aide always performs her functions under the supervision of a professional nurse. Home health aides are reimbursed by Medicare. Homemakers are not a service under Medicare. A homemaker may be a home health aide also and do a combination of activities. Light housekeeping and cooking are the services rendered. Homemakers also receive training and supervision by the employing agency.

Domiciliary care. Many states are adopting a domiciliary program as an alternative to a nursing home. A domiciliary client is usually an individual who can function at the intermediate-care level or better, requiring a minimum of supervision. The domiciliary program provides the supervision that the older adult needs to remain in the community. The program also serves as a resource for the individual discharged from a long-term-care facility.

Domiciliary care is provided in a private home that accommodates from one to three older adults. The domiciliary provider is a paid individual who is trained in the care of the older adult. A social worker and community health nurse assess the client upon entrance and at periodic intervals. The provider has been training in therapeutic diets, insulin injections, and adverse reactions such as shock, coma, and drug therapy. He supervises the older adult's independent functioning within the community. A network of health services and resources are available to the client. The provider and the domiciliary environment are continuously monitored. Additional education and training are given to the provider. When a crisis or a change in the older adult's physical condition occurs, the client is transferred to a hospital or long-term-care facility. He can return to domiciliary care when his condition improves.

The domiciliary model may vary from state to state and with the client's financial status. The state often pays the provider for his services. Domiciliary care is usually less expensive than long-term care. The domiciliary care approach is growing throughout the country and is an excellent alternative to long-term institutional care.

Spiritual life of the older adult. The older adult's spiritual resources can be a source of strength and peace. While the nurse tends to her clients physical and emotional needs, she can provide opportunities for spiritual expression also. Many of life's milestones are marked by religious ceremonies: christening, bar mitzvah, confirmation, marriage, and burial. The nurse can encourage the client to relate these occasions and associated memories as he reminisces.

Build upon the clients spiritual assets by encouraging full religious expression. Religious symbols and prayers offer daily comfort. Communal religious services provide social as well as spiritual opportunities. Arrange transportation and schedules so the client can attend religious activities and services conveniently. Have the agency chaplain visit with the client on the unit if the client prefers a one-to-one contact. Space should be available within the agency for a quiet or meditation room. The room could also serve as the center for religious services. Many agencies use taped services that are played over the in-house television system as one method of having services available to clients who are unable to leave their units. Also, services can be held on other than weekend days when the chaplain serves more than one agency and is not available every Saturday or Sunday.

Cultural mores sometime stereotype the woman as the sole religious participant; however, men also desire spiritual expression. The nurse can set an accepting climate for the spiritual needs of both sexes. Families of the client can be a part of the client's religious experience when they accompany the client to services and know the client's chaplain also.

Family healing. Researchers have been interested in the influence of the family and significant others on the health of the older adult. The scientific theory behind this phenomenon has not been specifically identified, but it has been observed that the ties that bind can also heal. Evidence is available that married people live longer than single, widowed, or divorced people. A widow during the first year of widowhood exhibits more physical and psychological symptoms than when married; the death rate of first-year widows is also higher than that of married women. The family role in the service of the individual has always been a part of the human story. Even in primitive tribes, the family rallied around the ill or frail member. The individual's problem was seen as a problem for the whole tribe. The tribesmen and family concentrated on curing the individual by using their rituals and catharsis systems. This ancient approach has been modified to bring family members of three and four generations together to support the terminally ill person. Wise (1979) reports some remission of the disease process and improvement in the client's condition after family contact. The love environment of the family supports the client, which aids the healing process. Such a family support system may be arranged for an older adult living in the community on long-term-care facility. Families often gather on birthdays, holidays, weddings, and Father's and Mother's Day. When he is included, the older adult is assured of his place in the family and can participate in the mutual exchange of love.

The older adult can use the family social event to do a life review and share family ancestry with the younger members as an oral historian.

When the client has no family himself, the families of other clients can be solicited to serve as his support system. They arrange a family and friend's reunion picnic or get-together at the facility. Many facilities do invite the immediate family or friends to holiday dinners and parties. A cocktail party is one activity that may attract delinquent families and friends. Clients without significant others may be introduced to substitutes in the form of family council, friendly visitors, staff, and fellow residents. The most important thing is the love the client finds at the facility. The nursing staff can be the bridge to extend the client's love from his previous life-style to his present life-style. Sincere interest and person-to-person contact make the difference.

Family and Friends Council. Admission of a client to a long-term-care facility may be a very traumatic experience, not only for the client but for the family as well. One mechanism to supply the necessary human support system is a facility Family and Friends Council. The state of Oregon has been very active in developing a state-wide council. Other states are using Oregon as a model for implementing such a program.

Oregon's Council, called *Friends and Relatives of Nursing Home Patients, Inc.,* is nonprofit and has been in operation since 1971 as the result of the governor's Nursing Home Task Force. The purpose stated in the charter is to "improve care for every nursing home and home-for-the-aged patient in Oregon." One of the goals is to have a relative or friend of every client receiving long-term-care in Oregon join the Council. However, membership is open to interested persons and organizations. The Council conducts regional meetings, local unit meetings and publishes a news letter discussing legislation affecting the older adult.

The Oregon Council's purpose, objectives, and activities have been heartily endorsed by the Oregon Health Care Association, the governor, the Health Division and Welfare Division of the state, the Consumer's League, the State Council of Senior Citizens, the Governor's Advisory Committee on Aging, and several organizations of health professionals. Oregon's Council has been in operation state-wide for 10 years, and older adult consumers of long-term care are reaping the benefits of the project. Oregon is a pioneer in establishing an advocacy program, recognizing that the best persons to speak for clients in long-term-care facilities are relatives and friends who care. The nurse may fill the place of the client's relative or friend in their absence. The nurse has functioned as the client's advocate for years and can now take a leadership position in establishing a Family and Friends Council at her facility. Assistance may be available from her own state Long-Term Care Advocacy Project, or by contacting the Oregon Council, whose address is found in Appendix D.

A Family and Friends Council is really a shared responsibility between the long-term-care facility and the client's family and friends. Each has the responsibility for the client and the shared goal of seeing that the client receives the best quality care available. The Family and Friends Council provides the mechanism to improve communications be-

tween the client's significant others and the administrator and staff of the long-term-care facility. The Council may function as the advocate for the older adult as well as for the facility. For example, in addition to promoting the rights of the residents, the Council may also increase the public awareness of the problems and achievements of the facility and its residents. The Council is readily available to help the resident and his family and friends make the transition from a community life-style to a long-term-care facility life-style. The client's family is not alone during the adjustment period. The new resident's family has the support of other family members who have gone through the same experience. The Council with facility representatives such as director of nursing, administrator, or other designated administrative personnel can give the new resident, his family and friends the counseling, guidance, and knowledge about aging needed to reduce fear of the unknown, isolation that occurs in a new social situation and promote a positive adjustment to a new life style that utilizes the client's assets to enhance maximum functioning. The Council may be the forum for the director of nursing to discuss the facility's philosophy of nursing care and individual goal planning, client care policies, reality orientation program, and other services provided. Nursing may use this opportunity to have the families and friends participate meaningfully in the management of care individually designed for the resident. When the resident's significant others know the ultimate goal is the attainment of the client's level of independence in activities of daily living, they can help the nursing staff achieve this goal. The client's family will be less likely to complain at the nurses' desk that the client should be fed his meals instead of using self-help utensils.

It is not uncommon for the client's family to experience feelings of guilt. Guilt feelings may be reduced when the common feelings associated with client admission are discussed frankly. Unresolved feelings are sometimes displayed as anger toward the agency and staff.

Family and friends are more likely to be satisfied that they selected the best possible facility when there are no secrets about nursing care, policies, and services. The client's family and friends are the best advocates within the community for the facility when they join with the facility in meeting the personal needs of the client. When the client and his family are satisfied consumers, they can, in turn, aid other families whose older adult member is coming into the facility.

On the other hand, if the family and the client are not satisfied with the services of the facility, they can discuss the situation with the nursing director or agency administrator, and the Council may be used as a mediator. The agency administrator may also use the Council to communicate with community agencies as well as to comply with various federal rules and regulations.

The Council helps administration, clients, friends, and families work together for the benefit of the clients who reside in the long-term-care facility.

How to implement a Family and Friends Council

1. The Director of Nursing explains the concept of a Family and Friends Council to the administrator. The advantages are discussed, and an agreement is made to assess the facility's interest in a Council. In those states that have a long-term-care advocacy project, the community organizers of the Long-Term-Care Advocacy Project will meet with interested groups and administrators to help develop a Council. The organizer can assist in planning meetings, developing an organizational structure, training and orientation, and resolving issues relating to the rights of administrators, relatives, and friends in the development or activities of a Council.

2. An in-service education program is held for the day evening, and night charge nurses and the admission officer to discuss the idea of the Family and Friends Council. Their interest and support are secured after questions are answered and advantages discussed openly.

3. The admission officer discusses the idea with clients and their families and friends at the preadmission interview. A record is kept of the number of people who would be interested in joining a Council.

4. The charge nurses discuss the Council idea with the clients and their families and friends who come to visit them at the long-term-care facility.

5. Several interested family members and friends are selected to hold a preplanning meeting with the administrator. It is important that he be included from the beginning and be informed of each step you take and the data collected in the process of forming a Council. This will help ensure direct communication with administration, his complete understanding of the project, and his cooperation and support of it.

6. An agenda is developed for the preplanning meeting. A preliminary statement is written regarding the purpose of the Family and Friends Council. Two or three objectives of the Council and recommended membership are listed. An initial agenda might look something like this:

Agenda
 I. Introduction to administrator and other invited family members and friends.
 II. Definition of the concept of a Family and Friends Council. (Discuss how it could be implemented and function at the facility.)
 III. Discussion of the purpose statement and objectives with the committee. (Get their input, and change, modify, and include additional objectives.)
 IV. Discussion of possible activities for the Council to engage in.
 V. Development of a plan for initiating a Council at the facility. (Decide on a meeting date, set up an agenda, and mail invitations to each client's family, friends, or guarantor.)

7. At the implementation meeting, the statements on purpose, objectives, memberships, and suggested activities are presented. These are discussed, and changes and additions are incorporated before accepting the statements. Some suggested activities that may have developed from the preplanning meeting follow:

- Preparation of an informational handbook about the Council, its purpose, objectives, membership, and activities.
- Preparation of a resident's handbook in conjunction with the administration if the facility does not have one. Information is included about visiting hours, meals, laundry, barber and hairdresser service, policies regarding smoking and food in rooms, the names of the department heads and how to contact each department for service, the Family and Friends Council and how to contact them for assistance with a problem, and social, recreational, and religious activities provided by the long-term-care facility.
- Preparation of an organizational chart of the facility that identifies administrative personnel, medical director, department heads, and consultant services. Preparation of a plan of the facility that identifies staff for the visitors.
- Interpretation of "Client's Rights" information to clients, their families, and friends.
- Development or expansion of volunteer service activities for clients.
- Fund-raising activities for special equipment,

activities, or additions to the long-term care facility.

- Regular meetings scheduled with the administrator to discuss policies and make recommendations, to share information and ask questions, to review the survey report of the facility, and offer assistance if needed in correcting deficiencies.
- Interest and support provided to clients who have no regular visitors, those serving as an alternate family member, or those sharing responsibility for clients when their family cannot be present because of vacations, emergencies, or other temporary absences on a mutual exchange basis.
- Providing human support to other clients or their families in times of crisis or transition.
- Participation in group activities for residents in the long-term-care facility.

8. An ad hoc committee is set up to develop by-laws and nominate offers for the Council. (The committee is given copies of by-laws and officers' duties collected from other Councils.)

9. A date is set up for the next Council meeting to vote on by-laws and officers.

10. The administrator communicates the Council's purpose, objectives, and activities to the board of directors, medical director, physicians, and department heads. (The director of nursing may take the leadership for structuring a plan to communicate information to the nursing staff, clients, and their relatives and friends. Personal communication is an acceptable route; in-service education meetings, minutes, and memos are also good means to gather suggestions, support, and additional participation from people who did not attend the first meeting.)

11. Minutes of the Council's meetings are posted on each unit, the client's bulletin board, and the employees' board. Send copies to the administrator, department heads, medical director, and others as needed.

12. The administrator or his representative is invited to every meeting to ensure open communication with him.

13. The agenda for second meeting is posted well in advance, and relatives and friends are personally invited during visiting hours. Clients are asked to call and remind their relatives and friends, postcards are sent, or someone is designated to call. This meeting must be publicized because the by-laws and officers will be voted on.)

14. A goal is to establish a news letter as another source of communication with members of the community and administration.

15. A regular monthly or bimonthly meeting pattern is established as needed. The activities of the Council are used for meeting topics and issues.

16. A time during meetings is scheduled periodically for the administrator to discuss policy issues, facility activities, problems with the staff, clients, relatives and friends and give a general report to the Council. The Council may also give positive and negative feedback to the administrator regarding the care the facility renders.

17. The Council arranges for conferences, orientation, and counseling of relatives and friends of newly admitted clients and other clients on request. These activities may be conducted by the professional nurse, medical director, or professional consultants of the facility, such as the social worker, the psychiatrist, or physical therapist. The interaction with these professionals will increase the relatives' and friends' sensitivity to aging and their knowledge of important aspects of long-term care.

18. Recruitment of new members to the Family and Friends Council is ongoing.

19. The function of the Council is periodically evaluated: its activities, contact with administration, successes, and any failures. Feedback is encouraged from Council members, clients, administrator, and facility employees.

Resident council. The resident council is an excellent vehicle for the older adult residing in a nursing home to have some control over his own destiny and increase self-esteem. Administration and nursing need to support and encourage resident participation in the council. Each member receives a sense of love and belonging from fellow residents. They will be able to govern their own group living by discussing and voting on policies and procedures for the long-term-care facility. The number of officers varies; however, a president, vice president, secretary, and treasurer for fundraising activities may be elected by the group. Committees are formed depending on the scope of the resident council's functions. Some councils have a representative for each nursing unit to orient new residents and help them adjust and settle into the long-term-care environment.

A dietary committee may work with the dietician in planning meals and resolving problems. The residents are engaging in consumer activities by discussing problems within the home, making recommendations, and working through solutions with administration and the head of the involved department. Administration and department heads should address recommendations immediately and give the residents rationales for negative responses.

The resident should be assured that he may speak freely at meetings and never be censured. Administration and representatives of personnel should not attend meetings unless they are invited by the residents. Resident councils at many facilities maintain open meetings, inviting administration and personnel representatives, because there is a mutual symbiotic relationship. Each group grows from the other's knowledge and understanding of the opposite side of a problem. Self-esteem is enhanced because the resident is not treated like a child; his adult role and consumer role are respected; he makes decisions about his new life-style.

Sensitivity training. Individualized nursing intervention is most effective when the nurse and her staff are sensitive to the older adult's perception of his world. The following exercise permits the staff to experience the older adult's world through role playing.

PLACE: Staff meeting
MATERIALS NEEDED
  Earplugs or cotton balls
  Eyeglasses coated with Vaseline
  Surgical gloves
  Small buttons to go in shoes to simulate sore feet and
    corns
  Wheel chair
  Posy restraints
  Geri chair
  Incontinency diaper or pants
SENSITIVITY ACTIVITIES
  Staff member tries to walk across room with impaired
    vision glasses.
  Cotton balls or earplugs are put into ears, and staff
    member must participate in discussion with simu-
    lated deafness.
  Staff member must walk around room with buttons in
    shoes to simulate pain causing impaired mobility.
  One of the staff members must wear under his clothing
    incontinence pants or diaper.
  Restrain a staff member in a Geri chair the length of
    the conference.
  Restrain a staff member in a Posy while in a wheel-
    chair for the length of the conference.
SENSITIVITY DISCUSSION: Discuss the physical discom-
  forts often experienced by the older adult and relate
  it to his feelings of:
    Helplessness
    Powerlessness
    Lowered self-esteem

Reducing relocation trauma. When relocation of the older adult is mentioned, it is often assumed that the move is to a nursing home. However, relocation is any change in the residential environment from one home or apartment in the community to another, from a community home or apartment to an institutional environment, and from one institutional setting to another. All these moves may be voluntary or involuntary. The most vulnerable moves are the involuntary ones to a dissimilar setting, such as one from a home or apartment to an institution.

Research has been done in the area of relocation from a community setting to an institutional setting. However, the literature is sparse regarding relocation from a home or apartment to a similar setting. Two studies have yielded evidence that involuntary moves within a similar setting result in a decrease in general activity and life satisfaction for the older adult.

There are many variables that contribute to the positive or negative adjustment in any relocation. The interrelationship among these variables within a social and cultural environment is still being investigated. Various assessment scales can predict the outcome of a relocation. The nurse and client's measurement of perceived physical and emotional health includes rating health, symptoms, general happiness and affect, subjective stress items, self-esteem, depression, and life satisfaction items. The social assessment area includes the presence of a confidant, degree of social isolation, the number of family and significant others available, and if the client shares his living arrangements with anyone. The client's own perception of the stress and difficulty of the move is an extremely important intervening variable. Those older adults with a low health status are more at risk during a relocation.

The older adult who is considering admission into a long-term-care facility is doing so usually because of some compromise to his health. Relocation brings with it a group of stages and developmental tasks and reactions to address. The three stages follow.

1. Decision-making or preparation stage
2. Moving-in or impact stage
3. Settling-in stage

During the decision-making stage, the client answers a series of questions:

Tasks	Possible reactions
Should he go to a long-term-care facility?	Helplessness
Which one?	Powerlessness
	Anxiety
How should he dispose of his belongings?	Depression
	Withdrawal
How can he take care of his business and legal affairs?	Grief
	Lowered self-esteem
How will he deal with regrets about going?	Crisis relating to anticipated loss, separation, rejection

Client and family counseling may help reduce the stress level of this stage.

Stage two, the moving-in or impact stage, requires the older adult to muster his energies and resources in adjusting to the following:

Tasks	Possible reactions
Admission procedure	Anger
New room and possible roommate	Helplessness
	Withdrawal
Staff	Role diffusion
Other clients/residents	Depression
Daily routines	Confusion
Emotional climate	Disorientation
Physical environment	Grief
	Idealization of lost environment
	Morbidity
	Mortality

It is during this stage that the client changes focus from the community to the institution. Morbidity and mortality are increased during this stage. Nursing intervention addresses helping the client adjust to the tasks of stage two. The client and nurse set up goals to accomplish the tasks. When the nurse is alert to the possible reactions and extends a sense of love and belonging to the client in her daily care, the client's adjustment is aided. A one-on-one contact between client and staff for at least 6 weeks helps reduce anxiety. Coping mechanisms that reduce distress are identified for the client, using ones that have been successful for him in the past. The nurse is alert that clients with fewer resources will exhibit more physical symptoms and depression. The nurse may help the client develop a network of social activities and relationships. The resident council and family council, as well as the client's own family and significant others, may support the client in his new environment and make moving in less traumatic.

The third stage, settling-in, is accomplished when the client feels comfortable in the facility. His functional limitations may hinder and slow the process. However, when he has recouped to some functional degree his self-esteem, dignity, and control of his destiny, the tasks will be accomplished.

Tasks	Possible reactions
Establishing new social relationships	The reactions are individual and depend on the adjustment during the previous stages, including how the client perceives the stress he has encountered and opportunities in the new situation.
Knowing the routines	
Becoming familiar with the physical environment	
Getting to know the staff	
Selecting a pattern of satisfying activities	
Establishing a purpose in life	
Relating the present to the total life experience	

SELECTED READING

The following selected reading, "Morbidity Patterns Among Recently Relocated Elderly" by Ellen G. Thomas, is a significant research study for the nurse working in a long-term-care facility. The research follows the admission of residents to long-term-care facilities and studies the second stage, moving-in or impact, of relocation. The client's reaction to the tasks of this stage, its effects on various body systems, and the signs and symptoms of encroaching morbidity are results of the study. Nursing may use this as a framework for anticipatory reactions and planning with the client nursing intervention.

Morbidity patterns among recently relocated elderly*

Ellen G. Thomas

Elderly persons frequently do not adapt readily to a new environment. This is evidenced by the appearance of an increase in the number of illnesses and unexpected deaths among recently relocated elderly persons following their admission to an institution.[1,2]

During the years that I was employed by the Commonwealth of Pennsylvania as a relocation specialist in its nursing home relocation program, it appeared that certain signs and symptoms of morbidity appeared rather frequently. The study conducted under the direction of Pastalan in conjunction with the project concentrated on the mortality rate among the relocatees.[3] The morbidities that occurred, whether merely adding to the relocatees' discomfort or as a predecessor to death, led me to wonder about their significance. A review of the literature of the state of the art of some of the problems confronted by others involved in relocation of the elderly, increased my curiosity.[4,5] Throughout

the literature, the mortality rates were regarded as an indicator of the trauma and stress involved in relocation. Clearly, the studies established the fact that relocation can precipitate increased mortality and help bring about a variety of morbidities.

More knowledge about morbidity patterns among recently relocated elderly is needed in order for health care professionals to plan appropriate and comprehensive care for persons during the relocation process. Morbidity following relocation is the focus of this study.

As an initial approach toward a better understanding of the morbidity patterns among recently relocated elderly, the research problem of the descriptive study reported here was, first, to differentiate norm morbidity from encroaching morbidity; and second, to identify patterns of encroaching morbidity, if indeed they existed, during the first four weeks following admission to a long term care facility.

For the purposes of this study, the following definitions were used for recently relocated elderly, relocation effect, morbidity, morbidity pattern, and stress.

Recently relocated elderly refers to a person who was age 65 or over, starting on the date of admission, and spent a four-week period in a nursing home.

Relocation effect pertains to the physiological and psychological changes that are assumed to have been precipitated by the stress of relocation and that may or may not have preceded serious morbidity or mortality.

Morbidity, that is, illnesses of the participants, was divided into two categories: (a) norm morbidity, an illness that is consciously experienced by the person and is confirmed by professional documentation at the time of admission, and (b) encroaching morbidity, an illness that appears after relocation, often by gradual steps, and is noted by observable signs or symptoms.

Morbidity pattern designates the observable features that characterized the health-illness state of the participant or group of participants, in relationship to baseline data collected by this investigator on the date of the subject's admission.

Stress refers to a physical or mental factor that caused bodily or mental tension and may have been a factor in illness causation.

The sample consisted of 30 elderly subjects as admitted sequentially to the skilled nursing section in nursing homes located throughout a three-county area in an eastern state. Six facilities were utilized. The number of skilled nursing care beds ranged from 72 to 185 per facility. The larger

*From Clinical and scientific sessions 1979. Published by and reprinted with permission of the American Nurses' Association, Kansas City, Mo.
Ellen G. Thomas MSN, RNC is instructor, College of Nursing, University of Illinois, Chicago, Illinois.

facilities offered a full range of services, but the services offered by the smallest home were limited. The major goal for all the homes was to promote health and foster independence. The six facilities had a combined total capacity of more than 1,000 beds.

The structural architecture of the facilities varied from brownstone mansions in a country setting to a remodeled hospital in the center of a large metropolitan area.

Criteria for participation were as follows:

1. The subject, or his significant other, had to be willing to be interviewed upon the day of admission.
2. The subject had to be able to talk.
3. The subject had to be age 65 or over.
4. The subject had to anticipate a confinement of at least three months in the new facility.

Data were gathered from May 22, 1978, through August 18, 1978. For any problem to be researchable, it must be observable and measurable. The following methods were utilized in this study. Baseline data, that is, the signs and symptoms that indicated norm morbidity, were obtained from the subjects through a two-part interview. The interview was conducted by this investigator within 24 hours of the subject's admission. Two standardized forms were used. The Cornell Medical Index Health Questionnaire (CMI) was used to obtain pertinent medical and psychiatric information. The Geriatric Social Readjustment Rating Scale (GSRRS), an outgrowth of the Holmes and Masuda life-event rating scale but modified to be used with an older population, was used to measure the amount of stress the subject had undergone in the five years prior to admission.[6,7,8] The subjects' current records were also used to collect portions of both norm and encroaching morbidity data.

It was assumed in the study that stressful situations contribute to the exacerbation of norm morbidity and to the precipitation of encroaching morbidity. A third instrument, the signs and symptoms of stress checklist (SOS), was developed by this investigator for use in this study. Whereas the GSRRS was used to measure the degree of stress prior to admission, the SOS was used by the nursing personnel to record the signs and symptoms demonstrated by a subject during the 28 consecutive days following the subject's admission to the new facility. Several sources were employed in developing the checklist, including a review of the literature on stress, consultation with professional nurses working in nursing homes, consultation with professional nurses functioning as relocation specialists in a nursing home setting, consultation with an authority in physiological mechanisms, and the investigator's own experiences as a relocation specialist.

There are three main areas of inquiry in the SOS, two of which are analogous to the structure of the CMI. They are, first, physiological signs and symptoms of stress, and second, signs and symptoms of mood and feeling patterns. Not all items on the CMI are related to stress; those items are not listed on the SOS. However, there are detectable signs and symptoms of stress not listed on the CMI that do appear on the SOS. The third category comprised those items. The signs and symptoms recorded on the SOS were the indicators of encroaching morbidity.

Before the data collection process could commence, both the nursing personnel and the subjects needed to be prepared. As indicated, the nursing personnel were the observers-recorders of the SOS data. They were prepared by means of inservice programs. The programs included an explanation of the research project, how the SOS form was to be used, how to obtain objective and subjec-

tive information, how to record it, and what types of interventions might be implemented. This investigator conducted six programs for each facility. Identical programs were presented to each of the three shifts on two separate days to accommodate the full staff. All staff members were trained prior to the first subject's admission.

All subjects had the research project explained to them and were given adequate time to decide whether or not to participate. If they chose to volunteer, they were required to sign a consent form, which stated that they understood the project. They also understood that they had the right to withdraw from participation at any time without fear of jeopardizing the quality of their care. In most instances, this process consumed more time than the actual interview.

Although preparation time was costly, it was well worth the price. It provided the investigator with the opportunity to establish good rapport with both staff and subjects. This was probably one of the most essential components leading to success of the research conducted.

In addition to the major research problem stated earlier, related problems were also considered. Specifically, the subquestions addressed were these: What signs and symptoms were present prior to relocation? What signs and symptoms appeared within 28 days following admission? Was there a difference between the signs and symptoms before and after admission? Did the amount of stress the relocatee experienced in the five years prior to admission influence the number of signs and symptoms that appeared within 28 days following admission? Did medication reactions account for any of the signs and symptoms? Did specific patterns of morbidity appear generally among the recently relocated elderly? What time of the day did the various signs and symptoms appear and disappear? How many days after relocation did the signs and symptoms appear or disappear?

Data were analyzed in two ways: tabulation according to major areas of investigation and classification of symptoms by body systems to identify morbidity patterns and trends. The Spearman rank order correlation coefficient was used to determine the degree of relationship between (a) the amount of prior stress and symptoms present on admission, (b) prior stress and the number of the symptoms appearing after admission, and (c) symptoms present at the time of admission and those following admission. In each case, no relationship was found. However, when the signs and symptoms of encroaching morbidity were divided into body systems, interesting patterns appeared.

Emergent patterns of signs and symptoms of stress in a selected group of categories, including body systems, which reported the greatest number of incidents, indicated that disturbances of the emotional state were most predominant before and after admission.

With the multiplicity of diagnoses among the frail elderly in the general population, it was not surprising to find that in this group of subjects (with a mean age of 82 and an average of nearly four diagnoses) who had degenerated to the point of requiring skilled nursing care, nearly 87 percent had diffuse medical problems. According to the CMI, if the subject answered yes to more than three of the questions on page 4 of the questionnaire, it indicated probable emotional problems. Among the 87 percent of the subjects with diffuse medical problems, more than 83 percent also reported emotional instability. It appears reasonable to assume that many of the medical problems were at least exacerbated, if not precipitated, by a psychological disturbance.

It is not within the scope of this paper to report all of the morbidity patterns that emerged. Only those signs and symptoms that were reported by at least 10 of the 30 subjects are included. On the CMI, which was used to measure norm morbidity, 16 symptoms were reported by 10 or more of the subjects. Seven of the 16 dealt with mood and feeling, that is, emotional problems. When broken down into specific areas of that category, 41 percent were reported to be "angry" and 27 percent were "depressed." The genitourinary system appeared to be most involved, with "frequency of urination during the day" and "occasional incontinence" most often reported. The digestive symptoms were divided about equally between "poor appetite" and "bad constipation."

The single physical symptom reported most frequently by the subjects was "ankles often badly swollen"; it was the only symptom indicating cardiovascular impairment. However, when compared to the overall report, cardiovascular problems were by far the most prevalent of the symptoms—with a total of 114 occurrences—reported by the subjects prior to or at the time of admission. Complaints, other than edema of the ankles, experienced by fewer than one-third of the subjects, included hypertension, vertigo, chest pain, palpitations, tachycardia, cold extremities, rapid respirations, and a feeling of "fullness in lungs."

The digestive system rated as the second highest problem area at the time of admission. In addition to "poor appetite" and "constipation," bloating, belching, indigestion, diarrhea, and occasional nausea and vomiting were reported.

Although genitourinary problems rated among the most frequently reported symptoms, the system was rated less problematic than mood and cardiovascular and digestive systems, in that order. However, the two most frequently recorded physical symptoms throughout the CMI were "frequent urination" and "loss of bladder control." These symptoms were reported by one-half of all respondents.

On the SOS, which was used to measure encroaching morbidity, 18 items were listed by 10 or more of the subjects. Following admission, and within the observational period, the single symptom experienced most frequently was confusion. Sixty percent of the subjects were reported to exhibit confusion, to a greater or lesser degree, during the observed period. Sleeplessness, loss of appetite, depression, and despondency were reported by at least one-half of the subjects at some time during the period. Fatigue, indicated by signs of "sluggishness" or "feelings of exhaustion," was common. "Crying/ feels like crying" and "feels hopeless and/or helpless" were not uncommon. Psychological disturbances, with 177 incidents reported, made the mood and feeling category the most highly involved. In fact, none of the subjects failed to report at least one incident of significant emotional disturbance during the 28-day period. Seventy-one percent of the cases occurred in the first week, and 37 percent of those were recorded on the first day following admission. The greatest number (30 percent) of the reported symptoms were recorded in the "depression" division.

Physical signs and symptoms in the top 18 items indicated that body areas most frequently reflecting the relocation effect following admission were, first, the digestive system; second, the cardiovascular system; and, third, the respiratory system. Looking back at the prevalence of norm morbidities, we see that, other than for mood and feelings, encroaching morbidities involved bodily systems differently. The digestive and cardiovascular systems exchanged places on the rating scale. The genitourinary system was replaced by the respiratory system.

The relationship between the

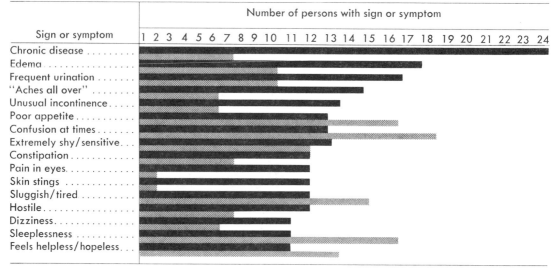

Note: This figure reports only those signs or symptoms reported by at least one third
of subjects.
*"Chronic disease" on CMI is analogous to "exacerbation of prior condition" on SOS.

■ CMI on admission.
▨ SOS during first 28 days following admission.

Fig. 1. Comparison of number of persons with signs and symptoms of norm morbidity and encroaching morbidity.

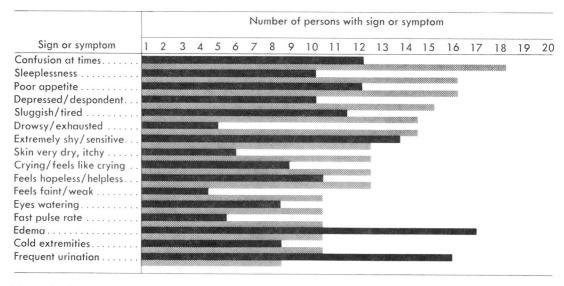

Note: This figure reports only those signs and symptoms that were reported by at least
one third of the subjects. Three symptoms have been deleted (see Fig. 1)
because they did not have analogous symptoms listed on the CMI.

■ CMI on admission
▨ SOS during first 28 days following admission.

Fig. 2. Comparison of number of persons with signs and symptoms of encroaching morbidity and norm morbidity.

signs and symptoms on the CMI and the SOS, that is, norm and encroaching morbidity, was not significant. This is illustrated by Figures 1 and 2.

Figure 1 is a reproduction of the signs and symptoms exhibited by at least 10 of the subjects upon admission (CMI). Below the number of persons exhibiting each sign and symptom reported on the CMI is the number of persons showing the same symptom on the SOS. Chronic disease, which was reported as the most frequently occurring symptom on admission, was compared with the number of exacerbations of the dis-

ease following admission. "Edema" and "frequent urination" ranked as the second and third most frequently appearing items on the CMI. However, the same two symptoms barely occurred for one-third of the subjects following admission.

In Figure 2, "exacerbation of chronic diseases" did not even appear among the top two-thirds of the reported symptoms following admission. "Aching all over" was common at the time of admission, but it dropped drastically following admission. The same was true of "frequency of urination" and "unusual in-

continence." "Poor appetite" was reported by fewer than half the subjects upon admission, but it increased to more than half following admission. This same phenomenon occurred with "confusion," which was the most predominant symptom after admission and was the slowest to disappear, if it disappeared at all. The same was true of sleeplessness.

Constipation, dizziness, and hostility symptoms each dropped half the number of occurrences following admission, but the time span for disappearances varied. Dizziness

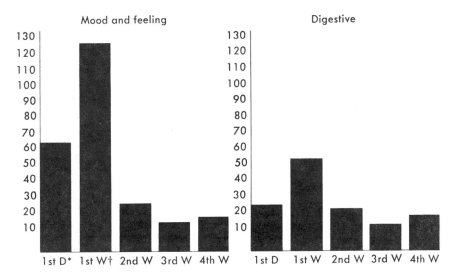

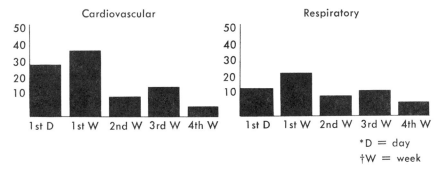

Fig. 3. Comparison of patterns of appearance of signs and symptoms of stress in four categories of the SOS, demonstrated by 30 elderly patients.

started to disappear soon after admission, whereas constipation and hostility occurred later during the 28-day period of observation. Feelings of hopelessness and helplessness *increased* following admission. This mood pattern of appearance and disappearance was widely scattered throughout the study period. "Pain in the eyes" and "stinging skin," prevalent on admission, were negligible following admission.

Edema, which was reported frequently at the time of admission, dropped from nearly two-thirds of the subjects reporting the symptom at that time to only one-third following admission. Cold extremities, watering eyes, crying, feelings of weakness or faintness, and rapid pulse rate, none of which were listed on the top CMI items, occurred in more than one-third of all subjects immediately following admission. Dry skin became more prevalent following ad-

mission, in most cases accompanied by frequent urination.

Figure 3 illustrates the emergent patterns of stress symptoms, that is, encroaching morbidity, in a selected group of systems reflecting the greatest number of incidents reported. Each system showed an increase in new symptoms in the first week, as compared with the date of admission. Appearance of new symptoms in all systems decreased in the second week and continued to do so in mood and digestive system, whereas the emergence of cardiovascular and respiratory signs increased. During the final week of observation, the patterns among the systems varied widely, with mood about constant, digestive symptoms increased, and cardiovascular and respiratory symptoms decreased tremendously.

Whereas Figure 3 illustrates only patterns of emergent new symptoms, Table 1 lists the duration of the most

frequently reported signs and symptoms. The mean number of days for duration of a symptom was 8.13 days. The disappearances of the symptoms did not show definitive patterns according to systems, as did their appearances. The time of day the symptoms appeared or disappeared did not reveal any significant findings. It had been assumed that circadian periodicity might be reflected in the configuration of the symptom patterns.

The young, healthy adult human has a tremendous ability to maintain, and readily regain, a constant state of physiochemical balance in his internal milieu regardless of changes in the external environment. The findings of this study augment the reality that the compromised body organs of debilitated elderly persons hinder their ability to adapt so easily.

Relocation is a powerful stressor for a person at any age; for the elder-

Table 1. Duration of the most frequently occurring signs and symptoms of stress among 30 elderly persons within 28 days following admission to a skilled nursing care facility

Sign or symptom reported on SOS	Number of persons whose signs or symptoms:		Mean[a] number of days persons showed sign or symptom
	Appeared during 28 days	Disappeared before 29th day	
Confusion at times	18	12	20
Sleeplessness	16	13	8
Poor appetite	16	15	6.5
Depressed, despondent	15	12	12
Sluggish, tired	14	9	11
Drowsy, exhausted	14	12	8
Mouth very dry	12	11	2.5
Skin very dry, itching	12	8	4
Crying/feels like crying	12	10	11
Feels hopeless, helpless	12	12	8
Feels faint or weak	11	10	8
Unsteady gait	11	11	10.5
Eyes watering	10	5	8
Fast pulse rate	10	9	7
Edema	10	7	4
Cold extremities	10	7	4
Bad breath	10	8	12
Frequent urination	10	8	12
TOTAL	223	179	146.5

[a]Subjects for whom the symptom did not disappear were not included in the sum of days from which the mean was derived.
$\overline{X} = 8.13$.

ly, it can be devastating. The implications for gerontological nursing practice resulting from the findings of this study, when added to findings in prior studies on relocation of the elderly, are many. The concept of stress as a basis for nursing practice is not a new idea.[9] However, using the knowledge of the physiological and psychological mechanisms of stress, as described by Selye and others, specifically to systematically detect encroaching morbidity presents a new appraoch.[10,11]

Perhaps an illustration will help present a clearer understanding of the concept and its usefulness. A young mother may be surprised to awaken one day and find her child has "*suddenly* come down with the measles." In retrospect, however, she will recall that during the several days prior to the appearance of the rash, Junior had exhibited altered patterns of eating and behavior. Perhaps he had even complained that the strong light hurt his eyes. Had she known he had been exposed to measles at school and had she been informed as to what early symptoms to watch for, she would not have been surprised. When a second child shows the telltale signs, she will know that her child was exposed and will recognize the signs early enough to offer care that might well prevent complications.

The analogy here is that health care workers caring for a recently relocated elderly patient should know that the patient has been exposed to a potent stressor (relocation) and continues to be exposed to further stressors, e.g. more losses, new faces, and ever-changing medications and additional treatments. How many times have you heard a staff member in a long term care facility say: say: "Golly, Mrs. S. had been adjusting so beautifully. *Suddenly* she be-

came very ill and died!" The point is that she undoubtedly did not suddenly get sick and die. The signs and symptoms of the encroaching illness were there all along. Taking a single symptom at a time does not seem significant. Collectively, however, several minor symptoms may have a greater impact on the relocatee than one single assault.

The gerontological nurse should, first, be aware of the potency of relocation for the recently relocated elderly patient. Second, the nurse should obtain a complete physical and psychological assessment, including usual coping mechanisms, when the patient is admitted. Third, she should have a sound working knowledge of the stress mechanism in general and, more specifically, as it operates for the older person. Fourth, and most important, the nurse should monitor the newly arrived patient for the signs and symptoms of stress, which are the indicators of encroaching morbidity. If each symptom was dealt with at its onset, the likelihood of the progression of morbidity could be halted, modified, or reversed before a chronic, disabling condition—or even death—could occur.

This study had many limitations, such as a small population, insufficiently trained data collectors, and a short observation period, and the data collection tools need modification. Nevertheless, it was a beginning. If nothing more, it at least indicates that patterns of encroaching morbidity following relocation do exist. Much more nursing research is needed in this clinical area. Through such research, perhaps a significant body of knowledge could lead to the development of a standardized nursing care plan for prevention of relocation trauma among recently relocated elderly.

REFERENCES

1. Kasl, S. V. Physical and Mental Effects of Involuntary Relocation and Institutionalization on the Elderly: A Review. *American Journal of Public Health* 62:2 (March 1972), 377-383.
2. Schultz, R., and G. Brebber. Relocation of the Aged: A Review and Theoretical Analysis. *Journal of Gerontology* 32:3 (May 1977), 323-333.
3. Pastalan, L. Report on Pennsylvania Nursing Home Relocation Program. Interim research findings. Ann Arbor, Mich.: University of Michigan, Institute of Gerontology, 1976.
4. Pablo, R. Y. Intra-Institutional Relocation: Its Impact on Long Term Care Patients. *Gerontologist* 17:5 (October 1977), 426-435.
5. Zweig, J., and J. Csank. Effects of Relocation on Chronically Ill Geriatric Patients on a Medical Unit: Mortality Rates. *Journal of American Geriatrics Society* 23 (May 1975), 132-136.
6. Amster, L., and H. Krauss. The Relationship Between Life Crises and Mental Deterioration in Old Age. *International Journal of Aging and Human Development* 5 (January 1974), 51-54.
7. Brodman, K., A. J. Erdmann, Jr., I. Lorge, and H. G. Wolff. The Cornell Medical Index: An Adjunct to the Medical Interview. *Journal of the American Medical Association* 140:6 (June 1949), 530-534.
8. Holmes, T. H., and M. Masuda. Life Change and Illness Susceptibility. Paper presented at a symposium of the American Association for the Advancement of Science, December 1970, Chicago, Illinois.
9. Dumas, R. G. Utilization of a Concept of Stress as a Basis for Nursing Practice. *ANA Clinical Sessions: American Nurses' Association, 1966, San Francisco.* New York: Appleton-Century-Crofts, 1967.
10. Selye, H. *The Stress of Life.* New York: McGraw-Hill Book Co., 1961.
11. Dohrenwend, B. S., and B. P. Dohrenwend. *Stressful Life Events: Their Nature and Effects.* New York: John Wiley & Sons, 1974.

SELF-ESTEEM

The next level on Maslow's hierarchy of needs is that of self-esteem (Fig. 11-4). The person with positive self-esteem feels that he is adequate and exhibits self confidence. He is able to accurately assess his assets and limitations. Physical attractiveness, interpersonal relationships, and work achievements are some sources of self-esteem. The emotionally healthy person likes and accepts himself and can deal with his own feelings. Some measure of independence in managing one's own activities is an important ingredient in self-esteem.

Nursing intervention can be geared to have the client involved in decisions regarding his care. Full independence in decision making can be encouraged wherever possible.

Emotional well-being is not necessarily a product of a few significant events. Rather, consistant small anticipated pleasures offer satisfaction. Nursing intervention directed at the recognition of small accomplishments such as the telling of a funny story or admiring a client's plant or her crocheting fuels the client's sense of self-esteem.

Reminiscence is a useful tool to encourage the client's positive self-esteem. When the nurse and other clients listen to the past joys and hurts, the client gains recognition and is seen as an individual. His past has value to others. Clients with positive self-esteem can accept and cope with stressful situations because they can tolerate moderate anxiety successfully. This flexibility helps him deal with uncomfortable situations realistically. He has more control over his environment. Nursing intervention can be directed towards reality orientation, health information, and counseling. With complete and accurate data regarding a situation, the older adult is in a better position to make decisions and maintain his independence.

Self-esteem project

One means to improve self-esteem is for the older adult to work and receive a salary. Most people have had a working role at one time in their life that was valued by receiving a salary. This role may be reinstated at the long-term-care center through the use of state funds. Each state is allowed a budget of "Green Thumb Money" to assist retired older adults who need supplemental in-

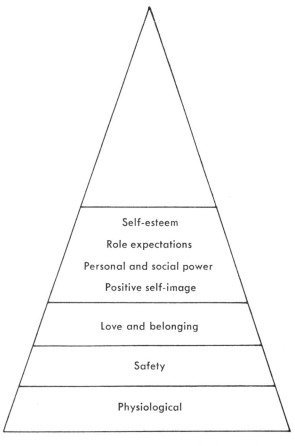

Fig. 11-4. Self-esteem needs—fourth level of Maslow's hierarchy.

come. They may work up to a total of 25 hours a week for pay. The working activity remotivates the older adult into a role of living. For example, Mr. Alexander has a part-time job working for an office supply firm. He is doing something useful by sorting pens and packaging them. He is of value to the pencil manufacturer because they need competent employees. The client now has money to buy himself some needed things, go out to lunch, and even buy some treats for his grandchildren. To the older adult it is a means for improving status and income. His self-esteem is enhanced because of his new working role and membership in a team project.

Recreational activities

Everyone needs some types of recreational activities to release tension, to take the mind off self, change gears, occupy time, and socialize. The client living in a long-term-care facility should be free to choose from a variety of activities scheduled throughout each week.

The ambulatory client living at home depends on family, friends, senior citizen clubs, his own hobbies, and television to supply recreation. Homebound clients may depend on an occupational therapist to supply him with materials for activities. Personal hobbies such as knitting and stamp collecting are something the client has with him no matter where the environment. The guiding principle in selecting recreational activities in the long-term-care facility is that it should be age appropriate for the client. For example, the client should not have to participate in third-grade level arts and crafts. The clients' unit should not look like a kindergarten with holiday mobiles hanging from the ceiling or on the windows. Very few older adults in the community senior citizen centers are doing this, so why should residents in nursing homes? The clients' environment should be adult-like. Recreational activities should maintain a close and open relationship with the outside community. Mrs. Blue was an ardent bridge player before admission into the nursing home. She could not find enough players at the home to make a bridge table. The director of nursing knew there was a senior citizen's center located close by and Tuesday was bridge day. Arrangements were made to take Mrs. Blue to the center on Tuesday afternoon for bridge. Word soon got around the nursing home, and Mrs. Blue had the company of four other clients on Tuesday. Everyone enjoyed the outing and socializing at the senior citizen's center. Arrangements were made to invite the senior citizens to play bridge in the nursing home. Mrs. Blue was excited to have guests see their home and thrilled to be able to extend an invitation to new friends. Other clients were invited to play cards other than bridge, so pinochle and canasta tables were set up. The outside world came into the nursing home, and a mutual sharing took place.

Those activities that the nursing home duplicates that are established in the community (church services for example) should be identified.

Have those residents who are able attend the church of their choice in the community. Be a change agent, and do not let barriers such as lack of transportation stop you. There is a difference between listening to a taped church service and actually attending one. The older adult should have every opportunity to continue this former role. It does take time from a busy nursing schedule to contact people and make arrangements for the activity. The rewards are great, both for the client and the nurse.

Start small and make plans for only a few clients. There may be friendly visitors, Family and Friends Council members, or people from the church who are interested in supplying the transportation. Explore every avenue for money for transportation within the community. Businessmen's associations may rent transportation for you. Contact nursing schools within the community and set up a learning experience for the student to take a resident out to the religious service. Expand the project to include students' taking clients shopping, to a library, to a movie, or out to lunch. Offer other health professional students and ministerial students a learning experience. Set up a work-study program for local high school students. Get them involved in resident activities. The two age groups often develop a good rapport, and the adolescents will add new fresh ideas to the existing program.

Nursing service generally has established a working relationship with the therapeutic activities director. Each nurse can assist her by suggesting different kinds of activities for the clients receiving various levels of nursing care. Nurses may support the activities programs by making sure clients are sent from their units on time. Favorable and unfavorable evaluations of programs that the client shares with the nursing staff can be discussed with the activities director.

The resident council may plan an activity schedule for a day. Clients' input is important to get them to participate in the programs. All possible assistance and support should be given to this group, so that the first projects are successful.

The council can then be encouraged to expand their efforts to activities for a week and even a month. An ad hoc committee may be assigned to work with the activity director. When the resident council's opinions and input are respected and implemented, they will experience a sense of love and belonging. Their self-esteem will be elevated also because they now have some control over activities that will be age appropriate, linking previous roles and skills.

Foster grandparent programs

Age barriers fall when the older adult is encouraged to reach out to children in foster grandparent programs. Day-care centers for children can be operated within the physical facility of the day-care center for the older adult. The client meets with a designated child at regular intervals, usually twice a week. The older adult and his foster child enjoy songs, crafts, and stories together. The aim of such a program is development of the mutual appreciation of youth and the older adult. Through these contacts, friendship and love are shared (Fig. 11-5). Self-esteem is enhanced in the client because he is useful and needed.

Occupational therapy

The nurse may complement her nursing intervention by arranging to have an occupational therapy consultation to restore, reinforce, and enhance skills and activities of daily living for the clients with "(1) sensory loss, (2) visual disturbances, (3) loss of muscle function, (4) loss of independence in activities of daily living (ADL), (5) impaired cognitive function, (6) psychosocial dysfunction, and (7) perceptual motor dysfunction," (Steinberg, 1976, p. 433).

The occupational therapist's expertise in suggesting appropriate activities for the client widens the client's options for recreational plans. The emphasis becomes rehabilitation of the individual rather than custodial care of an entire group.

Self-actualization

Self-actualization is the fullest possible expression of an individual's uniqueness (Fig. 11-6). Maslow believed that the self-actualization level

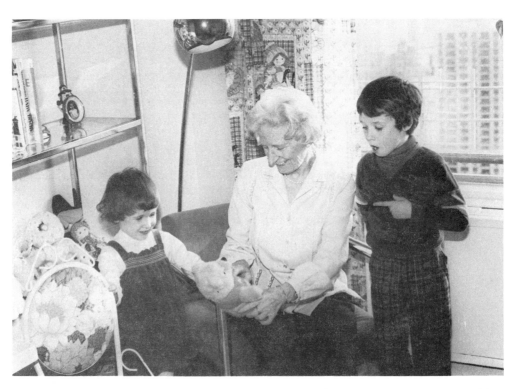

Fig. 11-5. This foster grandmother is listening as a young boy relates a story about his favorite teddy bear.

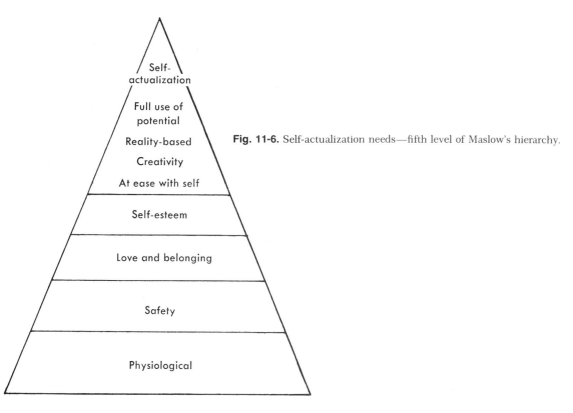

Fig. 11-6. Self-actualization needs—fifth level of Maslow's hierarchy.

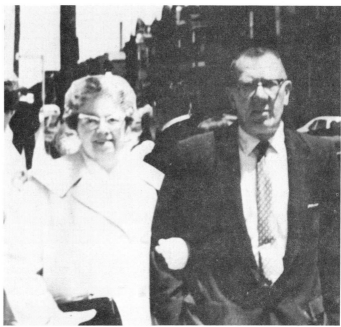

Fig. 11-7. Self-actualization requires maturity of years.

could not be achieved in youth, but only in adulthood. Self-actualization is a characteristic of a person mature in years who has had his physiological, safety, love and belonging, and self-esteem needs met successfully (Fig. 11-7). The self-actualized person is spontaneous, has a sense of humor, and is creative and democratic. The nurse can foster self-actualization in a client by establishing a milieu that offers new experiences, does not insist on conformity, and provides time and privacy to explore his personal inner experience. The older adult should be encouraged to make full use of his talents and potentials.

REFERENCES

Barnes, R., and Raskind, M.: Strategies for diagnosing and treating agitation in the aging, Geriatrics **35**:111, March 1980.

Blazer, D.: Working with the elderly patient's family, Geriatrics **33**:117, February 1978.

Blazer, D.: The diagnosis of depression in the elderly, J. Am. Geriatr. Soc. **28**:52, February 1980.

Blumenthal, M. D.: Depressive illness in old age: getting behind the mask, Geriatrics **35**:35, April 1980.

Brock, A. M.: Self-administration of drugs in the elderly, Nurs. Forum **18**(4):340, 1979.

Cheah, K. C., and Beard, O. W.: Psychiatric findings in the population of a geriatric evaluation unit: implications, J. Am. Geriatr. Soc. **28**:153, April 1980.

Craigmile, W. M., and others: Domiciliary care of the elderly, Nurs. Times **74**:Supp. 13-5, 2 February 1978.

Frisk, P. A., and Simonson, W.: The pharmacist's expanding role in home health care of geriatric patients, Geriatrics **32**:80, December 1977.

Gaitz, C. M.: Diagnosing mental illness in the elderly, J. Am. Geriatr. Soc. **28**:176, April 1980.

Gleckman, R. A. and Esposito, A. L.: Antibiotics in the elderly: skating on therapeutic thin ice, Geriatrics **35**:26, January 1980.

Goldberg, P.: Drugs and the elderly, Geriatr. Nurs. **1**:74, May-June 1980.

Heumann, L. F., and Lareau, L. S.: Local estimates of the functionally disabled elderly: toward a planning tool for housing and support service programs, Intl. J. Aging Hum. Dev. **10**(1):77, 1979-80.

Hunt, T. E.: Practical considerations in the rehabilitation of the aged, J. Am. Geriat. Soc. **28**:59, February 1980.

Jacobs, R. E.: Re-employment and unemployment in old age, J. Geriatric Psychiatry **11**(1):79-80, 1978.

Kral, V. A.: Psychosocial problems of the aged: a shared medical responsibility, J. Am. Geriat. Soc. **28**:68, February 1980.

Linn, B. S.: Age differences in the severity and outcome of burns, J. Am. Geriat. Soc. **28**:118, March 1980.

Lutwick, L. I.: Principles of antibiotic use in the elderly, Geriatrics **35**:54, February 1980.

Overstall, P. W., Johnson, A. L., and Exton-Smith, A. N.: Instability and falls of the elderly, Age Ageing Suppl:92, 1978.

Reuben, S., and Brynes, G. K.: Helping elderly patients in the transition to a nursing home, Geriatrics **32**:107, November 1977.

Simons, R. M.: Paget's disease in the head and neck, Gerontology **26**(3):155, 1980.

Steinberg, F. U., editor: Cowdry's the care of the geriatric patient, ed. 5, St. Louis, 1976, The C. V. Mosby Co.

Stevenson, I. H.: Drug metabolism in the elderly, Age-Ageing Suppl:131, 1978.

Stevenson, J.: Load, power, and margin in older adults, Geriatr. Nurs. **1**:52, May-June 1980.

Stout, R. W.: Falls and disorders of postural balance. Age-Ageing Suppl:134, 1978.

Stuart, M. R., and Mackey, K. J.: Mobile center links providers with isolated senior citizens, Hospitals **52**:101, 1 January 1978.

Treas, J.: Family support systems for the aged, Gerontologist **17**:486, December 1977.

Vinick, B. H.: Remarriage in old age, J. Geriatr. Psychiatry **11**(1):75, 1978.

Weisel, M. J., and Ullmann, A.: Volunteers boost spirits of elderly, Hospitals **54**:70, January 16, 1980.

Wise, H.: In Yates, J.: The ties that bind also heal, Prevention, October 1979.

IV

EVALUATION

12 Evaluation

IMPORTANCE OF EVALUATION

Evaluation is most important to the nurse. It is the mechanism the federal government requires for assuring quality care. In addition, a satisfactory evaluation of client care ensures reimbursement for the services given. Without these monies from government and third-party insurance sources, there is no budget to pay nurses. It is as complex and simple as that. No evaluation means no money for nursing; that is the reality of the health care system today.

An understanding of the mechanisms of required evaluation styles helps the nurse take the steps necessary to document the care she gives. This chapter presents evaluation styles of the three levels at which nurses are expected to participate.

The nurse has particular responsibilities in the evaluation of client care. The first area is the evaluation style seen in the fourth component of the nursing process that is used in the day-to-day activity of the nurse. The second area is evaluation in the larger focus of internal and external review of the nursing agency and the care it renders. On this level her notes are evaluated, and she may sit on the evaluation committees. Both areas of evaluation are closely related and affect the level of the quality of nursing care given to the client.

The nursing process evaluation component is essential for the audit process of the individual agency's self-review to document quality assurance. An audit means evaluation.

They both describe a review of the care given. The basic standards of care are established in the federal and state regulations and the ANA Standards of Nursing Practice (in the case of care for the older adult, this would be the Gerontological Standards of the ANA). The individual agency develops criteria to assess if the standards of care are met, and the staff and head nurses evaluate the individual care plans. As mentioned in Chapter 8, the ongoing client care undergoes both formative and sumative evaluation. While the client is still under care, the evaluation is called a process audit. Outcome evaluations or audits are done by the individual nurse, agency, and visiting surveyors when the care is complete as recorded on the chart and filed with the medical records department.

EVALUATIVE TERMS DEFINED

Quality assurance is a term used to describe a program in the health system that is constructed and executed to guarantee excellence in health care. Quality assurance places accountability with the health provider for the degree of excellence of care he or she renders to the client. The accountable health provider is answerable for his action or lack of action. When asked, the accountable person can explain the care given and take responsibility for the results of the care. The nurse is accountable for the nursing care she renders her client. She permits her decisions to be reviewed and documents the results of her care.

The notion of quality health care is a desirable goal. In order to measure the extent of the quality of care being given, some form of measurement should be available. Quality assurance is measured by using standards of care and the performance criteria derived from the standards. The standard describes a level of excellence that is regarded as a measure of adequate care. Criteria flow from the standard and represent the elements by which performance can be tested and judged (boxed material, p. 280).

Agency administration and personnel can measure the adequacy of client care in detail when they compare the standards and criteria with what exists in their institution. A norm is the average or usual way care is provided by a group of caregivers.

Quality assurance
Criteria flow from recognized standards of care

Standard: *Patient care policies*

The skilled nursing facility has written policies to govern the continuing skilled nursing care and related medical or other services provided.*

CRITERION: The agency has written policies related to client care.

CRITERION: The agency has an organized policy committee consisting of at least one physician and one registered nurse.

CRITERION: The policies are reviewed at least once annually.

CRITERION: The policy manual lists the range of services available to the clients.

CRITERION: The policies include provisions for client admission, transfer, and discharge.

*Standard from Federal Regulations for Skilled Long Term Care Facilities.

Standard: *Twenty-four-hour nursing service*

The facility provides 24-hour nursing services that are sufficient to meet total nursing needs and that are in accordance with the patient care policies developed.

CRITERION: The clients are bathed according to schedule.

CRITERION: The clients are dressed and well-groomed.

CRITERION: The clients' fingernails are clean and clipped.

CRITERION: The clients are up unless contraindicated.

CRITERION: Foley catheter bags and tubing are properly attached to beds and wheelchairs and are off floors.

CRITERION: Bowel and bladder training programs are in effect and documented.

Often the group norm does not measure up to the standards of care. In such a case, the standards and resulting criteria serve as a means to direct the group to improve the quality of the care being given. When care improves, the norm value rises and the typical care style is closer to the level of excellence described in the standard. An audit is a periodic, formal evaluation of the care documented as having been given to clients. The client charts are reviewed, and their contents are compared with the criteria listed with each standard. The audit summary states in which areas the clients received adequate care and which areas had deficits. Such a summary is called an *outcome audit*.

Formative, process, and *concurrent* are terms used when evaluation is done during care. When audit is done after client discharge, the following terms can be used: *summative, outcome,* and *retrospective*.

THREE LEVELS OF EVALUATION

Professional Standards Review Organizations (PSROs) are a part of the Medicare and Medicaid legislation and serve as the control mechanisms to monitor health care costs and client use of health care services. They are the evaluative arm of the Medicare and Medicaid legislation.

There are three levels in the evaluation of nursing care given to the client (Fig. 12-1). Level I is step four of the nursing process, called the *evaluation component*. It addresses the individual nurse's evaluation of the client's immediate care. Level II is broader and is seen as the *nursing audit*. The outcome audit reviews are done by the nursing service on large groups of client charts having the same diagnosis.

The third level is the most comprehensive of the evaluations and is done by the utilization review (UR) committee specifically for the federal government Medicare and Medicaid certification. The UR plans must be approved by the state agency for federal programs. An additional level III type of evaluation is the Joint Commission on Accreditation of Hospitals (JCAH) evaluation. The agency voluntarily requests a visit by the accounting committee. When an agency documents compliance with the JCAH quality assurance requirements, it is recognized as a JCAH-accredited hospital or agency. This title carries considerable status, because it identifies the agency as being a quality institution.

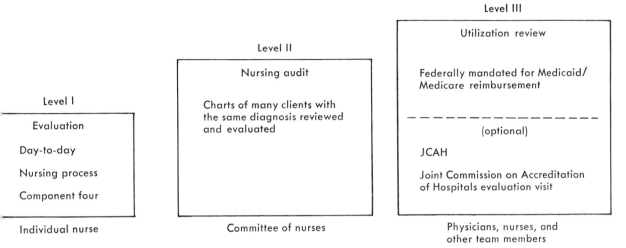

Fig. 12-1. Quality assurance program. Levels of evaluation. PSRO rules and regulations.

Level I: Evaluation as last step in nursing process

The nurse has collected her data, made a nursing diagnosis, formulated client goals, objectives and nursing orders, and implemented the care. On the date targeted for goal completion, she evaluates if the client's behavior is as the objectives states it should be. If she evaluates that the goals were met, then the care goals and objectives do not have to be changed. If the goals were not met, then she must begin the nursing process steps again. She collects more data to determine why the goals were not met. She then restates a nursing diagnosis, formulates alternative goals if necessary, or adjusts the objectives so the client is more likely to achieve the stated goals.

The client care plan that follows describes the goals set for Mr. Thomason. When the nurse returned to his house for the next visit, she evaluated his success in meeting the three goals that had been mutually set. The health assessment done on the second visit indicated that the leg ache and muscle fatigue had subsided to a moderate degree, the skin was pinker, the temperature of the skin was still cold, and some ankle swelling still remained. The skin of the legs and toes was intact with no evidence of cuts, bruising, or ulcerations. Mr. Thomason was able to explain to her what the function of veins is, and he described a varicose vein. He was also able to explain how his activities of the preceding week had improved his comfort level.

Client goals	Evaluation (audit)
1. Improved venous return from the legs	Not met
2. Protection from potential physical injury	Met
3. Knowledge regarding vascular system physiology	Met

Revised objectives

Mr. Thomason will:
    Apply elastic stockings before getting out of bed in the morning. Change worktable to a board on chair, and elevate legs on a hassock the entire time while working.
Target date for client objective: November 2

Nursing orders

Measure ankles.
Review the application of knee-high elastic stockings.
Observe a return demonstration of stocking application.
Demonstrate correct position of legs while sitting at workbench:
    Feet elevated on stepstool
    Legs and ankles kept uncrossed
    Use of lower chair with work board across arms of chair

Clearly stated client objectives and nursing orders enable the nurse to quickly evaluate her client's progress toward his goals. Because the nursing orders served as her nursing notes, the process is brief and complete. An external reviewer who visits this nurse's agency can read her nursing observations and decisions. Her care can be measured against standards of care and evaluated.

Level II: Nursing audit

A nursing audit is a systematic method of measuring the quality of patient care as it is reflected in the client charts. It is a particularly good way of meeting the increasing demand for accountability that has been placed upon the entire health care delivery system to provide optimal achievable care. A nursing audit is an action-oriented tool for measurement and evaluation of clinical observations of a group of similar clients to detect patterns of care.

A nursing audit is a means of meeting the demands for quality assurance from:

1. Courts: Continuing judicial decisions reaffirm the responsibility and authority of hospitals to establish mechanisms for ongoing evaluation of the quality of patient care services within the health care institutions.
2. Government: PSRO.
3. Third party payers: for example, insurance companies, Blue Cross/Blue Shield.
4. Joint Commission of Accreditation for Hospitals.
5. ANA Standards of Gerontological Nursing Practice.

It allows nurses to define roles and functions and to set standards for client care. In addition, an audit provides direction for in-service education programs; it demonstrates deficiencies in the agency's policies or procedures; and it offers a means of improving communications with other service departments, consultants, and the governing body.

What the audit does. An audit looks at outcomes. It measures the quality of care as reflected in the client's chart, and describes the client's progress toward health. The nursing audit detects patterns of care and provides a base for measurement of care given. By the use of consecutive charts, it gives a truer picture of the nursing care than random selection would provide. A cluster of the same diagnoses assembles a large quantity of related data that provide for an in-depth review of the documented care.

The audit committee collects data for possible nursing research. The committee's results help nursing service administrators document where more staff or equipment is needed in the delivery of nursing care. Sometimes new policies and procedures are developed from deficiencies noted in the results of the audit. The audit demonstrates accountability, and finally, it provides direction for improving client care and allows feedback to be given to other nursing committees.

Characteristics of a sound performance evaluation procedure

A. *Criteria to be established should:*
   1. Be objective.
      a. Nurses agree on measures for evaluating patient care.
      b. Criteria must be predetermined.
   2. Be clinically sound.
      a. Criteria are obtained by direct observation of the patient as opposed to comfort, safety, and environment checks.
      b. Criteria reflect local resources and clinical expertise.
   3. Include outcome.
      a. Client's health status at the time of discharge.
      b. Client's knowledge and ability to continue self-care or rehabilitation.
B. *Evaluation measures actual practice against criteria.*
   1. Shows the type of care given as measured against the criteria.
   2. Uses closed charts for retrospective measurement.
C. *Evaluation provides that actual practice findings be analyzed.*
   1. Those charts that do not meet the previously determined criteria are identified.
   2. Those identified charts must be reviewed to determine if the variation is a true deficiency.
   3. The mechanism must be flexible so that criteria are established for the individual agency.

The nursing audit results in identifying the appropriate corrective action that should be taken for the deficiencies identified and document it in the audit evaluation. The action is not always punitive and may be used for commendation. There are a number of actions that may be taken:

Referral of problem to in-service education

Recommendation for change in procedure or policy

Recommendation for change in physical environment or equipment

Recommendation for one-to-one counseling.

The corrective action is followed up to assure its implementation and appropriateness.

The results of the audit activity are reported to those individuals who have administrative responsibilities, such as the administrator, governing body, Director of Nursing, Nursing Care Coordinator, supervisors, in-service education, or staff and development persons.

Audit committee. The particular agency policy designates nursing personnel who constitute the audit committee. The members are nurses who are clinically competent and committed to client care.

The term of membership on the committee varies from agency to agency averaging 6 months to 1 year. The committee meetings are generally held once a month.

The committee selects audit topics, sets criteria, validates and interprets data, and recommends corrective action or appropriate responsible authority.

Audit topics. Tables 12-1 through 12-4 are examples of topics reviewed by one nursing audit committee. The particular audit topic is identified on the table heading. The Discharge Status column lists the outcome criteria or client behaviors expected in order for the Standard to be met. The Compliance Standard column indicates the percentages of cases that must meet the criteria for nursing care to be evaluated as satisfactory. The Exceptions column provides the nurses with the opportunity to list those reasons why clients could

Text continued on p. 289.

Table 12-1. Audit topic: cerebrovascular accident

OUTCOME

Criteria	Compliance standard	Exceptions	Instructions and definitions for data retrieval*
Skin intact	100%	None	No decubiti, no reddened areas, no ulcers over bony prominences
Able to ambulate	100%	Previously existing incapacity to ambulate	Use of walker or tripod cane in physical therapy record or nursing assessment form.
		Transferred to rehabilitation center or skilled nursing facility	
Able to perform activities of daily living (ADL)	100%	Transferred to rehabilitation center or skilled nursing facility	Documentation of skill on physical therapy notes or CVA summary record, or occupational therapist record Feed self Bowel and bladder training Bathe and dress self Ability to communicate
Client or family verbalizes understanding of limitations existing on discharge	100%	Transferred to rehabilitation center or skilled nursing facility; applicable only to existing limitations	Aphasia or speech limitations, motor limitations, exercises to minimize or improve function; EXAMPLE: plantarflexion, emotional lability, precipitating or aggravating factors, impaired comprehension, incontinence

*Information is found in nurses' notes, specific discharge summary sheet, or graphic sheet unless otherwise specified

Continued.

Table 12-1. Audit topic: cerebrovascular accident—cont'd

INDICATORS

Complications	Compliance standard	Critical preventive and responsive management	Instructions and definitions for data retrieval*
Extension of CVA	0%	Physician notified within 30 min of neurological deficit	Change in pupil size, nonreactive pupils, change from spasticity to flaccid paralysis, or change in level of consciousness
Pneumonia	0%	Signs and symptoms noted and reported to physician	Rales, chest pain, cough, temperature elevated above 101 F
		Up in chair within first 24 hr	
		Turn every 2 hr until turning independently	Graphic record
Urinary tract infection	0%	Signs and symptoms documented	Cloudy, concentrated, foul-smelling urine, temperature above 101 F; frequency, dysuria, urgency, pain, or burning
		Physician notified	
		Catheter care, bid, if catheter present and irrigated as ordered	
		Urine sent to lab for C & S, if ordered	Lab report for presence of bacteria
		Force fluids, unless contraindicated	Fluid balance record
Decubitus ulcer	0%	Signs and symptoms documented	Reddened or open area—ulceration
		Physician notified when redness noted	
		Turn every 2 hr; position off reddened area; massage area	Turning record
		Use of protective devices	Sheepskin flotation pads, alternating air mattress, elbow and heel protectors
		Use of treatment modalities	
Fecal impaction	0%	Signs and symptoms documented	No bowel movement for 3 days, digital exam, or frequent semiliquid stool
		Physician notified	
		Bowel movement pattern checked daily	Graphic sheet
		Impaction removed as ordered	Physician's order sheet
Contractures	0%	Signs and symptoms documented	Shortening of muscles causing flexion deformity of body part
		Physician notified	
		Footboards	
		Turned every 2 hr	Graphic sheet
		Active, passive, and active-resistive ROM exercises	Physical therapy

*For confirmation of complications, see face sheet, physician's progress notes, lab and x-ray reports, nurse's notes, assessment form, and graphic sheet

Table 12-2. Audit topic: chronic obstructive pulmonary disease

OUTCOME

Discharge status criteria	Compliance standard	Exceptions	Instructions and definitions for data retrieval*
Client or responsible person verbalizes knowledge of prescribed diet.	100%	Client on regular diet	Dietician record
Client or responsible person verbalizes knowledge of respiratory equipment for home use (care and use of equipment)	100%	None	Written information regarding use of equipment given to client or responsible person, in addition to verbalization and documentation
Client or responsible person verbalizes knowledge and understanding of specific discharge medications	100%	No discharge medications ordered	Physician's progress notes, pharmacist's record
Client and/or responsible person verbalizes understanding of importance of proper ventilation, humidity, refraining from smoking, and avoidance of irritants	100%	None	Written instructions given in addition to verbalization and documentation

INDICATORS

Complications	Compliance standard	Critical preventive and responsive management	Instructions and definitions for data retrieval
Pulmonary edema and heart failure	0%	Signs and symptoms noted and reported to physician immediately	Shortness of breath dyspnea, generalized rales, edema, tachycardia, distention of carotid arteries, confusion, fatigue, diaphoresis, frothy sputum
		Limited fluid intake 1000 ml/24 hr	Fluid balance record
		Daily weights	
		Limited sodium intake	Dietician record
		Rotating tourniquets if ordered	
		Vital signs (TPR and B/P) and lung sounds are monitored as needed	Blood pressure record
		Oxygen as ordered	Respiratory therapy record or nurses' notes
		High Fowler position	
		Emotional support	

*Information is found in nurses' notes, graphic sheet, or specific nursing discharge summary, unless otherwise specified

Continued.

Table 12-2. Audit topic: chronic obstructive pulmonary disease—cont'd

INDICATORS—cont'd

Complications	Compliance standard	Critical preventive and responsive management	Instructions and definitions for data retrieval
Ascites	0%	Signs and symptoms noted and reported to physician within 1 hour of onset	Pitting of lower extremities, enlarged scrotum, poor skin turgor, weight gain, shortness of breath
		Limit fluid intake, 1500 ml/24 hr	Fluid balance record
		Changed position and skin care for prevention of decubitus ulcers; air mattress and other prophylactic measures taken	
		Daily weights	
		Low sodium diet	
Respiratory acidosis	0%	Signs and symptoms noted and documented	Blood gas determinations (pH below 7.35, pO_2 below 60 mm Hg, Pco_2 above 60 mm Hg) cyanosis, lethargy, confusion, shortness of breath, and restlessness
		Monitored and reported blood gases to physician if ordered	Lab report
		Monitored vital signs	

Table 12-3. Audit topic: depression

OUTCOME

Audit criteria	Compliance standard	Exceptions	Instructions and definitions for data retrieval*
Client or responsible person verbalizes knowledge of medications related to condition	100%	None	Documented: "Patient or responsible person verbalizes knowledge of medications related to condition"
Client or responsible person verbalizes knowledge of signs and symptoms that are indicative of recurring depression	100%	None	Changes in sleep patterns, decreased drives, weight loss, slow talking and slow movements, change in bowel habits
Client demonstrates ability to communicate and interact with family and personnel at all levels within the facility	100%	None	Documented: "Less withdrawn—appropriate affect—talking with other patients and nursing staff—smiling—requiring less prn medication for anxiety and agitation"

*Information is found in nurses' notes, graphic sheet, or specific nursing discharge summary, unless otherwise specified

Table 12-3. Audit topic: depression—cont'd

INDICATORS

Complications	Compliance standard	Critical preventive and responsive management	Instructions and definitions for data retrieval
Suicidal attempt	0%	Remaining with patient when administering medications	Documented: "Nurse observes patient taking medications"
		All potentially dangerous effects removed on admission, and family instructed on the importance of eliminating potential dangers	Documented: "Family instructed on importance of eliminating all potentially dangerous objects"; Statement in admission nurses' notes and assessment form indicating "Potentially dangerous objects removed from room"
		Environmental checks daily	Documented: "Daily environmental checks made for potentially dangerous objects"
		Restraint as necessary	Documented: "Restraint applied"
		Sedation for apprehension as necessary	Documented: "Sedation given"
Hostility	0%	Restraint as necessary	Documented: "Restrained as necessary"
		Sedation as necessary	Documented: "Sedation given" and reason why
		Physician notified	Documented: "Physician notified of hostility"
		Verbalization of hostile feelings encouraged	Documented: "Verbalizes hostile feelings"
		Occupational therapy provided	Documented: "Occupational therapy provided" and indicate type: Drawing lines Drawing pictures Coloring pictures
		Observed for signs and symptoms of suicidal tendencies	Excuses made for not taking meds with nurse in attendance; increased requests for sedation; requests to be alone; requests for visit from clergyman; confessions of guilt and worthlessness; sudden unpected mood changes
		If signs and symptoms present, physician notified	Documented: "Physician notified of change of condition"
		Personnel assigned to remain with client	Documented: "Personnel assigned to remain with client for observation"
		Vital signs rescheduled every hour	Documented on blood pressure record

Table 12-4. Audit topic: insulin-dependent diabetic

CRITERIA

Discharge status	Compliance standard	Exceptions	Instructions and definitions for data retrieval*
Client or responsible person verbalizes knowledge and understanding of disease (signs, symptoms, etiology, control, and complications)	100%	None	Documented on diabetic discharge summary
Client or responsible person verbalizes knowledge and understanding of prescribed diet regimen	100%	None	Documented on dietician record and diabetic discharge summary; written instructions given
Client or responsible person verbalizes and demonstrates knowledge and understanding of urine testing	100%	None	Diabetic discharge summary
Client or responsible person demonstrates ability to administer and verbalizes knowledge of insulin administration (dosage, duration, peak, side effects, sites of injection)	100%	None	Diabetic discharge summary; written instructions given
Client and/or responsible person verbalizes knowledge and understanding of personal hygiene as prevention for future complications	100%	None	Diabetic discharge summary

INDICATORS

Complications	Compliance standard	Critical preventive and responsive management	Instructions and definitions for data retrieval
Insulin reaction	0%	Signs and symptoms documented	Lassitude, hunger, inability to concentrate, lethargy, drowsiness, weakness, shakiness, thirsty, headache, listlessness
		Physician notified within 30 min of onset of signs and symptoms	
		Amount of diet taken each meal documented	
		Accurate and fresh voided urine specimen tested (S & A) documented to anticipate change of insulin requirement	Diabetic discharge summary
		Blood glucose determination reported to physician if below 40 mg/100 ml blood	Lab sheet

*Information is found in nurses' notes, graphic sheet, or specific nursing discharge summary unless otherwise specified.

Table 12-4. Audit topic: insulin-dependent diabetic—cont'd

INDICATORS—cont'd

Complications	Compliance standard	Critical preventive and responsive management	Instructions and definitions for data retrieval
Diabetic coma	0%	Signs and symptoms documented	Thirsty, headache; listlessness; anorexia; drowsiness; vomiting; visual disturbances; hot, dry, flushed skin; Kussmaul breathing
		Physician notified within 30 min of onset of signs and symptoms	
		Amount of diet taken each meal documented	
		Blood glucose reported to physician if above 180 mg/100 ml blood	Lab report sheet
Ulcerations of feet and lower extremities	0%	Documentation of signs and symptoms	Discoloration, redness, tenderness, pain, numbness, sensitivity to touch, purulent drainage from ulceration
		Physician notified of signs and symptoms with 24 hr of onset of symptoms	
		Daily foot care; if ordered, podiatry treatment carried out	

not be expected to fulfill the stated criteria. The Instructions and Definitions for Data Retrieval column offers guidelines to the audit nurses regarding how criteria information can be obtained. Also in this column, terms are defined and proper documentation statements are presented. Complications that are frequently associated with the topic are listed in the next column. The Compliance Standard for Complications is the percentage of times the complication occurred. The Critical Prevention and Responsiveness Management states what the nursing activity was when the complication was noted in each case.

The selected examples of nursing audit reports provide nursing service with a detailed summary of the success of the nursing care given to clients with conditions frequently occurring in the older adult.

Nursing audit case study summary report. In addition to reviewing nursing care outcomes, nursing audits are also valuable tools in evaluating and upgrading the quality of written documentation of care (charting). A sample nursing audit form and case study follow.

This audit was done at a 131-bed skilled nursing facility and included two floors over a 6-month period.

The nurses evaluated the content of their charting to determine if it met standards of the federal regulations. It gave the nurses an opportunity to do a simple nursing audit before they began a more complex audit of direct client care. After charting deficiencies were identified, in-service education programs were conducted. A second audit was done, and again deficits in charting were noted. A form was developed listing all the essential information needed in the chart before the chart was ready for the Medical Records Department.

In June 19__ and January 19__, after an in-service program, a simple nursing audit was attempted by four charge nurses and the Coordinator of Staff Development under the guidance of the Assistant Administrator. The criteria were used from mechanics of the chart. The June sample consisted of five discharge charts, and January's sample was five current charts. The purpose of the audit was to introduce the nursing staff to the terminology, definition, and process of audit through this simple skill inventory of chart mechanics. Another purpose was to improve charting. The outcome summary follows.

Nursing audit

1. Criteria established (see samples, Tables 12-1 to 12-4)
2. Measurement of findings against criteria
   a. Deficiencies in June audit
      Mechanics of chart
      (1) Headings not filled and complete and legible
      (2) Nurses' notes not preceded by time
      (3) Nurses' notes not written at least every third day
      (4) Blank spaces left, and lines not drawn to prevent illegal entries
      (5) Lab slips not in correct sequence
      (6) Graphs not used for vital signs
      (7) BP, weight, stools, diet not recorded properly
      Nurses' notes
      (1) Results of prn and stat medication not noted
      (2) No record of any draining orifice
      (3) No record of any special feeding
      (4) No record of suction or syphon drainage
      (5) No use of oxygen
      (6) Nurse does not record when doctor is assisted
      (7) A descriptive note on untoward reaction not present
      (8) Surgical procedures not done
      (9) Discharge entry not always completed
      Corrective action taken
      (1) Continuing education programs
          (a) Charting
          (b) Clinical observations
          (c) More pertinent care plans
          (d) Medication procedure
          (e) Closer observation of client by nurse charting for subtle signs indicating change
      (2) New forms used for clarification
      (3) Charge nurses rotated to different floors to give them a fresh perspective
      (4) More complete shift change report, better communication
      (5) Closer observation of patient care
   b. Deficiencies in January audit
      Mechanics of chart
      (1) Headings continue to be filled out incompletely and illegibly
      (2) Time as to AM or PM not indicated

(3) Blank spaces left
(4) No nurses' notes every 3 days
(5) Improvement: Graphs are being used
Nurses' notes
(1) Need for charting reason for administering prn or stat medication
(2) Results must be noted
(3) Explanatory note not recorded when standing medication not administered
(4) Continue to ignore need of charting discharges
(5) Descriptive notes of untoward reaction not noted
(6) Surgical procedures do not apply
(7) Importance of keeping accurate clothing and valuables sheet
Evaluation of results
(1) Professional nurse needs further continuing education on importance of accurate charting to meet accountability demands of consumer, institution, and state/federal requirements.
(2) Charting methods should be studied and updated. Orient toward POR with use of SOAP as guideline for content of charting.
(3) Make charting more meaningful in relationship to plan of care for the client and quality care given.
(4) A new formulation for nursing audit directed to needs of ECF rather than acute care hospital. Emphasis on ADL-restorative and rehabilitative modules and documentation thereof.
(5) Audit based on criteria developed for care of the older adult client.
Corrective action taken
(1) In-service programs for future based on needs
    (a) Chart using SOAP principles
    (b) Clinical observations of the older adult client, differentiating between normal and abnormal signs and symptoms of aging
    (c) Write more relevant client care plans
    (d) Review medication procedure at 3- or 6-month intervals
    (e) Have client activities observed by the professional nurse and monitor daily
    (f) Closer observation by professional nurse of ancillary personnel
(2) Goal
    (a) Improvement of care plans leading to better care of client
    (b) Professional nurse to spend more time with clients assessing their needs; assessment necessary to improve care
    (c) Better communication between care providers
    (d) More complete documentation of clients' care

Mechanics of charting
Sample nursing audit form

Date: _____ Number: _____

	Yes	No	Does not apply

Criteria for charting

1. All record sheets and notes are properly identified.
   a. Headings filled out complete and legible ☐ ☐ ☐
   b. Stamped with addressograph ☐ ☐ ☐
   c. Correct dates entered ☐ ☐ ☐
   d. Signature of recorder included after each note and co-signature when indicated ☐ ☐ ☐
   e. All notes preceded by correct date and time, indicating AM and PM ☐ ☐ ☐
   f. Notes appear in correct sequence. No blank spaces left unless lines drawn to prevent illegal entries ☐ ☐ ☐
   g. Recordings are legible, and in ink or ball pen ☐ ☐ ☐
   h. At least one nurse's note every third day ☐ ☐ ☐
2. TPR and graphic record completed ☐ ☐ ☐
   a. Blanks filled in for calendar dates, and for hospital and postop days ☐ ☐ ☐
   b. Graphs of temps, pulse, and respirations clear and complete ☐ ☐ ☐
   c. BP, wt, stools, and diet recorded properly ☐ ☐ ☐
   d. Fluid intake and output record complete ☐ ☐ ☐
   e. All tests and treatments recorded properly ☐ ☐ ☐
   f. Lab slips in correct sequence ☐ ☐ ☐
3. Complete admission note written on nurse's notes ☐ ☐ ☐
4. Complete discharge note written on nurse's notes ☐ ☐ ☐
5. Include transfer note if indicated ☐ ☐ ☐
6. All identifying information appears on authorization permits, including signature of witness ☐ ☐ ☐

Nurses' notes

1. Condition of patient on admission
   a. Patient's physical abilities and limitations ☐ ☐ ☐
2. Medications
   a. Reason for administering prn or stat medication is noted ☐ ☐ ☐
   b. Results of prn and stat medication is noted ☐ ☐ ☐
   c. Explanatory note is recorded when any standing medication has not been administered ☐ ☐ ☐
   d. A note is recorded when intravenous solution containing medication is added or not completed. Amount absorbed is included ☐ ☐ ☐
3. Drainage from any orifice—note includes
   a. Source ☐ ☐ ☐
   b. Type ☐ ☐ ☐
   c. Consistency ☐ ☐ ☐
   d. Odor ☐ ☐ ☐
   e. Color ☐ ☐ ☐
4. Special feeding—note includes:
   a. Type ☐ ☐ ☐
   b. Ability to tolerate ☐ ☐ ☐
   c. Notation of time given ☐ ☐ ☐

Continued.

Mechanics of charting
Sample nursing audit form—cont'd

Nurses' notes—cont'd	Yes	No	Does not apply
5. Suction or siphon drainage—note includes:			
a. Type	☐	☐	☐
b. Description	☐	☐	☐
c. Amount of drainage	☐	☐	☐
6. Use of oxygen—note includes:			
a. Method of administration	☐	☐	☐
b. Duration	☐	☐	☐
c. Liter flow	☐	☐	☐
7. Treatments			
a. When nurse assists the doctor a note is written	☐	☐	☐
b. When an untoward reaction occurs, a descriptive note is written	☐	☐	☐
c. When the nurse performs a treatment, the note includes:			
(1) Time	☐	☐	☐
(2) Type	☐	☐	☐
(3) Results	☐	☐	☐
(4) Reactions	☐	☐	☐
8. Surgical procedures			
a. Preoperative check list	☐	☐	☐
b. Postoperative care			
(1) Vital signs	☐	☐	☐
(2) Drainage	☐	☐	☐
(3) Voiding	☐	☐	☐
(4) Fluid or food tolerance	☐	☐	☐
9. Personal property			
a. Clothing and valuables sheet	☐	☐	☐
10. Discharge			
a. This last entry includes:			
(1) Date	☐	☐	☐
(2) Time	☐	☐	☐
(3) Name of institution or home care	☐	☐	☐
b. If after 11:00 AM, reason for late discharge	☐	☐	☐
11. Ceased breathing			
a. Last observations	☐	☐	☐
b. Date	☐	☐	☐
c. Time pronounced dead	☐	☐	☐
d. Name of certifying physician is included	☐	☐	☐

Summary. A medical record audit form (see below) was developed by the audit committee. This form was placed on the front of each chart. It was completed by the charge nurse at each client's discharge. The Medical Records Department would not accept a discharge chart until the audit form was completed and signed by the charge nurse.

Level III: Utilization review plan

Federal regulations dictate that a utilization review (UR) planning committee be established at every skilled nursing facility having clients receiving benefits under Medicare and Medicaid. A UR plan must be submitted to the federal government. Sometimes the same plan can be adopted for use by both Medicare and Medicaid by those facilities that are providers of both kinds of services. The following UR plan focuses on providing Medicare services.

There are two elements to utilization review: (1) medical care evaluation studies that identify and analyze patterns of care in skilled nursing facility and (2) review of continued stay cases in the facility. The Utilization Review Committee certifies the appropriateness of the skilled care required to justify continued Medicare payments.

The plan is developed with the advice of professional personnel, including a physician and a registered nurse, and is approved for implementation by representatives of the facility's medical staff and governing body.

Medical record audit form

Patient admission number _____
☐ Recent admission ☐ Long-term resident
☐ Discharged patient

Criterion	Meets criterion	Variance	Not applicable	Comments
1. Admitting diagnoses				
2. Transfer agreement				
3. Written physician's orders on admission				
4. Summary of prior treatment				
5. Physical examination within 48 hr of admission				
6. Progress notes written by physician at each visit				
7. Progress notes (see individual state regulations)				
8. Physical examination annually				
9. Physician's orders signed and dated				
10. Verbal orders countersigned within 48 hr				
11. Nurse's notes at least every third day				
12. Patient's identifying data on every sheet				
13. Disposition				
14. Discharge diagnoses				
15. Discharge summary				

The physician members of the Utilization Review Committee have the specific responsibility for conducting utilization review and are accountable to the administrator of the facility.

The Utilization Review Committee meets as a whole regularly every 30 days. The Committee functions, in general, by reviewing and evaluating charts of all the Medicare clients. Its principal purpose is to identify and analyze factors that contribute to unnecessary or inappropriate use of the facilities and services and to make recommendations designed to minimize such use. This function is carried out by review of Medicare admissions, lengths of stay, and the professional services furnished with respect to their necessity and propriety. The Committee also performs medical care evaluation studies. Nurse members of the Committee contribute to the evaluation of the nursing components of care. The Committee is composed of two or more physicians, and often also includes representatives from nursing service and other disciplines. As the federal regulations now stand, however, only the physician has a vote on the Committee. No member of the Committee can have a significant financial interest, direct or indirect, in the institution. No physician has review responsibility for any client under his care.

Committee authority. The Committee has the authority to review the chart of any Medicare client on admission, while the client is currently under care, or on discharge and to discuss it with the physician or physicians concerned. The Committee does not have authority to take disciplinary action. The Committee regulates the extended use of the particular facility's Medicare beds. Findings and recommendations of the Utilization Review Committee are reported to the administrator of the facility, who has the authority and responsibility for considering and acting on them.

Functions of the committee. The UR Committee conducts utilization review by means of a review of the chart of each current Medicare client. The client's privacy is protected; he is not identified by name but by code number only. The name of the attending physician, date of admission, and Medicare benefits are included for extended duration cases with review of admissions, lengths of stay, and professional services furnished. The Committee reviews new Medicare admissions and previously approved clients classified as extended duration cases.

Identification of eligible clients. At the time of admission, the admitting officer of the facility notes if the client is eligible for Medicare coverage. The following guidelines are used.

1. Skilled nursing services or skilled rehabilitation services must be required.
2. Such services must be required on a daily basis.
3. The service can only be provided in a skilled nursing facility on an inpatient basis.

At the time of admission, the date of the extended stay review is attached to the front of the client's chart. In this way all involved personnel will have knowledge of the date of the review. The specified period of time cannot exceed 30 days after admission, regardless of the client's diagnosis or functional capability. The second and subsequent extended stay review dates are determined on the basis of a date 30 days after the initial review.

Utilization Review Committee method of conducting extended stay review (see utilization review worksheet, p. 295)

1. Extended stay review: conducted by the UR Committee will occur on or before the date assigned by the Admitting Officer. No physician member of the UR Committee shall review a continued stay case in which he is professionally involved. The review is based primarily on information provided in the client's record.
   a. Documentation of the assessment of the medical necessity for continued stay
   b. Medical plan for further care
   c. Appropriateness of professional services rendered
   d. Such additional supporting material as the committee may deem appropriate
   e. Meeting one of the following criteria to justify skilled nursing facility level of care on a daily basis:
      (1) Skilled nursing supervision and management of a complicated or extensive plan
      (2) Skilled observation, assessment, and monitoring of a complicated or unstable condition, or of the progress of a rehabilitation program
      (3) Skilled teaching services for self-maintenance after discharge
      (4) Intravenous or intramuscular medications or feedings
      (5) Levine tube or enterostomy feedings

(6) Nasopharyngeal or tracheotomy aspiration

(7) Insertion and sterile irrigation and replacement of catheters

(8) Application of dressings involving prescription medications and aseptic techniques

(9) Treatment of extensive decubitus ulcers or other widespread skin disorder

(10) Heat treatments specifically ordered by a physician and requiring skilled supervision

(11) Initiation of a regimen involving administration of medicinal gases

(12) Skilled performance or supervision of therapeutic exercises or activities

(13) Gait evaluation and training in which ability to walk has been impaired by a rehabilitatable neurological, muscular, or skeletal abnormality

(14) Skilled evaluation of the proper maintenance therapy for chronically debilitating illness

(15) Ultrasound, short-wave, or microwave therapy

(16) Skilled supervision of hot pack, hydrocollator, infrared, paraffin bath, or whirlpool therapy

(17) Skilled therapy for restoration of speech or hearing

2. *Adverse findings:* If the UR Committee finds that the criteria for extended stay are not met, the attending physician is notified and an opportunity is given for him to provide additional information relating to the client's need for extended stay.

a. If the attending physician does not respond within 48 hours or does not contest the findings of the committee, then the findings are final. Written notification of this final determination must be sent to the attending physician, the patient (or

---

Utilization review worksheet
Justification of level of care

ID No. _____ Room No. _____ Age _____

Adm date _____ Physician _____

Level of care: ☐ Skilled ☐ Int ☐ Res

Problems: _____

Major therapy: _____

Skilled criteria

☐ Supervision complicated/extensive plan/care

☐ Observation, assessment, monitoring of complicated unstable condition, progress of rehabilitation program

Specify: _____

☐ Teaching/learning for self-maintenance after discharge

Specify: _____

☐ IV fluids ☐ IV medications ☐ IM medications ☐ Clysis

☐ Levine tube or enterostomy feedings

☐ Nasopharyngeal or tracheotomy aspiration

☐ Foley catheter insertion, replacement or irrigation

☐ Dressings with medications, aseptic technique

☐ Decubitus ulcers, widespread skin disorder

☐ Supervised heat treatments

☐ Oxygen, inhalation therapy

☐ Gastrostomy feeding

☐ Ostomy care and teaching

☐ Physical therapy order

Specify: _____

☐ Rehabilitation order

Specify: _____

Continued.

Utilization review worksheet
Justification of level of care—cont'd

Utilization review committee action

Level justified: ☐ Yes ☐ No

If yes, state reason or recommendation: _____

_____

_____

_____

_____

_____

If no, attending physician specify reason for justification: _____

_____

_____

_____

_____

Final utilization review committee action: _____

_____

_____

_____

Extended stay review date: _____

Signature: _____, MD, Chairman, Utilization Review Committee

Date: _____

---

next of kin), and the facility administrator no later than 2 days after such final determination and in no event later than 3 working days after the end of the assigned extended stay period.

b. If the attending physician contests the findings of the committee who performed the initial review, or if he presents additional information relating to the patient's need for extended stay, the committee must review the case. If the members determine that the client's stay is not medically necessary or appropriate after considering all the evidence, their determination becomes final. Writ-

ten notification of this decision must be sent to the attending physician, client (or next of kin), and facility administrator no later than 2 days after such final decision and in no event, later than 3 working days after the end of the assigned extended stay period.

c. If, after referral of a questioned case to the committee the physician reviewer determines that extended stay is justified, the attending physician is notified and an appropriate date for subsequent extended stay review will be selected and noted on the patient's medical record.

Client care evaluation studies. Client care evaluation studies emphasize the identification and analysis of patterns of client care and suggest, where appropriate, possible changes for maintaining consistently high-quality client care and efficient use of services. One study is completed annually and there is a study in progress at all times. Studies are conducted using a scientific methodology:

1. Statement of purpose
2. Delimitations of the study
3. Need for the study
4. Definition of terms
5. Research design
6. Stages of research
7. Conclusions

The conclusions of the study may result in the need for further investigation, recommendations, or development of criteria that lead to further refinements in nursing care.

Maintenance and use of records. The Utilization Review Committee keeps regular minutes of its meetings and maintains adequate summaries of its activities. Reports are maintained that document recommendations and action taken as they relate to special studies of the Utilization Review Committee. Minutes of each committee meeting include at least the following:

1. Name of the facility
2. Date and duration of the meeting
3. Names of committee members present and absent
4. Description of the activities presently in progress to satisfy the requirements for care evaluation studies and a summary of extended duration cases reviewed

Records include the number of cases reviewed, case identification numbers, admission and review dates, and decisions reached, including the basis for each determination and the action taken for each case not approved for continued stay.

All records are regarded as confidential and are made available only to duly authorized representatives of the facility, its staff, and accrediting, licensing, or reviewing bodies.

Implementation of committee findings and recommendations. The facility is responsible for acting on the Utilization Review Committee recommendations for changes beneficial to clients, staff, the facility, and the community.

The facility notifies the Utilization Review Committee of the implementation of changes to improve the quality of care and promote more effective and efficient use of facilities and services.

Review facility's discharge planning program. The Utilization Review Committee annually reviews and reevaluates the overall discharge planning program that the facility has established through written discharge planning procedures. Discharge planning is presented in Chapter 8.

Administrative assistance. The facility provides administrative assistance to the Committee in the form of record maintenance, reports, statistical data and materials, and such clerical assistance as deemed necessary. Such assistance includes notifying the Committee of the initial review date for continued stay cases and providing the Committee with each Medicare client's discharge plan for continuing care after discharge that takes into account the individual's needs. The facility assigns responsibility for each of these activities to specific persons or positions.

Approval of utilization review plan. This utilization review plan has been approved by the facility's medical staff and governing board and constitutes the official plan and policies for utilization review of its facilities and services. It is available on request to state and federal representatives for the purpose of determining whether the plan and the facility meet the conditions prescribed for participation in the Medicare Program under the Social Security Act.

Reimbursement. Without state approval of the utilization review plan for the utilization of the agency's services, no Medicaid or Medicare money will be given to the agency. The agency is visited annually by a State surveyor to document the implementation of the plan.

The following evaluation criteria meet the federal standards for an agency's certification as a Medicaid or Medicare provider. It can be used for an agency's utilization review self-study.

Meeting licensure and certification criteria. Compliance with federal, state, and local laws for extended care facilities is required in order for the agency to be licensed and certified as a Medicare/Medicaid provider.

The primary purpose of extended care facilities is to provide nursing care to clients. Nursing is the one service that receives considerable attention in the evaluation survey of compliance with the rules and regulations for licensure and certification.

A nurse can use the audit techniques to evaluate the nursing service at her facility. Since she wants to base her audit on a recognized standard, she could choose the Medicare/Medicaid Skilled Nursing Facility Survey Report guidelines. The following pages represent criteria from these standards and were developed by the AID Health Care Centers, Inc., a nationwide firm that owns and manages long-term-care facilities and hospitals.

Use the checklist to audit the nursing in your agency. It will demonstrate areas of strengths and also point out areas that need further reassessment.

Text continued on p. 309.

Criteria for utilization review

	Yes	No	N/A
1. Is utilization review being performed by a PSRO that has assumed full responsibility for review? (NOTE: If yes, go on to discharge planning. If no, mark N/A.)	☐	☐	☐

Written plan of utilization review of activity

	Yes	No	N/A
2. Does the skilled nursing center have a currently applicable written description of its utilization review plan?	☐	☐	☐
3. Is this plan approved and stamped?	☐	☐	☐
By:			
4. The medical director?	☐	☐	☐
5. The governing body?	☐	☐	☐
6. Each federal program?	☐	☐	☐
Does the description include:			
7. The organization and composition of the committee or group responsible for its function?	☐	☐	☐
8. The frequency of meetings?	☐	☐	☐
9. Type of records to be kept?	☐	☐	☐
10. Methods and criteria (including norms where available) used to define periods of continuous extended duration and to assign or select subsequent dates for continued stay review?	☐	☐	☐
11. Method for selection and conduct of medical care evaluation studies?	☐	☐	☐
12. Relationship of URC plan to claims administration by a third party?	☐	☐	☐
13. Arrangements for committee reports and their dissemination?	☐	☐	☐
14. Responsibilities of the center's administrative staff?	☐	☐	☐
15. Does the plan cover both Medicare and Medicaid?	☐	☐	☐

Composition and organization of utilization review committee

	Yes	No	N/A
16. Is the UR function conducted by a staff committee of the center composed of two or more physicians, with participation of other professional personnel?	☐	☐	☐
17. Is the UR function conducted by a similarly composed group outside the center? (approved by local medical or osteopathic society or some or all hospitals and SNFs in the locality) (If no, mark N/A.)	☐	☐	☐
18. Is the UR function conducted by a group established and organized in a manner approved by the secretary that is capable of performing such functions?	☐	☐	☐
Are the medical care evaluation studies, educational duties of the review program and the review of long-stay cases performed by:			
19. The same committee or group? (If no, answer N/A.)	☐	☐	☐

Criteria for utilization review—cont'd

	Yes	No	N/A

Composition and organization of utilization review committee—cont'd

20. Two or more committees or groups? (If no, answer N/A.) ☐ ☐ ☐
21. The persons on the review committee or group are not employed by the center? ☐ ☐ ☐
22. These persons have no financial interest in the center? ☐ ☐ ☐
23. The persons on the review committee are not professionally involved in the care of the patient whose case is being reviewed? ☐ ☐ ☐

Medical care evaluation studies

24. Are medical care evaluation studies performed to promote the most effective and efficient use of available health facilities and services consistent with patient needs and professionally recognized standards of health care? ☐ ☐ ☐
25. Do studies emphasize identification and analysis of patterns of patient care and suggest, where appropriate, possible changes for maintaining high quality patient care and effective and efficient use of services? ☐ ☐ ☐
26. Does each study identify and analyze factors related to the patient care given in the center? ☐ ☐ ☐
27. When indicated, does the study result in recommendations for change beneficial to patients, staff, the center and the community? ☐ ☐ ☐

Do the studies, on a sample or other basis, include, but need not be limited to:
28. Admissions, duration of stay and ancillary services? ☐ ☐ ☐
29. Is at least one study in progress at any given time? ☐ ☐ ☐
30. Is at least one study completed per year? ☐ ☐ ☐

Will the study be accomplished by considering and analyzing data from any of the following sources:
31. Medical records or other appropriate data? ☐ ☐ ☐
32. External organizations, which compile statistics, design profiles, and produce comparative data? ☐ ☐ ☐
33. By cooperative endeavor with the PSRO, fiscal intermediary, providers of services or appropriate agencies? ☐ ☐ ☐
34. Does the committee or group document the results of each medical care evaluation study? ☐ ☐ ☐
35. Does this documentation show how results have been used to improve the quality of care and promote more effective use of facilities and services? ☐ ☐ ☐

Extended stay review

36. Is periodic review made of each current inpatient beneficiary care of continuous extensive duration and the length of which is defined in the utilization review plan to determine if further inpatient stay is necessary? ☐ ☐ ☐
37. Does the plan specify a different number of days for different diagnostic classes of days, for all cases? ☐ ☐ ☐
38. Does the period specified bear a reasonable relationship to current average length of stay statistics? ☐ ☐ N/A
39. Does the period not exceed 30 days after admission? ☐ ☐ ☐
40. Are the number of days and the diagnosis specified in the plan? ☐ ☐ ☐
41. Are there no exceptions to the 30 day limit? ☐ ☐ ☐

Continued.

Criteria for utilization review—cont'd

	Yes	No	N/A

Extended stay review—cont'd

42. If there are exceptions are these based on appropriate data or averages established by recognized guidelines? (If no, mark N/A.) ☐ ☐ ☐

43. Does the initial extended stay review take place prior to or at the end of the period of extended duration specified? ☐ ☐ ☐

44. Is the review based on the attending physician's reasons for and plan for continued stay and any other documentation the committee deems appropriate? ☐ ☐ ☐

45. Are cases screened also by a qualified non-physician representative of the committee? ☐ ☐ ☐

46. Are cases screened by the group? ☐ ☐ ☐

Further stay not medically necessary

47. Is final determination that further stay is not medically necessary made by at least two physician members of the committee or group? ☐ ☐ ☐

48. If the attending physician does not express his views or contest the findings or further stay not being medically necessary the determination is not then made by one physician? ☐ ☐ ☐

49. If the committee or group with physician member concurrence agrees that further stay is no longer medically necessary, do they then notify the attending physician and give him the opportunity to present his views before a final decision is made? ☐ ☐ ☐

When the final determination is made that further stay is no longer medically necessary, is written notification given to:

50. The center? ☐ ☐ ☐
51. The attending physician? ☐ ☐ ☐
52. The patient or his next of kin? ☐ ☐ ☐
53. Is this notification given no later than 2 days after the final determination? ☐ ☐ ☐
54. In the case of extended duration, is notification given no later than 3 working days after the end of the specified extended duration period? ☐ ☐ ☐
55. Does the reviewer use criteria established by the physician members of the committee? ☐ ☐ ☐
56. If nonphysician members are used, are cases referred to a physician if it appears that the patient no longer needs inpatient care? ☐ ☐ ☐
57. If nonphysician representatives are used to screen cases, are they experienced or trained in application of screening criteria? ☐ ☐ ☐
58. If an individual continues to need further inpatient skilled nursing care, is an appropriate stay approved, with reviews made at least every 30 days? ☐ ☐ ☐
59. Are these cases reviewed in like manner before the expiration of each new period? ☐ ☐ ☐
60. Are these reviews repeated as long as the stay continues beyond the scheduled review dates—and notice has not been given? ☐ ☐ ☐

Administrative responsibilities

61. Is the administrative staff directly and fully informed of the committee's activities? ☐ ☐ ☐
62. Does the administrative staff offer support and assistance? ☐ ☐ ☐
63. Does the administrator study and act upon recommendations made by the committee? ☐ ☐ ☐
64. Does he or she coordinate such functions with appropriate staff? ☐ ☐ ☐
65. Is there documentation of the administrator's action and support? ☐ ☐ ☐

Criteria for utilization review—cont'd

	Yes	No	N/A
Utilization and review records			
66. Are written records of committee activities maintained?	☐	☐	☐
67. Are appropriate reports, signed by the chairman, made regularly?	☐	☐	☐
68. To the medical staff?	☐	☐	☐
69. The administrative staff?	☐	☐	☐
70. The governing body?	☐	☐	☐
71. Other sponsors?	☐	☐	☐
Do committee minutes include:			
72. Name of committee?	☐	☐	☐
73. Date and duration of meeting?	☐	☐	☐
74. Names of committee members present and absent?	☐	☐	☐
75. Description of activities in progress to satisfy requirements for medical care evaluation studies?	☐	☐	☐
Do activities in progress for medical care evaluation studies include:			
76. Subject	☐	☐	☐
77. Reason for study?	☐	☐	☐
78. Dates of commencement?	☐	☐	☐
79. Expected completion?	☐	☐	☐
80. Summary of studies completed since last meeting?	☐	☐	☐
Do activities in progress for medical care evaluation studies include:			
81. Conclusions	☐	☐	☐
82. Follow-up on implementation or recommendations?	☐	☐	☐
Does the summary of the extended duration cases review include:			
83. Number of cases?	☐	☐	☐
84. Case identification number?	☐	☐	☐
85. Admission and review dates?	☐	☐	☐
86. Decisions reached?	☐	☐	☐
87. Basis for determination and action on nonapproved cases?	☐	☐	☐
88. Are full UR committee meetings held at least monthly (every 4 weeks)?	☐	☐	☐
Do internal records or methods used by UR committee for review of extended duration cases include:			
89. Complete medical record?	☐	☐	☐
90. Abstract of medical record?	☐	☐	☐
91. Face sheet of medical record?	☐	☐	☐
92. Utilization review checklist?	☐	☐	☐
93. Interview with attending physician?	☐	☐	☐
94. Observation of patient?	☐	☐	☐
95. Other? _____	☐	☐	☐
Do internal records or methods used by UR committee for medical care evaluation studies include:			
96. Complete medical record?	☐	☐	☐
97. Abstract of medical record?	☐	☐	☐

Continued.

Criteria for utilization review—cont'd

	Yes	No	N/A

Utilization and review records—cont'd

Do internal records or methods used by UR committee for medical care evaluation studies include:

	Yes	No	N/A
98. Face sheet of medical record?	☐	☐	☐
99. Utilization review checklist?	☐	☐	☐
100. Interview with attending physician?	☐	☐	☐
101. Observation of patient?	☐	☐	☐
102. Other? _____	☐	☐	☐
103. Does the center have an organized discharge planning program?	☐	☐	☐
104. Is this policy reviewed at least annually?	☐	☐	☐
105. Are the results of discharge planning available to the UR committee as well as alternate community resources?	☐	☐	☐
106. Is responsibility for discharge planning delegated in writing by the administrator to one or more members of the center's staff?	☐	☐	☐
107. Is consultation arranged if necessary?	☐	☐	☐
108. If center cannot provide services, are these arranged for with a health, social, or welfare agency?	☐	☐	☐

Discharge planning

Do the written discharge planning procedures describe:

	Yes	No	N/A
109. The function, authority and relationship of the discharge coordinator to the center?	☐	☐	☐
110. The time period in which each patient's need for discharge planning is determined? (preferably 7 days after admission)	☐	☐	☐
111. The maximum time period after which reevaluation of each patient's discharge plan is made?	☐	☐	☐
112. Local resources available to the facility, the patient and attending physician to assist in individual plans?	☐	☐	☐
113. Provisions for periodic review and reevaluaton of the center's discharge planning program?	☐	☐	☐
114. Does the center provide the person responsible for the patient's past discharge care with an appropriate summary of information—to ensure optimal continuity of care?	☐	☐	☐

Does the discharge summary include:

	Yes	No	N/A
115. Current information relative to diagnosis?	☐	☐	☐
116. Rehabilitation potential?	☐	☐	☐
117. Summary of the course of prior treatment?	☐	☐	☐
118. Physician's orders for the immediate care of the patient?	☐	☐	☐
119. Pertinent social information?	☐	☐	☐

Criteria for nursing support services

	Yes	No	N/A

Nursing services—pharmacy

1. Are all medications stored under lock and key? ☐ ☐ ☐
2. Are medication room cabinets and refrigerators clean? ☐ ☐ ☐
3. Are natcotics in separate double locked storage? ☐ ☐ ☐

Are medications labeled with:
4. Patient's name? ☐ ☐ ☐
5. Physician's name? ☐ ☐ ☐
6. Prescription number? ☐ ☐ ☐
7. Name and strength of drug? ☐ ☐ ☐
8. Date of issue? ☐ ☐ ☐
9. Expiration date if indicated? ☐ ☐ ☐
10. Name of pharmacy? ☐ ☐ ☐
11. Initial of dispensing pharmacist? ☐ ☐ ☐
12. Is the individual narcotic record being maintained? ☐ ☐ ☐
13. Is the narcotic control book being co-signed at the shift change? ☐ ☐ ☐
14. Does the center have an emergency drug kit? ☐ ☐ ☐
15. Is PDR at each nusing station current? ☐ ☐ ☐
16. Are medicines reordered as needed? ☐ ☐ ☐

Nursing services—medical records

17. Are charts neat and all organized in the same manner? ☐ ☐ ☐
18. Has a professional person in the center been assigned the job of checking charts for completeness before filing? ☐ ☐ ☐
19. Are nursing notes current and meaningful? ☐ ☐ ☐
20. Are medications properly charted?? ☐ ☐ ☐
21. Are medications not given properly charted with reason not given? ☐ ☐ ☐
22. Is lab work performed as ordered and reported to a physician? ☐ ☐ ☐
23. Is there a documented procedure for notifying physician if anything unusual results? ☐ ☐ ☐
24. Does the nursing staff document any teaching of family and patients? ☐ ☐ ☐
25. Are physicians orders current (not over 30 days)? ☐ ☐ ☐
26. Are telephone orders being countersigned on the physician's order sheet? ☐ ☐ ☐
27. Do charts contain a record of all physician visits? ☐ ☐ ☐
28. Are histories and physicals on all charts, and are they current? ☐ ☐ ☐
29. Are restraints charted properly, that is, what patient did while out of restraints? ☐ ☐ ☐
30. Are patients weighed monthly and are TPRs and BPs being taken monthly and charted? ☐ ☐ ☐
31. Is intake-and-output procedure instituted where necessary and charted? ☐ ☐ ☐
32. Does each chart contain a meaningful patient plan of care, with appropriate time frames? ☐ ☐ ☐
33. Is discharge planning evidenced? ☐ ☐ ☐
34. Are admissions and discharges completed and paper work in order? ☐ ☐ ☐

Nursing services—dietary

35. Are nourishment carts being passed on time? ☐ ☐ ☐
36. Do most of the patients eat their meals in the dining room? ☐ ☐ ☐
37. Are patients fed in their rooms only if they so desire or are ill? ☐ ☐ ☐
38. Are patients fed as needed? ☐ ☐ ☐
39. Are meals and snacks served as ordered? ☐ ☐ ☐
40. Are adaptive feeding devices used when necessary? ☐ ☐ ☐

Continued.

Criteria for nursing support services—cont'd

Nursing services—policies and meetings	Yes	No	N/A

Policies

	Yes	No	N/A
41. Are nursing procedure manuals at nursing stations and are they being used?	☐	☐	☐
42. Is there a philosophy for the nursing department?	☐	☐	☐
43. Is there a written isolation procedure in the policy and procedures manual?	☐	☐	☐
44. Are all personnel neatly dressed and in correct uniform as specified?	☐	☐	☐
45. Have new employees been oriented to company policies and job procedures?	☐	☐	☐

Meetings

	Yes	No	N/A
46. Are patient care conferences being held at least twice a month?	☐	☐	☐
Is there evidence on record of participation in in-service training by:			
47. ADA dietitian?	☐	☐	☐
48. Pharmacist?	☐	☐	☐
49. Dentist?	☐	☐	☐
50. Physician?	☐	☐	☐
51. Social service?	☐	☐	☐
52. Are there nursing personnel conferences at change of shift?	☐	☐	☐
53. Is there a policy and procedure in the nursing manual for every procedure used in the center?	☐	☐	☐

Criteria for nursing services

	Yes	No

Director of Nursing Services

	Yes	No
1. Is the Director of Nursing Services a currently licensed registered nurse who is employed full time?	☐	☐
2. Does the Director of Nursing serve only one facility?	☐	☐
3. Does the Director of Nursing have in writing full administrative authority?	☐	☐
4. Is she responsible and accountable for the functions, activities and training of the nursing services staff?	☐	☐
5. Does a qualified registered nurse serve as assistant if the Director of Nursing Services has other institutional responsibilities?	☐	☐
Is the Director of Nursing Services responsible for the following:		
6. Development and maintenance of nursing service objectives?	☐	☐
7. Standards of nursing service practice?	☐	☐
8. Nursing policy and procedure manuals?	☐	☐
9. Written job descriptions for each level of nursing personnel?	☐	☐
10. Scheduling of daily rounds to see all patients?	☐	☐
11. Methods for coordination of nursing services with other patient services?	☐	☐
12. Recommending the number and levels of nursing personnel to be employed?	☐	☐
13. Nursing staff development?	☐	☐
14. Does the Director of Nursing know the names of patients in the center?	☐	☐

Criteria for nursing services—cont'd

	Yes	No

Charge nurse

15. Is a registered nurse or a qualified licensed practical nurse designated as Charge Nurse by the Director of Nursing Services for each shift? ☐ ☐

16. Is the Charge Nurse responsible for supervision of the total nursing activity in the center during each shift? ☐ ☐

17. If the center has 60 patients or more, is it a policy that the Director of Nursing does not serve as Charge Nurse? ☐ ☐

18. Does the Charge Nurse delegate responsibility to nursing personnel, including assistants for the direct nursing care of specific patients during each shift? ☐ ☐

19. Is this done on the basis of staff qualifications, size and physical layout of the center, characteristics of the patient load and emotional, social, and nursing care needs of patients? ☐ ☐

20. Are specific assignments to nursing assistants provided in writing? ☐ ☐

Twenty-four hour nursing service

21. Does the center provide 24-hour nursing services that are sufficient to meet total nursing needs and are in accordance with the patient care policy? ☐ ☐

Are the policies designed to ensure that each patient receives the following:

22. Treatments, medications, and diet as prescribed? ☐ ☐

23. Rehabilitative nursing care as needed? ☐ ☐

24. Proper care to prevent decubitus ulcers with deformities? ☐ ☐

25. Kept comfortable, clean, and well groomed? ☐ ☐

26. Protected from accidents, injury, and infection? ☐ ☐

27. Encouraged, assisted, and trained in self care and group activities? ☐ ☐

28. Are nursing personnel, including at least one registered nurse on the day tour of duty, licensed practical nurses, nurses aides, orderlies, and ward clerks, assigned to duties consistent with their education and experience? ☐ ☐

29. Are these duties based on the characteristics of the patient load? ☐ ☐

30. Do the time schedules indicate the number and classification of nursing personnel including relief personnel who worked on each unit for each tour of duty? ☐ ☐

31. Does staffing meet needs and state and federal requirements? ☐ ☐

32. Is a written patient care plan for each patient developed and maintained by nursing service consonant with the attending physician's plan of medical care? ☐ ☐

33. Is this patient care plan implemented upon admission? ☐ ☐

34. Does the plan indicate care to be given and long- and short-term goals to be accomplished? ☐ ☐

35. Does the plan indicate which professional service is responsible for each element of care? ☐ ☐

36. Is the patient care plan reviewed, evaluated and updated as necessary by all professional personnel involved in the care of the patient? ☐ ☐

37. Does the plan of care have specific time frames for each discipline or element of care? ☐ ☐

Rehabilitative nursing care

38. Are nursing personnel trained in rehabilitative nursing? ☐ ☐

39. Does the center have an active program of rehabilitative nursing care? ☐ ☐

40. Is this program an integral part of nursing service, and is it directed toward helping each patient achieve and maintain an optimal level of self-care and independence? ☐ ☐

41. Are rehabilitative nursing care services performed daily for those patients who require such services? ☐ ☐

42. Are these services recorded routinely? ☐ ☐

Continued.

Criteria for nursing services—cont'd

	Yes	No

Rehabilitative nursing care—cont'd

43. Are nursing personnel aware of the nutritional needs and food and fluid intake of patients? □ □
44. Do they assist promptly where necessary in the feeding of patients? □ □
45. Is a procedure established to inform the dietetic service of the physician's diet orders and of patient's dietetic problems? □ □
46. Is food and fluid intake of patients observed? □ □
47. Are deviations from normal recorded and reported to the Charge Nurse and the physician? □ □

Administration of drugs

48. Are drugs and biologicals administered only by physicians, licensed and nursing personnel, or by other personnel who have completed a state-approved training program in medication administration? □ □
49. Are procedures established by the pharmaceutical service committee to ensure that drugs are checked against physician's orders? □ □
50. Is the patient identified before the administration of the drug? □ □
51. Does each patient have an individual medication record? □ □
52. Is the dose of the drug administered to that patient properly recorded by the person who administers the drug? □ □
53. Are drugs and biologicals administered as soon as possible after doses are prepared? □ □
54. Are drugs and biologicals administered by the same person who prepares the doses for administration except under unit dose distribution systems? □ □

Conformance with physician's drug orders

55. Are drugs administered in accordance with the written instruction of the attending physician? □ □
56. Are the drugs that are not specifically limited as to the time or number of doses when ordered to be controlled by automatic stop orders or other methods in accordance with written policies? □ □
57. Are physician's verbal orders for drugs given only to a licensed nurse, pharmacist, or physician? □ □
58. Are verbal orders immediately recorded and signed by the person receiving the order? □ □
59. Are such orders countersigned by the attending physician within 48 hours? □ □
60. Is the attending physician notified of an automatic stop order before the last dose so that the physician may decide if the administration of the drug or biological is to be continued? □ □
61. Is there a policy for distribution of drugs when a patient is allowed to leave the facility for a weekend or overnight? □ □
62. Does this policy state who is responsible for dispensing these drugs? □ □

Storage of drugs and biologicals

63. Are procedures for storing and disposing of drugs and biologicals established by the pharmaceutical services committee? □ □
64. Are all drugs and biologicals stored in locked compartments under proper temperature control? □ □
65. Do only authorized personnel have access to the keys? □ □
66. Are controlled schedule II drugs and other drugs subject to abuse stored in separately locked, permanently affixed compartments? □ □
67. Is emergency drug box approved by the pharmaceutical services committee? □ □
68. Is pharmacist responsible, in writing, to check emergency drug box? □ □

Criteria for patient care

	Yes	No

Nursing and patient care

1. Do all patients have ID arm bracelets or appropriate means of identification? ☐ ☐
2. Are patients up when possible? ☐ ☐
3. Are patients dressed and well-groomed? ☐ ☐
4. Are patient's fingernails clean and clipped? ☐ ☐
5. Are lap robes used? ☐ ☐
6. Are patients being bathed according to schedule? ☐ ☐
7. Is there documentation of time oral hygiene is to be given? ☐ ☐
8. Is there a documented oral hygiene procedure? ☐ ☐
9. Are the male patients being shaved regularly? ☐ ☐
10. Are beds made up before lunch? ☐ ☐
11. Are Foley catheter bags properly attached to beds and wheelchairs and off floors? ☐ ☐
12. Are catheters off floors? ☐ ☐
13. Are Foley catheters draining well? ☐ ☐
14. Are catheters irrigated and maintained according to procedure? ☐ ☐
15. Is bowel and bladder training program in effect and documented? ☐ ☐
16. Are bedpans, emesis basins, and urinals being sterilized regularly? ☐ ☐
17. Do any patients have pressure sores at this time? ☐ ☐
18. Did the patient have these pressure sores when admitted? ☐ ☐
19. Are families aware of patient's condition on admission? ☐ ☐
20. Are restraints used discriminately? ☐ ☐
21. Are foot rests being used? ☐ ☐
22. Are IVs and clysis used as ordered? ☐ ☐
23. Do only trained nursing personnel draw blood or start IVs? ☐ ☐
24. Is there documentation of this training? ☐ ☐
25. Is special supportive equipment used as ordered, such as braces and prosthetics? ☐ ☐
26. Do patients appear happy and content? ☐ ☐
27. Do patients who are able, communicate or intermingle? ☐ ☐
28. Is there evidence of meaningful activity? ☐ ☐
29. Does the unit try to promote a healthy, happy, dignified patient environment? ☐ ☐
30. Is the staffing level at least 2.5 hours/ppd? ☐ ☐
31. Are licensed professionals involved in direct patient care? ☐ ☐
32. Is there evidence of follow through of patient plan of care? ☐ ☐
33. Is transportation arranged and timely for patients who cannot get to medical appointments and so on alone? ☐ ☐
34. Does the unit have adequate supplies? ☐ ☐

Is participation by patients documented and evidenced in the following:
35. Physical therapy? ☐ ☐
36. Activities of daily living? ☐ ☐
37. Accelerated restorative nursing program? ☐ ☐
38. Stroke groups? ☐ ☐
39. Reality orientation? ☐ ☐
40. Remotivation? ☐ ☐
41. Is patient's right to dignity and privacy respected? ☐ ☐
42. Are cubicle curtains drawn when appropriate? ☐ ☐
43. Does administrator know names of patients? ☐ ☐
44. Does Director of Nursing know name of patients? ☐ ☐
45. Are patients called by surname or by name requested? ☐ ☐
46. Is anyone assigned (or does someone volunteer) to stay with dying patients in final hours? ☐ ☐
47. Does nursing staff knock before entering a patient room? ☐ ☐
48. Are the majority of patients sitting in lounge areas? ☐ ☐
49. Are the majority of patients watching television? ☐ ☐
50. Does there appear to be a meaningful one-to-one relationship between staff and patients? ☐ ☐
51. Are patients treated as adults and not on an infantile or childlike level? ☐ ☐

Criteria for specialized rehabilitation services

	Yes	No
Organization and staffing		
1. Are rehabilitative services provided by qualified therapists?	☐	☐
2. Are qualified assistants under the supervision of qualified therapists?	☐	☐
3. Are administrative and patient care policies and procedures available for rehabilitative services?	☐	☐
4. Have they been developed by therapists and representatives of the medical, administrative, and nursing staffs?	☐	☐
Plan of care		
5. Does attending physician initiate plan of care with input from nursing and therapists?	☐	☐
6. Is therapy provided only on written order of attending physician?	☐	☐
7. Does physician review progress report in 2 weeks?	☐	☐
8. Is patient's progress reviewed at least monthly?	☐	☐
9. Is plan of care reevaluated at least every 30 days by physician and therapist?	☐	☐
Documentation of service		
Are the following in the patient's record—dated and signed by the attending physician and appropriate therapist:		
10. Physicians orders?	☐	☐
11. Plan of rehabilitative care?	☐	☐
12. Services rendered?	☐	☐
13. Evaluations of progress?	☐	☐
14. Any other pertinent data?	☐	☐
15. If the facility provides outpatient physical therapy services, does it meet applicable health and safety regulations?	☐	☐

Quality assurances

A. Level I: Evaluation of client care
   1. Nursing standards of care met
   2. Client goals met in client care plan
   3. Client care conferences: client and family interviewed regarding care rendered
   4. Client's environment observed
   5. Documentation in chart
   6. Reassess client's:
      a. Data base
      b. Care plan
      c. Nursing orders
      d. Nursing intervention
   7. Modify, amplify, or abandon plan and start process over
B. Level II: Nursing audit
   1. Select audit topic
   2. Develop criteria from standards
   3. Evaluate findings; take corrective action
   4. Follow up on action taken
   5. Report audit findings
C. Level III: Utilization review/PSRO
   1. Evaluation mechanisms
      a. Admission certification
      b. Continued stay review
      c. Discharge planning
      d. Evaluation studies
   2. Compliance with federal and state and local laws for agency licensure and certification as Medicare/Medicaid provider
   3. JCAH accreditation
   4. Evaluate findings: take corrective action
   5. Follow up on action taken
   6. Report audit findings

SUMMARY

Evaluation of client care is important to nursing, because it documents quality care and is the basis for reimbursement from Medicare, Medicaid, and third-party payers.

Nurses participate in evaluation on three levels. Level I is the day-to-day evaluation of client care as part of the nursing process. Level II involves nursing committee audits of groups of clients' charts seeking common nursing care needs and evaluation of the care given. Level III involves the nurse in the evaluation of her agency's care by outside organizations. These external reviewers can be from the federal, state, or local governments or from the Joint Commission on Accreditation of Hospitals. The written nurse's note is one measure by which the nurse's agency is evaluated.

The utilization review plan of an agency evaluates the patterns of care within the facility and documents the justification of client stay. Medicare and Medicaid reimbursement is based entirely on the outcome of the utilization review report.

Nursing is an active participant in each level of evaluation. Familiarity with the mechanisms of the evaluation/audit process enables the nurse to present the most accurate documentation of the care she provides.

REFERENCES

Accreditation Manual for Hospitals, Chicago, 1980, Joint Commission on Accreditation of Hospitals.

Accreditation Manual for Long Term Care, Chicago, 1980, Joint Commission on Accreditation of Hospitals.

Aimsworth, M. D.: Quality assurance in long-term care, Germantown, Md., 1978, Aspen Co.

Altieri, A. J.: Developing quality long-term care, Geriatrics **32:**126, July 1977.

Egelston, E. M.: New J.C.A.H. standards on quality assurance, Nurs. Res. **29:**113, March/April 1980.

Engle, J., and Barkauskas, V.: The evaluation of a public health nursing performance evaluation tool, J. Nurs. Admin. **13:**8, April 1979.

Flynn, B. C., and Ray, D. W.: Quality assurance in community health nursing, Nurs. Outlook, October 1979, p. 650.

Froebe, D. J., and Bain, J. R.: Quality assurance programs and controls in nursing, St. Louis, 1976, The C. V. Mosby Co.

Gallant, B. W., and McLane, A. M.: Outcome criteria: a process for validation at the unit level, J. Nurs. Admin. January 1979, p. 14.

Howe, M. J.: Developing instruments for measurements of criteria: a clinical nursing practice perspective, Nurs. Res. **29:**100, March-April, 1980.

Phaneuf, M. C.: Future direction for evaluation and evaluation research in health care: the nursing perspective, Nurs. Res. **29:**123, March/April 1980.

Plant, J.: Various approaches proposed to assess quality in long-term care, Hospitals **51:**93, 1 September 1977.

Schmadl, J. C.: Quality assurance: examination of the concept, Nurs. Outlook, July 1979, p. 462.

Williamson, J. W.: Information management in quality assurance, Nurs. Res. **29:**78, March/April 1980.

Woody, M. F.: An evaluator's perspective, Nurs. Res. **29:**74, March/April 1980.

A On being a good listener*

Reuel L. Howe

THE NATURE OF LISTENING

Listening is an art, a skill and a discipline. As in the case of other skills, it requires control—intellectual, emotional and behavioral. The individual must understand what is involved in listening and in developing the necessary self mastery to be silent and listen by subordinating his own ego and substituting a sense of humility.

Listening obviously is based on hearing and understanding of what others say to us. Hearing becomes listening only when we pay attention to what is said and follow it very closely.

Listening is a personal, private and intimate relationship, particularly if people are talking about personal, private and intimate problems. Consequently, listening is as different with different individuals as individuals differ in terms of their individual differences.

SITUATIONS INVOLVING LISTENING

In interviewing. Listening is involved in a wide range of interviewing situations. Some of these are:

- *In the counseling interview*—where we work with the individual on his problems that he brings.
- *In the performance interview*—where we assess how well the work is being done and what problems and needs are encountered in getting it done.
- *In the disciplinary interview*—where problems of observance of rules and regulations and standards of performance may be involved.
- *In the coaching interview*—where we help an

individual develop in terms of his work and responsibilities.

In other individual face-to-face situations. Wherever we are dealing with people face-to-face, day-to-day on a wide range of problems, we must listen to them in order for us to understand them, their problems and needs.

The better we understand them, the more willing and able they are to understand us.

In individual-to-group situations. Wherever an individual is dealing with a group, he must listen to them or they will lose interest both in him and the problems under consideration. The listening process here is basically the same as listening with an individual although the ways of handling the comments and contributions from the group may differ.

OBJECTIVES IN LISTENING

The objectives when we listen to people are both basic and simple.

- We want people to talk freely and frankly.
- We want them to cover matters and problems that are important to them.
- We want them to furnish as much information as they can.
- We want them to get greater insight and understanding of their problem as they talk it out.
- We want them to try to see the causes and reasons for their problems and to figure out what can be done about them.

SOME DOS AND DON'TS OF LISTENING

In listening we should try *to do* the following:
- Show interest.
- Be understanding of the other person.

---

*By permission of Forward Movement Publications, 412 Sycamore Street, Cincinnati, Ohio 45205.

- Express empathy.
- Single out the problem if there is one.
- Listen for causes to the problem.
- Help the speaker associate the problem with the cause.
- Encourage the speaker to develop competence and motivation to solve his own problems.
- Cultivate the ability to be silent when silence is needed.
- Successful people usually know how to remain silent and keep their counsel.

In listening, *don't do* the following:

- Argue.
- Interrupt.
- Pass judgment too quickly or in advance.
- Give advice unless it's requested.
- Jump to conclusions.
- Let the speaker's sentiments react too directly on your own.

THE URGENT NEED FOR LISTENING TO UNDERSTAND THE COMPLEXITY OF PROBLEMS INVOLVING PEOPLE AND SITUATIONS

We think we *understand people* and all the difficulties involved when frequently we don't even listen intently to them.

We think we *understand a situation* when we see only part of the situation and experience even less of it.

We think we *understand the problems people face* when we may have only a surface acquaintance with their elements and relevance, and in actuality we may be dealing merely with symptoms and not causes.

We should realize that *listening* is a *key* to *knowing* and *understanding*.

- One way to *know more* is *to listen more* and to get more information upon which they are based.
- A man's judgments and decisions are only as good as the information upon which they are based.
- We need to discard the *"allness"* orientation, namely, that we know or have *all* the answers.
- We can never know all about anything.
- We need to approach people and their problems with greater humility and recognition of the complexities involved.

- We need to *listen* with greater *intensity*.
- We need to *observe* with greater *acuity*.
- We need to *react* to other people with greater *empathy*.
- We need to *synthesize* what they say, think, and feel with greater *understanding*.

Recognizing the *difficulty* and *complexity* of people, situations, and problems enables us to become better listeners.

- We can listen not just for words and sounds but for what lies behind them.
- We can listen for facts, meanings, and reactions.
- We can listen for feelings, sentiments, and emotions.
- We can seek to distinguish between an actual event and people's interpretations of that event.
- We can be aware of overtones, what they mean and convey, as well as undertones, their meaning and relevance. For example, we can listen in terms of whether the speaker is conveying pessimism versus enthusiasm in terms of what he is saying, or whether he really has a positive versus negative approach in terms of what he proposes to do.
- We can be aware of the signal reaction—responding automatically in terms of previous thought and habit patterns.
- We can remember, in understanding people and their problems, that words are only *symbols* for things but they are not the things themselves. Words do not mean—people mean. The meaning is not in the words, it is in what the person means when he uses the word. Indeed, for the 500 most commonly used words in the English language that appear in the Oxford Dictionary there are over 14,070 different meanings or an average of 28 separate meanings per word. What people mean is not necessarily conveyed solely by the words put in many other subtle ways. As the old Arab adage goes, "Listen to what men *say*, but find out how they *feel*." We should remember that we listen to people, their words and meaning through a baffle or screen made up of our own attitudes, values, beliefs, and preconceived notions and judgments. Thus, in listening to others, we tend to add

something to what they say in terms of what we think, feel, and believe. We must try to minimize this.

SPECIFIC LISTENING TECHNIQUES

Clarify—to get at additional facts; to explore all sides of the problem.

Restate—to show you are interested, and listening and understand.

Reflect—to help evaluate the feelings expressed.

Summarize—to bring discussion in focus; to keep open for any additional aspects of the problem.

B A brief explanation of Medicare*

A BRIEF EXPLANATION OF MEDICARE

Medicare is a federal health insurance program that helps millions of Americans 65 and older, and many severely disabled people under 65, to pay the high cost of health care. It is administered by the Health Care Financing Administration. Medicare has two parts—hospital insurance and medical insurance.

The hospital insurance part of Medicare helps pay for inpatient hospital care and for certain follow-up care after you leave the hospital.

The medical insurance part of Medicare helps pay for your doctor's services, outpatient hospital services, and many other medical items and services not covered under hospital insurance.

WHO CAN GET MEDICARE

Practically everyone 65 or older is eligible for Medicare. Also eligible are:

- Disabled people under 65 who have been entitled to Social Security disability benefits for 24 consecutive months or railroad retirement benefits, based on disability, for 29 consecutive months; and
- People insured under Social Security or the railroad retirement system who need dialysis treatments or a kidney transplant because of permanent kidney failure. Wives, husbands, or children of insured people also may be eligible if they need maintenance dialysis or a transplant.

HOW YOU GET MEDICARE HOSPITAL INSURANCE PROTECTION

You do not have to retire to get hospital insurance protection. If you keep working, you'll have this protection at age 65 if you have worked long enough under Social Security or railroad retirement. To find out whether you are eligible for hospital insurance and to make sure you get the full protection of Medicare starting with the month you reach 65, please check with your Social Security office about 3 months before you reach 65.

People 65 or older who have not worked long enough to be entitled to hospital insurance can buy this protection. The basic premium is $69 a month through June 30, 1980. It will increase to $77 a month for the 12-month period starting July 1, 1980. To buy hospital insurance, you also have to enroll and pay the monthly premium for medical insurance. You can apply at any Social Security office.

Everyone 65 or older who is entitled to monthly Social Security or railroad retirement benefits gets hospital insurance without paying monthly premiums. If you are now receiving Social Security or railroad retirement checks, you will receive information about Medicare in the mail a few months before you are 65.

If you are a disabled person who has been entitled to Social Security disability benefits for 24 consecutive months or more, you will get hospital insurance automatically. You will receive information about Medicare in the mail several months before your coverage becomes effective. (People who receive railroad disability annuities or retirement benefits because of a disability should contact a railroad retirement office about the special requirements they must meet to get Medicare.)

If you are a widow 50 or older and have been severely disabled at least 2 years but haven't filed a claim based on your disability because you were getting Social Security checks as a mother caring for young or disabled children, you should contact your Social Security office to see if you're eligible for Medicare.

---

*U.S. Department of Health, Education, and Welfare Social Security Administration, Health Care Financing Administration, SSA Publication No. 10043, January 1980.

You, your spouse, or your dependent child who needs kidney dialysis or a kidney transplant may be eligible for hospital insurance and medical insurance regardless of age. You can get further information from any Social Security office.

MEDICARE HOSPITAL INSURANCE BENEFITS

Your hospital insurance helps pay the cost of medically necessary covered services for the following care:

- Up to 90 days of inpatient care in any participating hospital in each benefit period.* For the first 60 days, it pays for all covered services except for the first $180. For the 61st through the 90th day, it pays for all covered services except for $45 a day.
- A "reserve" of 60 additional inpatient hospital days. You can use these extra days if you ever need more than 90 days of hospital care in any benefit period. Each reserve day you use permanently reduces the total number of reserve days you have left. For each of these additional days you use, hospital insurance pays for all covered services except for $90 a day.
- Up to 100 days of care in each benefit period in a participating skilled nursing facility, a specially qualified facility which is staffed and equipped to furnish skilled nursing care, skilled rehabilitation care, and many related health services. In each benefit period, hospital insurance pays for all covered services for the first 20 days and all but $22.50 a day for up to 80 more days if *all* of the following five conditions are met:
  1. You have been in a hospital at least 3 days in a row (not counting the day of discharge) before your transfer to the skilled nursing facility.
  2. You are transferred to the skilled nursing

facility because you require care for a condition that was treated in the hospital.
  3. You are admitted to the facility within a short time (generally within 14 days) after you leave the hospital.
  4. You actually receive medically necessary skilled nursing or skilled rehabilitation services on a daily basis.
  5. The facility's Utilization Review Committee or the Professional Standards Review Organization in the area does not disapprove your stay.

- Up to 100 home health "visits" from a home health agency after the start of one benefit period and before the start of another. Payment for these visits can be made for up to 12 months after your most recent discharge from a hospital or participating skilled nursing facility if *all* six of the following conditions are met:
  1. You were in a qualifying hospital for at least 3 days in a row (not counting the day of discharge).
  2. The home health care is for further treatment of a condition that was treated in the hospital or skilled nursing facility.
  3. The care you need includes part-time skilled nursing care, physical therapy, or speech therapy.
  4. You are confined to your home.
  5. A doctor determines you need home health care and sets up a home health plan for you within 14 days after your discharge from a hospital or participating skilled nursing facility.
  6. The home health agency providing services is participating in Medicare.

WHAT MEDICARE HOSPITAL INSURANCE COVERS

Covered services in a hospital or skilled nursing facility include the cost of a semiprivate room (2 to 4 beds) and meals (including special diets), regular nursing services, and the cost of special care units such as an intensive care unit of a hospital. They also include the cost of drugs, supplies, appliances, equipment, and any other services ordinarily furnished to inpatients of hospitals or skilled nursing facilities.

---

*A benefit period is a way of measuring your use of services under Medicare hospital insurance. Your first benefit period starts the first time you enter a hospital after your hospital insurance begins. When you have been out of a hospital or other facility primarily providing skilled nursing or rehabilitation services—whether or not it participates in Medicare—for 60 days in a row (including the day of discharge), a new benefit period starts the next time you go into a hospital. There is no limit to the number of benefit periods you can have.

Covered services from a home health agency include part-time skilled nursing care, physical therapy, and speech therapy. When you need one or more of these services, hospital insurance also covers part-time services of home health aides, occupational therapy, medical social services, medical supplies (except drugs and biologicals), and medical equipment provided by the agency.

WHAT MEDICARE HOSPITAL INSURANCE DOES NOT COVER

Hospital insurance is basic protection against the high cost of illness after you are 65 or while you are severely disabled, but it will not pay all of your health care bills. Hospital insurance cannot pay for:

- Services or supplies that are not necessary for the diagnosis or treatment of an illness of injury.
- Doctor bills. (They are covered, however, if you have Medicare medical insurance.)
- Private duty nurses.
- The first 3 pints of blood you receive in a benefit period. (You do not have to pay for the first 3 pints if they are replaced through a blood plan or you have someone donate blood for you.)
- Convenience items requested by you, such as a telephone or television in your room.
- Care that is mainly custodial, such as help with bathing, eating, dressing, walking, or taking medicine.
- Homemaker services or meals delivered to your home.

SERVICES RECEIVED OUTSIDE THE U.S.

Payments under Medicare will usually be made *only* for services in the 50 States, the District of Columbia, Puerto Rico, the Virgin Islands, Guam, and American Samoa. However, when you live in the U.S. and a qualified Canadian or Mexican hospital is closer to your home than the nearest U.S. hospital that can provide the care you need, hospital insurance will help pay for the covered services you receive in the Canadian or Mexican hospital.

Also, if you are in the U.S. when an emergency occurs and a qualified Canadian or Mexican hospital is closer than the nearest U.S. hospital that could provide the care you need, then hospital insurance can help pay for the emergency care.

Hospital insurance can also help pay for care in a Canadian hospital if you are traveling through Canada directly to or from Alaska and another state and an emergency occurs that requires that you be admitted to a Canadian hospital.

HOW YOU GET MEDICARE MEDICAL INSURANCE

Anyone who is 65 or older *or* who is eligible for hospital insurance can get Medicare medical insurance. If you want medical insurance protection, you pay a monthly premium for it. The basic premium is $8.70 a month through June 30, 1980. It will increase to $9.60 a month for the 12-month period starting July 1, 1980.

If you are receiving Social Security benefits or retirement benefits under the railroad retirement system, you will be automatically enrolled for medical insurance—unless you say you don't want it—at the same time you become entitled to hospital insurance. You will receive information in the mail about 3 months before you become entitled to hospital insurance. The information you receive will tell you exactly what to do if you do not want medical insurance.

Automatic enrollment for medical insurance does not apply to people:

- Who are 65 but who have not worked long enough to be eligible for hospital insurance
- With permanent kidney failure
- Living in Puerto Rico and foreign countries

These people must apply for medical insurance at a Social Security office if they want it.

Medical insurance has a 7-month initial enrollment period. This period begins 3 months before the month you first become eligible for medical insurance and ends 3 months after that month. If you turn down medical insurance and then decide you want it after your 7-month initial enrollment period ends, you can sign up during a general enrollment period—January 1 through March 31 of each year. If you enroll during a general enrollment period, however, your protection won't start until the following July, and your premium will be 10 percent higher for each 12-month period you could have been enrolled but were not.

If you decide to cancel your medical insurance, your coverage and premium payments will stop at the end of the calendar quarter following the quarter in which your written cancellation notice is filed. You can reenroll in medical insurance only once after canceling your protection. We suggest you get in touch with a Social Security office if you are considering cancellation.

MEDICARE MEDICAL INSURANCE BENEFITS

Medical insurance will help pay for the following services when they are determined to be medically necessary:

- Physicians' services no matter where you receive them in the United States—in the doctor's office, the hospital, your home, or elsewhere—including medical supplies usually furnished by a doctor in his or her office, services of the office nurse, and drugs administered as part of your doctor's treatment that you cannot administer yourself. There is a limit on payment for covered psychiatric services furnished outside a hospital (see next section). Physicians' services outside the U.S. are covered only if they are furnished in connection with covered care in a Canadian or Mexican hospital (see previous section).
- Outpatient hospital services for diagnosis and treatment, such as care in an emergency room or outpatient clinic of a hospital.
- Up to 100 home health "visits" each calendar year, if *all* the following four conditions are met:
  1. You need part-time skilled nursing care or physical or speech therapy.
  2. A doctor determines you need the services and sets up a plan for home health care.
  3. You are confined to your home.
  4. The home health agency providing services is participating in Medicare.

  These visits are in addition to the 100 post-hospital home health visits covered under Medicare hospital insurance. Medical insurance covers the same home health services as hospital insurance (see pp. 314-315).
- Outpatient physical therapy and speech pathology services you receive as part of your treatment in a doctor's office or as an outpa-

tient of a participating hospital, skilled nursing facility, or home health agency; or an approved clinic, rehabilitation agency, or public health agency, if the services are furnished under a plan established and periodically reviewed by a doctor.
- A number of other medical and health services prescribed by your doctor such as diagnostic services; x-ray or other radiation treatments; surgical dressings, splints, casts, braces; artificial limbs and eyes; certain colostomy care supplies; and rental or purchase of medically necessary durable medical equipment such as a wheelchair or oxygen equipment for use in your home.
- Certain ambulance services.
- Limited services by chiropractors.
- Home and office services by licensed and Medicare-certified physical therapists, with certain payment limitations.

HOW MUCH MEDICARE MEDICAL INSURANCE PAYS

Each year, as soon as you have $60 (the annual deductible) in reasonable charges for covered medical expenses, medical insurance will pay 80 percent of the reasonable charges for any additional covered services you receive during the rest of the year.

There are four exceptions to this general rule:
- While you are a hospital inpatient, medical insurance pays 100 percent of the reasonable charges for services by doctors in the fields of pathology and radiology—whether or not you have met the annual deductible.
- After you meet the annual deductible medical insurance pays the reasonable costs for home health services.
- Medical insurance payment for services of independent physical therapists is limited to a maximum of $80 in reasonable charges during any one year.
- Physicians' psychiatric services outside a hospital are covered under a special payment rule and medical insurance payment is limited to a maximum of $250 during any one year.

Medical insurance payments are based on reasonable charges, which are determined by Medicare carriers—health insurance organizations selected by the federal government to handle medical insurance claims. Reasonable charges are based on the customary charges of the physician or supplier furnishing covered services but cannot be higher than the prevailing charges—the charges most commonly made by other physicians or suppliers in your area for these services.

Reasonable charges are updated annually, but increases in prevailing charges from year to year are limited by an "economic index" formula based on actual increases in the cost of maintaining a practice and raises in general earnings levels.

Because of the way reasonable charges are determined under the law, they may be lower than the actual charges made by doctors and suppliers.

WHAT MEDICARE MEDICAL INSURANCE DOES NOT COVER

Medical insurance does not cover some services or supplies. For example, it cannot pay for:

- Services or supplies that are not necessary for the diagnosis or treatment of an illness or injury.
- Routine physical checkups and tests directly related to such examinations.
- Prescription drugs and patent medicines.
- Glasses and eye examinations to fit glasses.
- Hearing aids and examinations for hearing aids.
- Dentures and routine dental care.
- Homemaker services and meals delivered to your home.
- Full-time nursing care in your home.

- Orthopedic shoes.
- Personal comfort items.
- The first 3 pints of blood you receive in each calendar year. (You do not have to pay for the first 3 pints if they are replaced through a blood plan or you have someone donate blood for you.)

FINANCING MEDICARE

The hospital insurance part of Medicare is financed by contributions from employees, their employers, and self-employed people. Each group pays the same rate. The contribution rate is 1.05 percent of the first $25,900 of yearly earnings for 1980.

Medical insurance is financed by the monthly premiums paid by people who have enrolled for it and by the federal government. When medical insurance costs increase because of higher charges for medical services, the premium you pay may be increased, but only if Social Security cash benefits were increased during the previous year. The premium increase cannot be more than the percentage increase in cash benefits during the previous year. The federal government pays over two thirds of the total premium cost for medical insurance.

FOR MORE INFORMATION

Call any social security office for more detailed information about Medicare or any other social security program. The people there will be glad to help you.

C Directory of state agencies on aging and regional offices

As a result of the Older Americans Act of 1965, advocate offices for the older adult have been established in each state and territory. These offices offer older adults and health and other professionals information about services and programs designed for the older adult. They also serve as advocates for the older adult and coordinate activities on their behalf.

Call or write these offices when referral information is needed. They can direct you or your client to the source of help in your area.

Alabama
Commission on Aging
740 Madison Ave.,
Montgomery, Ala. 36104
Tel. (205) 269-8171

Alaska
Office on Aging
Department of Health & Social Services
Pouch H
Juneau, Alaska 99801
Tel. (907) 586-6153

American Samoa
Government of American Samoa
Office of the Government
Pago Pago, Samoa 96920

Arizona
Bureau on Aging
Department of Economic Security
Suite 800, South Tower
2721 North Central
Phoenix, Ariz. 85004
Tel. (602) 271-4446

Arkansas
Office on Aging
P. O. Box 2179
Hendrix Hall
4313 West Markham
Little Rock, Ark. 72203
Tel. (501) 371-2441

California
Office on Aging
Health & Welfare Agency
455 Capitol Mall, Suite 500
Sacramento, Calif. 95814
Tel. (916) 322-3887

Colorado
Division of Services for the Aging
Department of Social Services,
1575 Sherman St.
Denver, Colo. 80203
Tel. (303) 892-2651

Connecticut
Department of Aging
90 Washington St., Rm. 312
Hartford, Conn. 06115
Tel. (203) 566-2480

Delaware
Division of Aging
Department of Health & Social Services
2407 Lancaster Avenue,
Wilmington, Del. 19805
Tel. (302) 571-3480

District of Columbia
Office of Services to the Aged
Department of Human Resources
1329 E. St., N.W. (Munsey Bldg.)
Washington, D.C. 20004
Tel. (202) 638-2406

Florida
Division on Aging
Department of Health & Rehabilitation Services
1317 Winewood Blvd., Bldg. 3
Tallahassee, Fla. 32301
Tel. (904) 488-4797

Georgia
Office on Aging
Department of Human Resources
618 Ponce de Leon Ave.
Atlanta, Ga. 30308
Tel. (404) 894-5333

Guam
Office of Aging
Social Services Administration
Government of Guam
P. O. Box 2816
Agana, Guam 96910

Hawaii
Commission on Aging
1149 Bethel St., Room 311
Honolulu, Hawaii 96813

Idaho
Office on Aging
Department of Special Services
Capitol Annex No. 7
509 N. 5th St., Room 100
Boise, Idaho 83720
Tel. (208) 384-3833

Illinois
Department on Aging
2401 W. Jefferson St.
Springfield, Ill. 62706
Tel. (217) 782-5773

Indiana
Commission on the Aging & the Aged
Graphic Arts Bldg.
215 North Senate Ave.
Indianapolis, Ind. 46202
Tel. (317) 633-5948

Iowa
Commission on the Aging
415 West 10th (Jewett Bldg.)
Des Moines, Iowa 50319
Tel. (515) 281-5187

Kansas
Services for the Aging Section
Division of Social Services
Social & Rehabilitation Services Department
State Office Building,
Topeka, Kan. 66612
Tel. (913) 296-3465

Kentucky
Aging Program Unit
Department for Human Resources
403 Wapping St.
Frankfort, Ky. 40601
Tel. (502) 564-4238

Louisiana
Bureau of Aging Service
Division of Human Resources
Health & Social Rehabilitation
Services Administration,
P. O. Box 44282, Capital Station,
Baton Rouge, La. 70804
Tel. (504) 389-6713

Maine
Bureau of Maine's Elderly
Department of Health & Welfare,
State House
Augusta, Me. 04330
Tel. (207) 622-6171;
   ask for 289-2561.

Maryland
Office on Aging
1004 State Office Building
301 W. Preston St.
Baltimore, Md. 21201
Tel. (301) 383-5064

Massachusetts
Executive Office of Elder Affairs
State Office Building
18 Tremont St.
Boston, Mass. 02109
Tel. (617) 727-7751

Michigan
Offices of Services to the Aging
1026 East Michigan
Lansing, Mich. 48912
Tel. (517) 373-8230

Minnesota
Governor's Citizens Council on Aging
Suite 204, Metro Square Bldg.
7th & Robert Sts.
St. Paul, Minn. 55101
Tel. (612) 296-2544

Mississippi
Council on Aging
P. O. Box 5136, Fondren Station
2906 N. State St.
Jackson, Miss. 39216
Tel. (601) 354-6590

Missouri
Office of Aging
Division of Special Services,
Department of Social Services
The Broadway State Office Bldg.
Jefferson City, Mo. 65101
Tel. (314) 751-2075

Montana
Aging Services Bureau
Department of Social & Rehabilitative Services,
P. O. Box 1723
Helena, Mont. 59601
Tel. (406) 449-3124

Nebraska
Commission on Aging
State House Station 94784
300 S. 17th Street
Lincoln, Neb. 68509
Tel. (402) 471-2307

Nevada
Division of Aging
Department of Human Resources
Room 300, Nye Bldg.
201 S. Fall St.
Carson City, Nev. 89701
Tel. (702) 882-7855

New Hampshire
Council on Aging
P. O. Box 786
14 Depot St.
Concord, N.H. 03301
Tel. (603) 271-2751

New Jersey
Office on Aging
Department of Community Affairs
P. O. Box 2768
363 West State St.
Trenton, N.J. 08625
Tel. (609) 292-3765

New Mexico
State Commission on Aging
Villagra Bldg.
408 Galisteo Street
Sante Fe, N. Mex. 87501
Tel. (505) 827-5258

New York
Office for the Aging
N.Y. State Executive Department
855 Central Avenue
Albany, N.Y. 12206
Tel. (518) 457-7321

New York City
Office for the Aging
Room 5036
2 World Trade Center
New York, N.Y. 10047
Tel. (212) 488-6405

North Carolina
Governor's Coordinating Council on Aging,
Administration Building
213 Hillsborough St.
Raleigh, N.C. 27603
Tel. (919) 829-3983

North Dakota
Aging Services
Social Services Board
State Capitol Building
Bismarck, N.D. 58501
Tel. (701) 224-2577

Ohio
Commission on Aging
34 North High St., 3rd floor
Columbus, Ohio 43215
Tel. (614) 466-5500

Oklahoma
Special Unit of Aging
Department of Institutions, Soc. and Rehab. Serv.
Box 25352, Capitol Station
Sequoyah Memorial Bldg.
Oklahoma City, Okla. 73125
Tel. (405) 521-2281

Oregon
Program on Aging
Human Resources Department
315 Public Service Building
Salem, Oreg. 97310
Tel. (503) 378-4728

Pennsylvania
Office for the Aging
Department of Public Welfare
Capital Associates Building
7th & Forster Sts.
Harrisburg, Pa. 17120
Tel. (717) 787-5350

Puerto Rico
Gericulture Commission
Department of Social Services
Apartado 11697
Santurce, Puerto Rico 00910
Tel. (809) 725-8015
(Overseas Operator)

Rhode Island
Division on Aging
Department of Community Affairs
150 Washington St.
Providence, R.I. 02903
Tel. (401) 528-1000
Ask for 277-2858

South Carolina
Commission on Aging
915 Main St.
Columbia, S.C. 29201
Tel. (803) 758-2576

South Dakota
Program on Aging
Department of Social Services
St. Charles Hotel
Pierre, S.D. 57501
Tel. (605) 224-3656

Tennessee
Commission on Aging
S & P Bldg., Room 102
306 Gay St.
Nashville, Tenn. 37201
Tel. (615) 741-2056

Texas
Governor's Committee on Aging
Southwest Tower, 8th Floor
211 East 7th Street
Austin, Tex. 78711
Tel. (512) 475-2717

Trust Terr. of the Pacific
Office of Aging
Community Development Div.
Gov. of the Trust Territory of the Pacific Islands
Saipan, Mariana Islands 96950

Utah
Division of Aging
Department of Social Services
345 South 6th East
Salt Lake City, Utah 84102
Tel. (801) 328-6422

Vermont
Office on Aging
Department of Human Services
56 State St.
Montpelier, Vt. 05602
Tel. (802) 828-3471

Virginia
Office on Aging
Division of State Planning and Community Affairs
9 North 12th Street
Richmond, Va. 23219
Tel. (804) 770-7894

Virgin Islands
Commission on Aging
P. O. Box 539, Charlotte Amalie
St. Thomas, Virgin Islands 00801
Tel. (809) 774-5884

Washington
Office on Aging
Department of Social and Health Services,
P. O. Box 1788—M.S. 45-2
410 W. Fifth
Olympia, Wash. 98504
Tel. (206) 753-2502

West Virginia
Commission on Aging
State Capitol, Room 420-26
1800 Washington St.
Charleston, W. Va. 25305
Tel. (304) 348-3317

Wisconsin
Division on Aging
Department of Health & Social Services
State Office Building, Room 686
1 West Wilson St.
Madison, Wis. 53702
Tel. (608) 266-2536

Wyoming
Aging Services
Department of Health & Social Services
Division of Public Assistance & Social Services
State Office Building
Cheyenne, Wyo. 82002
Tel. (307) 777-7561

REGION 1
(Conn., Maine, Mass., N.H., R.I., Vt.)
J. F. Kennedy Federal Bldg.
Government Center, Room 2007
Boston, Mass. 02203
Tel. (617) 223-6885

REGION II
(N.J., N.Y., Puerto Rico, Virgin Islands)
26 Federal Plaza, Rm. 4106
Broadway & North Sts.
New York, N.Y. 10007
Tel. (212) 264-4592

REGION III
(Del., D.C., Md., Pa., Va., W. Va.)
P. O. Box 13716
36th & Market Sts., 5th Fl.
Philadelphia, Pa. 19101
Tel. (215) 597-6891

REGION IV
(Ala., Fla., Ga., Ky., Miss., N.C., S.C., Tenn.)
50 Seventh St. N.E. Rm. 326
Atlanta, Ga. 30323
Tel. (404) 526-3482

REGION V
(Ill., Ind., Mich., Minn., Ohio, Wis.)
29th Floor
300 S. Wacker Drive
Chicago, Ill. 60606
Tel. (312) 353-4695

REGION VI
(Ark., La., N. Mex., Okla., Tex.)
Fidelity Union Tower Bldg.
Room 500
1507 Pacific Avenue
Dallas, Tex. 75201
Tel. (214) 749-7286

REGION VII
(Iowa, Kans., Mo., Nebr.)
12 Grand Building, 5th Fl.
12th & Grand
Kansas City, Mo. 64106
Tel. (816) 374-2955

REGION VIII
(Colo., Mont., N. Dak., S. Dak., Utah, Wyo.)
19th and Stout Sts., Rm. 7027
Federal Office Building
Denver, Colo. 80202
Tel. (303) 837-2951

REGION IX
(Ariz., Calif., Hawaii, Nev., Samoa, Guam, T.T.)
50 Fulton St., Room 204
406 Federal Office Building
San Francisco, Calif. 94102
Tel. (415) 556-6003

REGION X
(Alaska, Idaho, Oreg., Wash.)
Dexter Horton Building, Room 1490
710 2nd Avenue
Seattle, Wash. 98104
Tel. (206) 442-5341

Index